Health Crisis Mana

Ridwan Shabsigh
Editor

Health Crisis Management in Acute Care Hospitals

Lessons Learned from COVID-19 and Beyond

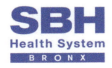

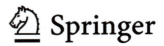

Editor
Ridwan Shabsigh
Department of Surgery
SBH Health System
Bronx, NY, USA

Department of Urology
Weill Cornell Medical College of Cornell University
New York, NY, USA

CUNY School of Medicine
New York, NY, USA

ISBN 978-3-030-95805-3   ISBN 978-3-030-95806-0 (eBook)
https://doi.org/10.1007/978-3-030-95806-0

© SBH Health System 2022
This work is subject to copyright. All rights are solely and exclusively licensed by the Publisher, whether the whole or part of the material is concerned, specifically the rights of translation, reprinting, reuse of illustrations, recitation, broadcasting, reproduction on microfilms or in any other physical way, and transmission or information storage and retrieval, electronic adaptation, computer software, or by similar or dissimilar methodology now known or hereafter developed.
The use of general descriptive names, registered names, trademarks, service marks, etc. in this publication does not imply, even in the absence of a specific statement, that such names are exempt from the relevant protective laws and regulations and therefore free for general use.
The publisher, the authors and the editors are safe to assume that the advice and information in this book are believed to be true and accurate at the date of publication. Neither the publisher nor the authors or the editors give a warranty, expressed or implied, with respect to the material contained herein or for any errors or omissions that may have been made. The publisher remains neutral with regard to jurisdictional claims in published maps and institutional affiliations.

This Springer imprint is published by the registered company Springer Nature Switzerland AG
The registered company address is: Gewerbestrasse 11, 6330 Cham, Switzerland

This book is wholeheartedly dedicated, as a humble gesture of love, respect, and appreciation, to all healthcare workers around the entire world, who worked tirelessly to help patients and save lives during the overwhelming COVID-19 pandemic.

Tribute

The editor and the authors of this book pay sincere tribute to all healthcare workers who lost their lives during the COVID-19 pandemic, and to their families and loved ones. Special tribute is given to the five heroes of the SBH Health System family, who lost their lives during the COVID-19 pandemic:

Warren Bates, *technician, telecommunications*

Corazon Espinosa, RN, *registered nurse, psychiatry*

Maria Grace E. Laureta, RN, *registered nurse, ICU*

Nelson Then, *EKG technician, radiology*

***Ronald Verrier**, **MD**, critical care surgeon and director of general surgery residency program*
We commend and honor their dedication to healthcare and their commitment to improving the lives of so many. Our thoughts and best wishes go to their families and loved ones.

Foreword

It would not be over-optimistic to state that, out of the suffering of millions of people, the sadness over the loss of so many lives, the economic harm, and the sociopolitical disruption, all brought about by the COVID-19 pandemic, we emerged more resilient and better capable of handling future health crises than ever in the history of humankind. This optimism is fully justified by the richness of the lessons learned from the crisis, the immense improvements made to healthcare systems all over the world, and the great advancements in medical science, such as the ability to rapidly develop and distribute new testing technology, novel vaccines, and therapeutics. It is well established that acute-care hospitals stand at the frontline of healthcare delivery in peacetime; however, during times of disaster, the proper functioning of an acute-care hospital is a major indispensable part of a successful response to a health crisis. Currently, hospitals need to plan and prepare for a number of scenarios including future surges of COVID-19, new variants of it, other future infectious/viral pandemics, or any other public health crises. Such planning and preparation could benefit tremendously from the rich lessons learned during the COVID-19 pandemic over the past 2 years.

This book brings together the rich experiences of the SBH Health System, presented in 20 chapters. The various chapters include frontline healthcare workers' accounts and case studies, in addition to charts, figures, tables, boxes, and vignettes. The need for such practical guidance and the timeliness of this book cannot be overstated. It is our hope that this book will energize worldwide dialogue and advance the establishment of best practices for the improvement of any hospital system's ability to enhance their preparedness and management of any and all future health crises.

SBH Health System   David Perlstein
Bronx, NY, USA

Prologue

The COVID-19 crisis came as an unpleasant surprise and a shock to many healthcare systems and hospitals especially in the crisis epicenter of New York City. The Bronx was one of the hardest-hit boroughs of New York City with significant negative impact of the COVID-19 pandemic on its indigent population. SBH Health System (formerly known as St. Barnabas Hospital) is an integrated system of an acute-care hospital, ambulatory care center, trauma center, dialysis center, stroke center, and other services and facilities serving the community of the Bronx. The story of SBH in preparing for and managing the rapidly escalating surge of severely ill patients at the onset of the COVID-19 crisis is a treasure of lessons in health crisis preparedness and management at all levels, clinical, administrative, and financial.

This book draws lessons from the success of SBH Health System in tackling the dramatically fast unfolding pandemic from the perspective of the system as a whole and from each of the specific departments which all played a significant role in managing the local crisis of the largest threat to human health the world has seen in recent years. Such lessons may benefit us and other health systems and hospitals elsewhere in planning and preparing for similar crises in the future.

Within a short 3-week period, the SBH Health System increased its in-patient capacity by 50%. However, during the same short time span, it increased its critical care capacity by more than 500%, providing critical care to severely ill patients on ventilators. This book chronicles step by step the drastic adaptations that were made and describes how this incredible accomplishment was undertaken in such a short time, to ultimately save the lives of many patients. Accounts from the frontline healthcare workers and clinical and administrative leaders alike describe important aspects of crisis management, such as team building, multi-departmental coordination, effective communications, dynamic decision-making in response to rapidly changing situations, keeping up the morale, caring for the healthcare workers themselves, and managing the supply chain and essential resources.

Case studies are presented from positive and negative experiences to draw lessons on what worked and what didn't and how challenges were addressed. This is a prescriptive book in a "how it works" and "how to do it" style. The fact that the book is authored by those who worked directly in the field, witnessing firsthand the distressing reality of the clinical devastation caused by the rapid surge in the pandemic and living every decision and adaptation every day that dynamically changed the provision of care helping minimize loss of life, makes for a unique perspective.

The uniqueness of the experience of SBH Health System is enhanced by the fact that it is a capital-constrained "safety net" hospital serving the poorest population in New York City. The worldwide trend is toward tighter healthcare budgets with demands for higher efficiency and productivity. Within this low-budget safety-net hospital, we faced unique and often amplified challenges. There is a lot to be learned from the SBH Health System crisis management, including how efficient management, team building, management of limited resources, and collaborative workplace culture make the foundation of success in the face of the crisis of the century.

Many senior healthcare administrators, chairpersons of clinical departments, and frontline workers are eager to learn lessons from health systems that experienced the severe surge of such an unprecedented crisis. From this book the reader will learn how to effectively plan and prepare for a health crisis in a speedy and efficient manner. Such planning and preparation involve clinical departments, critical care teams, nursing, respiratory therapy, physical therapy, nutrition, pharmacy, laboratory, information technology, facilities, biomedical engineering, supply chain, senior administration, and others. Therefore, healthcare workers at all levels will be eager to learn about the procedures, policies, and operations that were implemented in the successful crisis management at SBH Health System. Similarly, this book will be of interest to public health officials and planners, disaster management planners and educators, healthcare educators, and universities that teach public health administration and planning to learn how capital-constrained healthcare systems can adapt and cope with such a health crisis. The book also touches on the recovery from a health crisis and the "new norm" emerging from the COVID-19 pandemic. We hope this book provides useful lessons to ultimately help improve patient care when confronting health crises.

Ridwan Shabsigh

Acknowledgments and Appreciations

As editor-in-chief of this book, I would like to express my highest acknowledgment and warmest appreciation to a number of individuals who worked hard to help bring this work to completion. My dear friends and colleagues at SBH Health System helped tremendously as effective chapter authors and co-authors. They shared their firsthand experiences from the COVID-19 pandemic and presented valuable lessons learned for the planning, preparation, and management of future health crises. Without them and their passionate efforts, this book would have never been possible.

My special appreciation goes to Dr. Joanne (Jo) Nettleship and her team for their exceptional efforts in critically editing and effectively finalizing this work in the face of tight production timelines and delivery deadlines. The hard work of Dr. Nettleship brought high quality and professionalism into the production of this book.

Ridwan Shabsigh

Contents

1. **Background, the Hospital System, the Patient Community, and the Bronx** 1
   Steven Clark and Ridwan Shabsigh

2. **COVID-19 Crisis Timeline: The Warning and the Surge** 9
   Ridwan Shabsigh and Daniel Kelly

3. **Preparation, Planning, and the Command Center** 23
   Eric C. Appelbaum, Daniel P. Lombardi, Manisha Kulshreshtha, Mary M. Bolbrock, Zane S. Last, and Morena Lasso

4. **Internal Medicine, Infection Control, and Occupational Health Services** 37
   Edward E. Telzak and Judith Berger

5. **Critical Care** 53
   Christopher A. Grantham, Dmitriy Karev, Robert D. Karpinos, Rocco J. Lafaro, Edward E. Telzak, Ralph Rahme, and Ridwan Shabsigh

6. **Emergency Medicine** 99
   Daniel G. Murphy, Jeffrey D. Lazar, and Brian J. Dolan

7. **Nursing** 123
   Robert Church, Raymundo M. Apellido, Angela Babaev, Alma Calandria, Mary B. Carmel, Brian J. Dolan, Donna L. Douglas, Ann C. Hennessy, Pauline A. Lattery, Clover Mclennon, and Courtney White

8. **Clinical Nutrition and Food Services** 137
   Cecilia Moy

9. **Rehabilitation** 151
   Jovito S. Sabino, Josephine S. Dolera, and Glenn H. Constante

10	**Respiratory Therapy and Proning** 165
	Angela Babaev, Tracey Martin-Johnson, and Mark Klion
11	**Pharmacy**... 183
	Ruth E. Cassidy
12	**Laboratory**.. 201
	Richard R. Hwang and Muhammad F. Durrani
13	**Radiology**... 217
	Brian Bobby Chiong, Steven B. Epstein, and Razia Rehmani
14	**Supply Chain, Material Management, and Finance** 227
	Marilyn L. G. Gates, Louis M. Santomauro, Steven M. Beltis, Patricio F. Villacreses, Ricardo Negron, Mark Sollazzo, Don Hester, Steven Berger, and Mary Grochowski
15	**Information Technology, Healthcare Data and Analytics, and Clinical Engineering** 241
	Jitendra Barmecha
16	**Medical Students and the Medical School** 259
	Nancy Sohler, Lisa Auerbach, and Erica S. Friedman
17	**Dynamic Decision-Making and Effective Communications** 277
	Ridwan Shabsigh, Eric C. Appelbaum, and Robert D. Karpinos
18	**Collaborative Culture and Lean Daily Management** 291
	David Perlstein, Daniel P. Lombardi, and Ridwan Shabsigh
19	**Soft Skills, Emotional and Social Intelligence, and Resilience** 301
	Lizica C. Troneci and Ridwan Shabsigh
20	**Recovery From Crisis**....................................... 315
	Ridwan Shabsigh and Joanne E. Nettleship

Index.. 333

Contributors

Raymundo M. Apellido Intensive Care Units, SBH Health System, Bronx, NY, USA

Eric C. Appelbaum SBH Health System, Bronx, NY, USA

Lisa Auerbach CUNY School of Medicine, New York, NY, USA

Angela Babaev Department of Nursing, SBH Health System, Bronx, NY, USA

CUNY School of Medicine, New York, NY, USA

Bloomfield College, Bloomfield, NJ, USA

Jitendra Barmecha SBH Health System, Bronx, NY, USA

CUNY School of Medicine, New York, NY, USA

Steven M. Beltis Purchasing Department, SBH Health System, Bronx, NY, USA

Judith Berger CUNY School of Medicine, New York, NY, USA

Infection Control, Division of Infectious Disease, Department of Medicine, Occupational Health Services, SBH Health System, Bronx, NY, USA

Steven Berger SBH Health System, Bronx, NY, USA

Mary M. Bolbrock Quality and Risk Management, SBH Health System, Bronx, NY, USA

Alma Calandria Department of Nursing, SBH Health System, Bronx, NY, USA

Mary B. Carmel Department of Nursing, SBH Health System, Bronx, NY, USA

Ruth E. Cassidy Clinical Support Services and Pharmacy, SBH Health System, Bronx, NY, USA

Brian Bobby Chiong Department of Radiology, SBH Health System, Bronx, NY, USA

CUNY School of Medicine, New York, NY, USA

Robert Church Department of Nursing, SBH Health System, Bronx, NY, USA

Steven Clark Marketing and Communications, SBH Health System, Bronx, NY, USA

Glenn H. Constante Physical Therapy, SBH Health System, Bronx, NY, USA

Brian J. Dolan Department of Emergency Medicine and Department of Nursing, SBH Health System, Bronx, NY, USA

Josephine S. Dolera Rehabilitation Services, SBH Health System, Bronx, NY, USA

Donna L. Douglas Perioperative Services, SBH Health System, Bronx, NY, USA

Muhammad F. Durrani Laboratory Services, SBH Health System, Bronx, NY, USA

Steven B. Epstein Department of Radiology, SBH Health System, Bronx, NY, USA

Erica S. Friedman CUNY School of Medicine, New York, NY, USA

Marilyn L. G. Gates Value Analysis, SBH Health System, Premier/Nexera, Bronx, NY, USA

Christopher A. Grantham Medical Intensive Care Unit, Department of Medicine, SBH Health System, Bronx, NY, USA

CUNY School of Medicine, New York, NY, USA

Mary Grochowski Department of Finance, SBH Health System, Bronx, NY, USA

Ann C. Hennessy Department of Nursing, SBH Health System, Bronx, NY, USA

Don Hester Supply Chain, SBH Health System, Bronx, NY, USA

Richard R. Hwang Laboratory Services, SBH Health System, Bronx, NY, USA

CUNY School of Medicine, New York, NY, USA

Dmitriy Karev CUNY School of Medicine, New York, NY, USA

Division of Trauma and Surgical Critical Care, Department of Surgery, SBH Health System, Bronx, NY, USA

Robert D. Karpinos Perioperative Services and Department of Anesthesiology, SBH Health System, Bronx, NY, USA

CUNY School of Medicine, New York, NY, USA

Daniel Kelly Department of Biosciences & Chemistry, Faculty of Health & Wellbeing, Sheffield Hallam University, Sheffield, UK

Mark Klion Division of Orthopedics, Department of Surgery, SBH Health System, Bronx, NY, USA

Manisha Kulshreshtha SBH Health System, Bronx, NY, USA

CUNY School of Medicine, New York, NY, USA

Contributors

Rocco J. Lafaro CUNY School of Medicine, New York, NY, USA

Division of Cardiothoracic Surgery, Department of Surgery, SBH Health System, Bronx, NY, USA

Morena Lasso SBH Health System, Bronx, NY, USA

Zane S. Last Healthcare Analytics and Business Intelligence, SBH Health System, New York, NY, USA

Pauline A. Lattery Department of Nursing, SBH Health System, Bronx, NY, USA

Jeffrey D. Lazar Department of Emergency Medicine, SBH Health System, Bronx, NY, USA

CUNY School of Medicine, New York, NY, USA

Daniel P. Lombardi SBH Health System, Bronx, NY, USA

Tracey Martin-Johnson Respiratory Therapy, SBH Health System, Bronx, NY, USA

Clover Mclennon Department of Nursing, SBH Health System, Bronx, NY, USA

Cecilia Moy Department of Food and Nutrition, SBH Health System, Bronx, NY, USA

Daniel G. Murphy Department of Emergency Medicine, SBH Health System, Bronx, NY, USA

CUNY School of Medicine, New York, NY, USA

Ricardo Negron SBH Health System, Bronx, NY, USA

Joanne E. Nettleship Astra Health, Sheffield, UK

David Perlstein SBH Health System, Bronx, NY, USA

Ralph Rahme CUNY School of Medicine, New York, NY, USA

Division of Neurosurgery, Department of Surgery, SBH Health System, Bronx, NY, USA

Razia Rehmani Neuro and Musculoskeletal Imaging, Department of Radiology, SBH Health System, Bronx, NY, USA

Jovito S. Sabino Rehabilitation Services, SBH Health System, Bronx, NY, USA

Louis M. Santomauro Supply Chain, SBH Health System, Bronx, NY, USA

Ridwan Shabsigh Department of Surgery, SBH Health System, Bronx, NY, USA

Department of Urology, Weill Cornell Medical College of Cornell University, New York, NY, USA

CUNY School of Medicine, New York, NY, USA

Nancy Sohler CUNY School of Medicine, New York, NY, USA

Mark Sollazzo Materials Management, SBH Health System, Bronx, NY, USA

Edward E. Telzak Department of Medicine, SBH Health System, Bronx, NY, USA
Department of Medicine, CUNY School of Medicine, New York, NY, USA
Albert Einstein College of Medicine, Bronx, NY, USA

Lizica C. Troneci Department of Psychiatry, SBH Health System, Bronx, NY, USA
CUNY School of Medicine, New York, NY, USA

Patricio F. Villacreses Supply Chain, SBH Health System, Bronx, NY, USA

Courtney White Department of Nursing, SBH Health System, Bronx, NY, USA

Chapter 1
Background, the Hospital System, the Patient Community, and the Bronx

Steven Clark and Ridwan Shabsigh

The Bronx

Beginning in early 2020, the Belmont and East Tremont neighborhoods of the Bronx found themselves squarely in the destructive path of the nation's worst pandemic in a century. The reasons for this would soon become apparent. This is a community of color. According to the American Community Survey's 2019 data, its population is 56.4% Latino and 29% Black. Many suffer from comorbidities [1]. It is New York City's (NYC) epicenter for chronic disease – diabetes, asthma, obesity, and cardiovascular and renal disease. Mortality rates from heart disease, stroke, and diabetes far exceed citywide or national averages. This is also a haven for HIV, drug use, and gun violence. It is a Health Resources and Services Administration (HRSA)-designated medically underserved area and Healthcare Provider Shortage Area.

Every day, those who live here confront what is known as the social determinants of health (SDOH). As defined by the US Department of Health and Human Services in its Healthy People 2030 initiative, SDOHs are "conditions in the environments where people are born, live, learn, work, play, worship and age that affect a wide range of health, functioning and quality-of-life outcomes and risks." [2]. Here, in the Bronx, residents face food, housing, education, and economic insecurity due to such factors as lack of safe housing, job opportunities, safe places, access to healthy and

---

S. Clark (✉)
Marketing and Communications, SBH Health System, Bronx, NY, USA
e-mail: sclark@sbhny.org

R. Shabsigh
Department of Surgery, SBH Health System, Bronx, NY, USA

Department of Urology, Weill Cornell Medical College of Cornell University, New York, NY, USA

CUNY School of Medicine, New York, NY, USA

© The Author(s), under exclusive license to Springer Nature Switzerland AG 2022
R. Shabsigh (ed.), *Health Crisis Management in Acute Care Hospitals*, https://doi.org/10.1007/978-3-030-95806-0_1

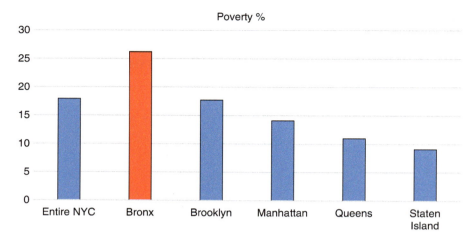

Fig. 1.1 The Bronx borough has the highest poverty rate in entire New York City far surpassing every other borough. (Data from the US Census Bureau [1])

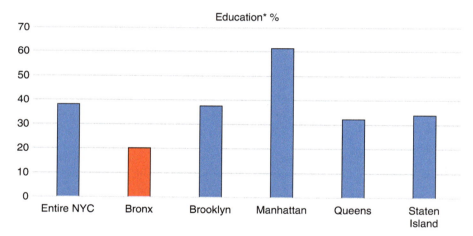

Fig. 1.2 The Bronx borough has the lowest education rate in entire New York City far below every other borough. (Data from the US Census Bureau [1]). * Percentage of people with bachelor degree or higher)

nutritious foods, and language and literacy skills. Three major problems – poverty, low education, and poor health – exist the most and the highest in the Bronx part of New York City (Figs. 1.1, 1.2, and 1.3). The Bronx has the poorest socioeconomic determinants of health in New York City and one of the lowest in the United States.

The organization, Feeding America, estimates that 17.5% of Bronx residents suffer from food insecurity [3]. NYC's 2018 Food Metric Report found that more than 230,000 of its predominantly Black and Latino residents lack access to nutritious, affordable food [4]. Instead of fresh produce, the delis, fast food restaurants, grocery stores, and bodegas that line many of the local streets here load up on their

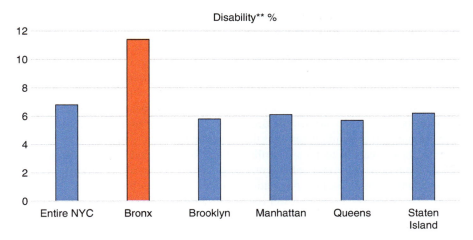

Fig. 1.3 The Bronx borough has the highest disability rate in entire New York City far surpassing every other borough. (Data from the US Census Bureau [1]). ** Percentage of people with a disability under 65 years)

higher ticket items: high-fat and high-sugar foods. Signs outside retailers hawking pizza, fried chicken, burgers, and sodas predominate, with those selling fresh produce all but invisible.

The Bronx has the lowest levels of socioeconomics, health, and education in New York City along with diminished access to healthy and nutritious foods, thus representing the poorest socioeconomic determinants of health, placing it at the highest risk when facing a health crisis, such as COVID-19 pandemic.

These key, distinguishing demographics set the stage for understanding the compounded deep impact of the COVID-19 health crisis on the Bronx population and the extraordinary task that faced St. Barnabas Hospital (SBH) Health System. Unlike in the more affluent sections of New York City, people in the Bronx tend to live in smaller apartments, making isolation and social distancing all but impossible, which can mean a higher likelihood of virus transmission. In far greater numbers, they are more likely to take public transportation to work and have a far less opportunity of being able to work from home. All these conditions led to a considerably higher, far more serious incidence of COVID-19 illness, and in hindsight, as result of this perfect storm of circumstances, it is hardly surprising that the Bronx community was, among those areas in the United States, hit hardest by COVID-19.

The SBH Patient Community During COVID-19

According to data provided by the New York City Health Department [5], neighborhoods with high concentrations of Blacks and Latinos, as well as low-income residents, have experienced the highest incidence of coronavirus infections, hospitalizations, and deaths. Its findings reported that Black and Latino New Yorkers died at twice the rate of White residents – when the data was adjusted for age – which coincided with national figures that showed that Blacks were infected and died at disproportionately high rates. "The data, which shows death rates in each of the city's zip codes, underscores the deep disparities already unearthed by the outbreak," reported *The New York Times*, in an article that appeared in April 2020 [6]. "While the majority of the deaths across the city have been older residents, race and income have proven to be the largest factors in determining who lives and who dies."

In the best of circumstances, the Bronx ranks at the bottom in virtually all health care measures. It perennially ranks as the 62nd and last county in New York State in terms of health care outcomes according to the Robert Wood Johnson Foundation [7]. According to the American Community Survey [8], it is the nation's poorest urban county with 28% of the population living in poverty compared to 15.9% citywide. The poverty rate is even lower in the Belmont/East Tremont section, the community that surrounds St. Barnabas Hospital, which is 31%. The Bronx's median household income is $37,397 (compared to $56,942 in Brooklyn, $64,509 in Queens, $79,201 in Staten Island, and $85,071 in Manhattan). The age-adjusted mortality rate in the Bronx is 20.5% higher than the rest of New York City – the premature mortality rate, for those under the age of 75, is 38.7% higher.

Conversely, the Bronx had been the fastest growing borough in New York City, having experienced an economic boom prior to the onset of the virus. New housing had grown dramatically, with population in 2017 increasing faster here by 10.4% since 2000, according to the Office of the New York State Comptroller [9], than anywhere else in New York City, and private sector jobs had grown by 20%. Unemployment had dropped to a low of 4.6%. That all changed with the advent of the coronavirus. According to the US Bureau of Labor Statistics, unemployment climbed to 15.1% in the Bronx by December 2020, after peaking at 25% in July of that year [10].

While the Bronx did not have the highest rate of COVID-19 among the city's boroughs, its outcomes were more severe, with the highest hospitalization and death rates (Box 1.1).

Box 1.1 Key Considerations Related to the Severity of COVID-19 Outcomes in the Bronx
- *Prior to COVID-19, the life expectancy of a Manhattan resident was 85, compared to 75 in the Bronx, with the Bronx having far higher rates of preexisting conditions like asthma, heart disease, and obesity – all underlying conditions that increase the risk of severe COVID-19 illness.*
- *The Bronx's population is 85% Black or Hispanic, whereas in Manhattan 64% of the population is White.*
- *The incidence of obesity is 15% in Manhattan and 29% in the Bronx.*
- *Almost 60% of Bronx residents pay more than they can afford for housing, which has led to multigenerational housing arrangements and more residents in public housing.*

> - *On average, two people live in a single unit in Manhattan and 2.8 in the Bronx.*
> - *Residents in the Bronx deal with lower-quality housing infrastructure, with maintenance problems that include leaks, rats, cracks, and plumbing issues.*
> - *While 61% of those living in Manhattan say they could work from home during the pandemic, only 9% of those in the Bronx say they have that luxury.*
> - *During the pandemic, subway ridership was down 75% in Manhattan but only 55% in the Bronx.*

All this notwithstanding, when the pandemic struck, SBH – like other health systems through much of the world – was ill prepared to confront this lethal and largely mysterious virus. This meant fighting this disease with no playbook and little advanced knowledge or expectations on what was to come. Yet, as the reader will find out in the forthcoming chapters, SBH healthcare workers became fast learners. Amid incredibly difficult conditions, they learned a great deal over the subsequent months in terms of safety protocols, treatments, and technologies. SBH Health System proved that it was up to the challenge.

SBH Health System

St. Barnabas Hospital is a safety net hospital. While the term "safety net hospital" itself does not have a universal definition, it is generally meant to refer to those primarily urban hospitals with high levels of Medicaid and uninsured patients. As such, this means that no patient is turned away because of their inability to pay or their immigration status. At SBH, an estimated 80% of patients are uninsured or covered by Medicaid, with most of the remaining patients insured through Medicare. The hospital staff of 3000 reflects the community SBH Health System cares for, with a high percentage of Blacks and Hispanics.

The hospital has served the Bronx for more than 150 years. It is a 422-bed, not-for-profit, nonsectarian acute care community hospital with a level 2 trauma center authorized to treat the most critically ill and severely injured patients, a level 3 NCQA patient-centered medical home, a state-designated stroke center, and freestanding hemodialysis treatment center. Its ambulatory care center offers a full range of pediatric, adolescent, and adult primary care and specialty services. SBH provides a wide range of mental health services to children, adults, and geriatric patients through SBH Behavioral Health.

SBH is an academic institution, annually training an estimated 250 residents in the specialties of internal medicine, emergency medicine, surgery, psychiatry, pediatrics, osteopathic manipulative medicine, podiatry, general and pediatric dentistry, and orthodontics. Clinical affiliations are with the CUNY School of Medicine, New York Institute of Technology College of Osteopathic Medicine, and the Albert Einstein College of Medicine.

In late 2020, SBH opened its newest addition, the SBH Health and Wellness Center. Located across the street from the hospital, the center is part of a $156 million, 450,000 square-foot project that also includes 314 units of affordable housing. It includes a medical fitness center, a culinary education center, and teaching kitchen and a rooftop farm, as well as an urgent care center and clinical services. A food pantry provides fresh and free produce for those in need, as does a "Farmacy" program for those in the community who are referred by their providers. The vision behind the new center was to support community access to a healthier life, keep people healthy and out of the hospital, and address the Social Determinants of Health. Early results have been very positive.

SBH recognizes that in order to address the health care disparities, collaboration with community partners and expanding the scope of services to focus on prevention and wellness programs are essential. To this end, SBH took the lead in creating Bronx Partners for Healthy Communities (BPHC), a group of more than 200 Bronx community-based organizations working together to improve the health care delivery and outcomes. BPHC has allowed SBH and its partners to develop and implement innovative programs that address both the medical and social needs of our community.

In its Community Service Plan, SBH adopted three priority areas: *1. Prevent chronic disease by the screening of food insecurity.* The focus is on reduction of obesity in children. In a community survey, food and nutrition ranked #2 for "priority health issues" and access to healthier food ranked #1 in both "most helpful actions for the community" and "priority health issues" for individuals. *2. Promote healthy and safe environments.* The focus is on reducing violence by targeting prevention programs to high-risk populations. This has included implementation of the Bronx Rises Against Violence (B.R.A.G.) program, which provides support for those young patients hospitalized due to violence. *3. Promote healthy women, infants, and children.* The mission here is to increase breastfeeding, with SBH recently designated as a Baby Friendly Hospital.

SBH During the Initial COVID-19 Surge: First Thoughts

The SBH Health System came under immense strain in March 2020 from when patients with COVID-19 symptoms first appeared in the emergency room at the system's flagship institution, St. Barnabas Hospital. *"It hit us so fast and so hard…we had to use everything at our disposal to get where we were,"* said Dr. Manisha Kulshreshtha, Senior Vice President, Medical Director at SBH, in an episode of SBH Bronx Health Talk, the hospital's podcast. *"We did not expect them to come in and die so quickly. It was almost like an avalanche of patients. We did not expect that and had to gear up. We had a plan with phases A, B, C, D and we thought we'd go in steps. I think very quickly, within a day or two, we went from phase A to phase D."*

Throughout this book, recommendations for health crisis planning and preparation and management of health crisis from the perspective of several key departments within an acute care hospital are presented. Such recommendations come from lessons learned by the SBH Health System in the Bronx, New York, USA, and the individuals and teams directly involved with managing the crisis during the COVID-19 pandemic surge in the Spring of 2020. While widely applicable to other acute care hospitals around the world, the recommendations and the lessons come from the very unique context of SBH and its extreme circumstances that warrants understating of the special situation of the population which SBH serves.

References

1. The United States census bureau. https://www.census.gov/programs-surveys/acs/data.html. Accessed 26 June 2021.
2. Office of Disease Prevention and Health Promotion: U.S. Department of Health and Human Services. Social Determinants of Health. https://health.gov/healthypeople/objectives-and-data/social-determinants-health#:~:text=What%20are%20social%20determinants%20of,of%2Dlife%20outcomes%20and%20risks. Accessed 14 July 2021.
3. Feeding America. Map the Meal Gap, technical note on 2018. https://map.feedingamerica.org/. Accessed 11 June 2021.
4. New York City Food Policy. Food metrics report 2018. https://www1.nyc.gov/assets/foodpolicy/downloads/pdf/2018-Food-Metrics-Report.pdf. Accessed 14 June 2021.
5. NYC Health. NYC Department of Health and Mental Hygiene. https://www1.nyc.gov/site/doh/index.page. Accessed 18 June 2021.
6. The New York Times. Coronavirus deaths. https://www.nytimes.com/2020/05/18/nyregion/coronavirus-deaths-nyc.html. Accessed 18 Aug 2020.
7. Robert Wood Johnson Foundation. https://www.rwjf.org/. Accessed 23 June 2021.
8. The United States census bureau. American Community Survey (ACS). https://www.census.gov/programs-surveys/acs. Accessed 14 June- 2021.
9. Office of the New York State Comptroller, June 2021. https://www.osc.state.ny.us/.
10. U.S. Bureau of Labor Statistics. Civilian unemployment rate. https://www.bls.gov/charts/employment-situation/civilian-unemployment-rate.htm. Accessed 14 June 2021.

Chapter 2
COVID-19 Crisis Timeline: The Warning and the Surge

Ridwan Shabsigh and Daniel Kelly

Defining the COVID-19 Pandemic

A pandemic is defined as an epidemic of an infectious disease (in case of COVID-19, a viral disease) that has spread across a large region or worldwide, affecting a large number of people. Over the past 100 years, viral and bacterial infections have shown the ability to spread locally, regionally, and even globally, crossing borders and barriers, causing disability and death in an increasingly globalized world [1]. Pandemics frequently strain healthcare resources and sometimes overwhelm them. After localized sporadic cases, an initial outbreak occurs. Following the outbreak, a pandemic is characterized by three phases: a rapidly escalating surge, a peak, and a slow or very slow de-escalation. Not infrequently, pandemics also feature a second or even multiple surges after the first one. Such surges of a crisis, and particularly initial surges, can potentially overwhelm healthcare institutions and resources, especially in large densely populated urban areas and communities of low socioeconomic status.

Infectious health crises, compared to earthquakes, hurricanes, and other health crises, have the unique ability to infect and disable not only the patients but also the healthcare workers themselves, thus multiplying the potential of overwhelming healthcare institutions with the loss of staffing. Resultantly, infectious health crises

---

R. Shabsigh (✉)
Department of Surgery, SBH Health System, Bronx, NY, USA

Department of Urology, Weill Cornell Medical College of Cornell University, New York, NY, USA

CUNY School of Medicine, New York, NY, USA
e-mail: rshabsigh@sbhny.org

D. Kelly
Department of Biosciences & Chemistry, Faculty of Health & Wellbeing, Sheffield Hallam University, Sheffield, UK

© The Author(s), under exclusive license to Springer Nature Switzerland AG 2022
R. Shabsigh (ed.), *Health Crisis Management in Acute Care Hospitals*, https://doi.org/10.1007/978-3-030-95806-0_2

place special demands for the protection of healthcare workers and the preservation of healthcare institutions' ability to continue to function. Best practices in such protection as well as prevention and patient treatment require the rapid sharing of knowledge and a united approach to understanding and developing novel treatments for newly emerged pandemic diseases. A global health crisis requires a global response. This can be achieved through the strengthening of the global health system focusing on improving collaboration and coordination across organizations (e.g., the WHO, Gavi, CEPI, national centers for disease control, and pharmaceutical manufacturers) [2].

Origins of COVID-19

The origins of the SARS-CoV-2 virus, which causes COVID-19, are still not definitively known. Many of the early cases of COVID-19 were linked to the Huanan market in Wuhan [3, 4], indicating a possibility that an animal source at that location may be responsible for zoonotic transfer of the virus. Indeed, it is likely that bats were the original animal hosts for the progenitor virus due to the similarity of SARS-CoV-2 to bat SARS-CoV-like coronaviruses [4], although an intermediate host may exist between bats and humans. It is possible that the virus adapted into its current infectious and transmissible form either in the animal host before jumping to humans or by first transferring to humans and subsequently evolving via natural selection during undetected human-to-human transmission [5].

Basics of SARS-CoV-2: The Coronavirus

SARS-CoV-2 is a member of the coronavirus family, Coronaviridae, related to those that were previously responsible for the outbreaks of severe acute respiratory syndrome (SARS) from 2002 to 2004 predominantly in East Asia and Middle East respiratory syndrome (MERS) in 2012. It has a similar structure and genome to the other coronaviruses and possesses the spherical shape with spike proteins protruding from its surface which gives its typical appearance (Fig. 2.1). While the coronaviruses are made up of four structural proteins, including the spike (S), membrane, envelope, and nucleocapsid proteins, it is the S protein which is recognized as particularly important for attachment to and penetration into host cells. There are two functional domains of the S protein known as S1 which binds with the host cell receptor and S2 which mediates the fusion of the virus with the host cell membrane.

Indeed, the entry of SARS-CoV-2 into host cells depends on the recognition and binding of S protein to angiotensin-converting enzyme 2 (ACE2) receptor of the host cells, indicating that organs and tissues that have high expression of ACE2 receptor, particularly the lung alveolar epithelial cells and also enterocytes of the small intestine, are the primary targets of SARS-CoV-2 [6]. Interestingly, S protein

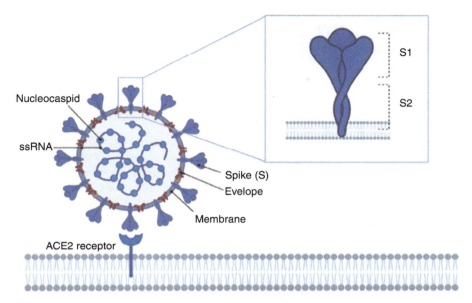

Fig. 2.1 SARS-CoV-2 structure. The virus has a spherical shape with spike proteins protruding from its surface which gives its typical appearance. It is made up of four structural proteins, including the spike (S), membrane, envelope, and nucleocapsid proteins. The S protein has two functional domains known as S1 and S2. S1 is recognized and binds to angiotensin-converting enzyme 2 (ACE2) receptor on host cells allowing penetration of the virus and host cell infection. Created with BioRender.com

of SARS-CoV-2 is demonstrated to possess a 10- to 20-fold higher affinity to ACE2 receptor than that of SARS-CoV and likely contributes to the quick spreading of the virus [7]. Once inside the cell, the virus undergoes replication to form new viral particles which can invade the adjacent epithelial cells while at the same time generating new infective viral particles for release out of the host via respiratory droplets enabling community transmission. This reinitiates the cycle in new cells and hosts.

Within the host, SARS-CoV-2 activates an inflammatory immune response, particularly in the lungs where the virus most commonly resides, through the production of a milieu of cytokines and chemokines and the activation of lymphocytes. Often this initial response is insufficient, so the host amplifies the response to defend against the infection. It is this amplification of the inflammatory immune response that gives rise to the so-called "cytokine storm" which further acts to recruit neutrophils, CD4 helper T cells, and CD8 cytotoxic T cells to the site. These cells are responsible for fighting off the virus, but consequently the heightened inflammation and excessive immune cell accumulation can injure the lung. Alveolar epithelial cells undergo apoptosis (programmed cell death) and release new viral particles which infect adjacent cells to continue the cycle. Diffuse alveolar damage ensues, and alveolar flooding can occur as a result of insufficient resorption and capillary leakage of plasma proteins and fluid. All of these features inhibit normal respiratory function of the lungs and eventually culminate in an acute respiratory distress syndrome (ARDS).

Symptoms

The SARS-CoV-2 virus mainly spreads from person to person via respiratory droplet transmission, which occurs when a person is in close contact with someone who is actively coughing or sneezing. Once the virus is contracted, an initial early viral response phase ensues before an inflammatory second phase follows, resulting in an overall biphasic pattern of illness. The incubation period of COVID-19, which is the time period from exposure to the virus to symptom onset, is 5–6 days, but can be up to 14 days. During this period, also known as the "pre-symptomatic" period, the infected individuals can be contagious and transmit the virus to healthy individuals in the population.

Throughout both phases of the disease, most symptoms are mild typically presenting as an influenza-like illness, which includes fever, cough, malaise, myalgia, headache, and taste and smell disturbance. However, approximately one in five patients infected with the virus progress to the severe pneumonia-like disease known as ARDS which displays extreme symptoms like high fever, severe cough, and shortness of breath. These symptoms, particularly difficulties in breathing, require the patient to be hospitalized and in many cases, where high-risk comorbidities are present, can result in death.

Classification as a Pandemic

In December 2019, Wuhan city of Hubei province of China was overwhelmed by a series of acute atypical respiratory infections which soon later were discovered to be caused by a novel coronavirus, SARS-CoV-2, and therefore the disease has been named COVID-19. COVID-19 was broadcast as a public health emergency on January 30, 2020, and on March 11, 2020, the World Health Organization (WHO) declared the novel coronavirus outbreak a global pandemic [8]. Following accumulated data that more than 118,000 cases were reported in 114 countries and 4291 deaths worldwide, Dr. Tedros Adhanom Ghebreyesus, the WHO Director-General, made clear his deep concerns regarding the alarming levels of spread and disease severity. Although some argue that COVID-19 is not a pandemic, but a syndemic—a concept to describe how epidemic disease clusters with preexisting conditions, interacts with them, and is driven by larger political, economic, and social factors [9]—it is universally acknowledged that this disease has caused a global health crisis, like no other before it.

COVID-19 Pandemic in the USA and Its Epicenter New York City: Timeline of the Crisis

A remarkable feature of this particular threat was the fact that this was a completely new virus with lack of knowledge of its pathophysiology and clinical effects and an absence of diagnostics, therapeutics, and vaccines at the time. After the subsequent news of the COVID-19 spread through China, Italy, and Europe, detection of cases started occurring in the USA at a very rapidly accelerating rate, most notably in its epicenter, New York City. According to the New York City Department of Health, the first confirmed case in New York City was on February 29, 2020, and although earlier cases in the USA had been confirmed, the numbers in New York City began to rise faster than other states and became the worse affected area in the country. Figures 2.2, 2.3, 2.4, 2.5, and 2.6 show the rapid surge in cases, hospitalizations, mortality, emergency room visits, and hospital admissions through the emergency rooms in New York City.

There are several observations that can be noted from the data of the crisis as it happened in March, April, and May 2020. The first observation of the timeline of the crisis is the rapid escalating increase of all categories of patients, emergency room visits, in-patient admissions, and critically ill patients requiring ventilation,

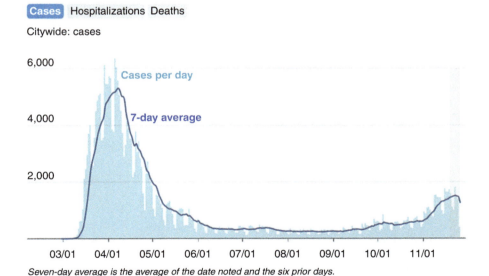

Seven-day average is the average of the date noted and the six prior days.
Gray bar indicates data from most recent days are incomplete.

Fig. 2.2 The number of COVID-19 cases per day and the 7-day average over the period of March–November 2020. Axes correspond to New York citywide cases (*y* axis) and the chronological date indicated by the first of each month (*x* axis). (Source New York City Department of Health website accessed on 11/29/2020 https://www1.nyc.gov/site/doh/covid/covid-19-data-trends.page)

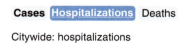

Citywide: hospitalizations

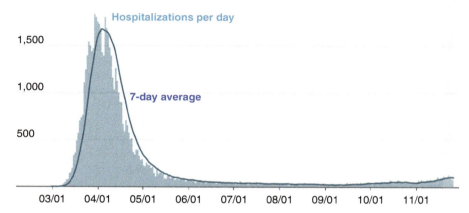

Seven-day average is the average of the date noted and the six prior days.
Gray bar indicates data from most recent days are incomplete.
Get the data • Created with Datawrapper

Fig. 2.3 The number of COVID-19 hospitalizations per day and the 7-day average for March–November 2020. (Source New York City Department of Health website accessed on 11/29/2020 https://www1.nyc.gov/site/doh/covid/covid-19-data-trends.page)

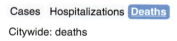

Citywide: deaths

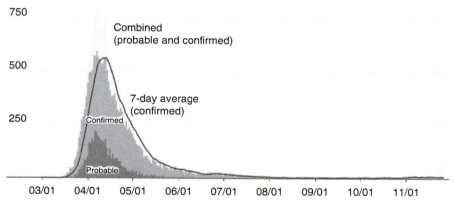

Seven-day average is the average of the date noted and the six prior days.
Gray bar indicates data from most recent days are incomplete.
Get the data • Created with Datawrapper

Fig. 2.4 The probable, confirmed, and total number of COVID-19 deaths per day and the 7-day average for March–November 2020. (Source New York City Department of Health website accessed on 11/29/2020 https://www1.nyc.gov/site/doh/covid/covid-19-data-trends.page)

2 COVID-19 Crisis Timeline: The Warning and the Surge

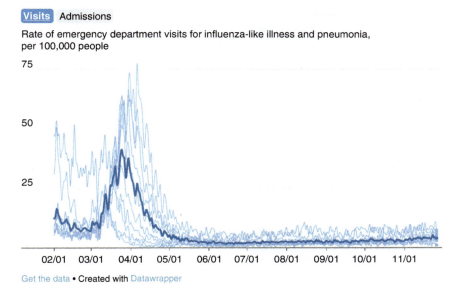

Fig. 2.5 The rate of emergency department visits in New York City hospitals for influenza-like illness and pneumonia per 100,000 people, March–November 2020. (Source New York City Department of Health website accessed on 11/29/2020 https://www1.nyc.gov/site/doh/covid/covid-19-data-trends.page)

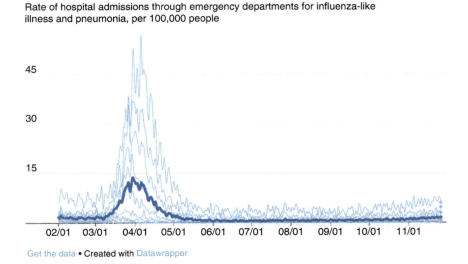

Fig. 2.6 The rate of hospital admissions through emergency departments in New York City hospitals for influenza-like illness and pneumonia per 100,000 people, March–November 2020. (Source New York City Department of Health website accessed on 11/29/2020 https://www1.nyc.gov/site/doh/covid/covid-19-data-trends.page)

dialysis, and other intensive care measures (Figs. 2.3 and 2.5). The second observation is the accumulative effect of the rapid successive waves of patients coming to hospitals, resulting in a rapidly reached peak of the surge in the first week of April 2020. As severely ill patients accumulate in all parts of a hospital and at all levels of care, regular, intermediate and intensive, the effect is an acute severe strain on the human and material resources of a hospital.

The third observation is that disease progression occurs in a substantial number of patients after admission, requiring transfer from regular care to intermediate or intensive care. This progression of disease has an additional additive and accumulative straining effect on top of the critically ill patients arriving in the emergency room and transferred directly to intensive care. The fourth observation is that the majority of patients have a long length of stay (LOS) in the hospital until either recovery and discharge or death. Such long LOS slows down the recovery from the crisis and prolongs the strain on the human and material resources of a hospital. The strain on the human resources is particularly profound as the demand for care outstrips the capacity for provision (Fig. 2.7).

The fifth observation is the high mortality of the infectious pandemic. This high mortality has significant psychological impact on families and on the frontline hospital staff as well. The high mortality also requires substantial logistical effort to keep patient workflow in process and to free resources for other patients. In

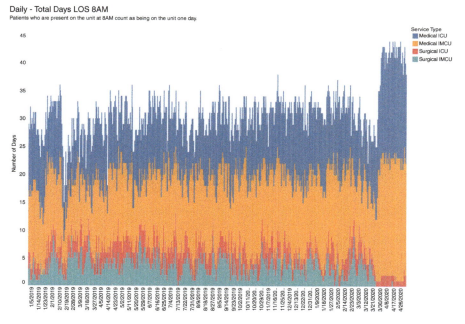

Fig. 2.7 The severe increase in length of stay (LOS) in critical care units during the surge of the COVID-19 pandemic in late March and throughout April 2020 in comparison to LOS prior to COVID-19 pandemic at SBH Health System

addition, prior to death, there is a high demand for palliative care services and communications with families.

The sixth observation is that the peak of the surge of the crisis was reached much earlier than the warning at the declaration of crisis had suggested. The epidemiologists of the various health authorities predicted the peak of the surge to occur 6 weeks after declaration of the crisis. In reality, the surge occurred in half that time, 3 weeks after the declaration of the crisis, catching all New York City hospitals by surprise and shock. As a consequence, and the seventh observation, at the time of the first surge, no hospital in the greater New York City metropolitan area was adequately prepared for the magnitude of the COVID-19 health crisis. The magnitude and the rapidity of the surge of the COVID-19 crisis were above and beyond the expectations and capacities of the usual and customary hospital disaster planning. Modern healthcare is expensive. Therefore, most hospitals function with tight lean staffing and capacities during peaceful regular times, with little reserve and ability to expand rapidly. With a crisis hitting all hospitals in a large geographic area, it is unrealistic to expect broad-scale inter-hospital mutual help and support.

The eighth observation is the disruptive effect of the crisis on regular hospital functions and services, such as non-COVID-19 emergencies, elective surgery, ambulatory clinics, trauma care, cancer care, and care and follow-up of patients with chronic diseases other than COVID-19, such as diabetes, asthma, and mental health disorders. This disruption undoubtedly resulted in deterioration and worsening of chronic disease such as diabetes and heart failure and delayed diagnosis and treatment of cancers potentially causing progression of cancer and consequently late presentation of cases at higher clinical stages of disease. Furthermore, this places special requirements for resumption of regular services after the crisis and a substantial burden of services after the crisis.

Timeline of the Response at SBH Health System

The first phase of the response of the SBH Health System was triggered by the public news of the spreading COVID-19 pandemic in addition to information coming from the State and City Departments of Health. The leadership and senior administration officials of the hospital started early preparations for the crisis. Once it was clear that the pandemic had broken out significantly in the greater New York City metropolitan area, the Departments of Health of New York State and New York City issued orders to all hospitals to increase bed capacity by 50% and prepare for a surge of the crisis.

Significantly, the first patient admitted to SBH Health System was on March 13, 2020. Table 2.1 shows a timeline of some of the key events that followed at the hospital during this surge of the crisis, highlighting the rapid escalation of the number and severity of illness of the admitted patients. The SBH Health System responded quickly with several adjustments to normal practice across all departments. These included primarily setting up a crisis command center with multiple daily briefings, meetings, and communications. Multiple multidisciplinary crisis teams and

Table 2.1 Timeline of the key events at SBH Health System during the surge of the COVID-19 crisis

Date (m/d/y)	Event
3/4/2020	Hospital leadership COVID-19 emergency management call started 3 times/week
3/13/2021	First symptomatic COVID-19 patient admitted to SBH Health System
3/16/2020	Health crisis declared with predicted peak in the third or fourth week of April
3/17/2020	All elective surgeries canceled
3/18/2020	Multidisciplinary critical care committee established
3/23/2020	Hospital command center opened
3/26/2020	First body collection-point refrigerated truck on site
4/2/2020	Second body collection-point refrigerated truck on site
4/6/2020	Peak of surge reached lasting 6 days
4/7/2020	Intermittent partial diversion from the hospital emergency room over 7 days
4/9/2020	Peak of number of ventilated COVID-19 in-patients
4/12/2020	Peak of total COVID-19 in-patients, ventilated and non-ventilated
4/13/2020	Start of slow decline in total COVID-19 in-patients; slower decline in critical care patient
4/16/2020	Quietest day in ED in the past 4 weeks with only 1 ventilated patient in the ED
5/1/2020	Continuation of slow decline of COVID-19 admissions and number of in-patients

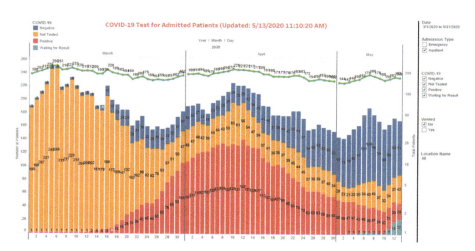

Fig. 2.8 The surge in COVID-19 patient admissions in March, April, and early May, 2020, at SBH Health System

workgroups were also set up from all clinical and administrative departments, to plan, prepare, and manage the anticipated health crisis and the surge of the pandemic. The teams of medical critical care, surgical critical care, and anesthesiology were combined into one critical care team to cope with the influx of severely ill patients. Figures 2.8 and 2.9 show the surge of in-patient admissions and the surge of critically ill mechanically ventilated patients at SBH Health System. A critical care committee and multidisciplinary tiered teams were set up to serve the rapidly rising needs for

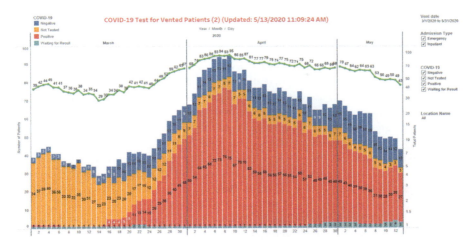

Fig. 2.9 The surge in COVID-19 critically ill ventilated patients in March, April, and early May, 2020, at SBH Health System

critical care services of acceleratingly increasing numbers admitted with severe respiratory failure and other multiorgan failure. Daily briefings and meetings were conducted and frequent communications were established. Human and material resources were mobilized maximally to allow provision of care in areas under increased demand, and to aid in this, all elective surgeries were canceled on March 17, 2020.

Once the peak of the surge started to pass from April 13, 2020, the various teams returned very slowly, carefully, and gradually to regular functions. Ultimately, elective surgery was resumed, and other functions were restarted, albeit with new rules and processes, including infection prevention measures. The details of the hospital response are recounted in the subsequent chapters of this book with explanations specific to each clinical or administrative department described along with the lessons learned from critical reflection. These highly valuable lessons may guide preparation, planning, and management of future crises, here at SBH Health System and potentially elsewhere at hospitals and healthcare providers across the world.

Although the above describes in detail the acute first surge of the COVID-19 crisis, it should be emphasized that the crisis continued well beyond the surge with slow recovery and second and third surges, albeit less intense than the first surge. The recovery from the crisis has taken a long time and major efforts.

> **International Vignette: Sex Differences in the Morbidity and Mortality of COVID-19**
>
> *The current COVID-19 pandemic has a male bias in morbidity/severity and mortality. This is consistent with previous coronavirus pandemics such as SARS- CoV and MERS-CoV, and viral infections in general. Data from previous coronavirus epidemics such as SARS-CoV (2002) and Middle Eastern*

respiratory syndrome coronavirus (MERS, 2012) showed differences in their manifestation based on sex, with men being consistently more severely affected than women. Reports of COVID-19 suggest a sex imbalance, with men at a higher risk of more severe disease and increased mortality.

Publicly available data from the Global Health 50/50 research initiative showed an increased mortality in men, despite similar numbers of COVID-19 cases in men and women. In addition to mortality, hospitalizations and admissions to intensive care units (ICU) showed men more affected than women. A review of data in several countries showed that there were 50% more men requiring hospitalization compared to women, with ICU admission being three- to fourfold higher. A meta-analysis of 15 independent studies found men had an odds ratio of 1.31 to develop a severe COVID-19 infection compared to women. Early reports by the Centers for Disease Control and Prevention (CDC) observed higher hospitalization rates for men.

There are, however, some limitations to this data particularly as the interaction between age and sex remains unclear. It was reported that the relative risk of dying from COVID-19 was consistently elevated in men across all age groups with the differences increasing until the age range 60–69 years. Thereafter, the sex difference in survival decreases and was at its lowest for ages ≥80.

The sex disparities in COVID-19 morbidity and mortality are multifactorial. They may potentially be caused by the sex differences in comorbidities and behaviors. There is a need to collect sex and age-disaggregated data to better understand disease pathology, study the sex differences, and guide clinical care. Furthermore, the consistencies with previous coronavirus pandemics may suggest that the public health policies and risk stratification should take sex into consideration for future pandemics. Additionally, more research is needed to clarify inflammatory and immunity disparities to close some knowledge gaps in these concerns.

Alwani M, Yassin A, Al-Zoubi RM, Aboumarzouk OM, Nettleship J, Kelly D, Al-Qudimat AR, Shabsigh R. Sex-based differences in severity and mortality in COVID-19. Rev Med Virol. 2021 Mar 1: https://doi.org/10.1002/rmv.2223. Epub ahead of print. PMID: 33646622; PMCID: PMC8014761.

Prof. Dr. Dr. Aksam A. Yassin MD PhD EdD FEBU
Senior Consultant Urologist/Andrologist,
Director of Men's Health & Vice-Chair of Surgery for Research
Hamad Medical Corporation, Doha/Qatar
Professor of Clinical Urology, Weill Cornell Medical School New York & Qatar Dresden International University, Dresden Germany
Editor, Journal of Men's Health

Key Lessons Learned from the Surge at SBH

An infectious health crisis can surge rapidly from a small outbreak to an overwhelming epidemic or even a pandemic. This surge may include an increase of all categories of patients, emergency room visits, in-patient admissions, and critically ill patients with multiorgan failure. There is an accumulative effect of the waves of patients coming to the hospital, with a severe strain on the human and material resources. Long hospitalization of the majority of patients slows the recovery from the crisis. Consequently, there is undoubtedly a disruptive effect of a health crisis on regular hospital functions and services, such as elective surgery, ambulatory clinics, cancer care, mental health, and care and follow-up of patients with diseases other than infectious crisis. This places special requirements for resumption of regular services after the crisis and a substantial burden of services after the crisis; therefore, strategic plans to minimize this recovery burden are needed.

A collaborative culture and teamwork are very important for any hospital system at the time of a health crisis to overcome extreme adversity. Furthermore, it is important for a hospital to establish collaborative relationships with other health institutions for future health crises.

It became clear that there are a number of vulnerabilities, during peaceful regular times, in hospital systems that could hamper crisis efforts, including low capacities, shortages in equipment and supplies, shortages in staffing, and inadequacies of the physical facilities. In particular, redundancy of suppliers of essential items is very prudent and the hospital should include into its planning mitigation of the difficulty in accessing and affording such resources.

In reflection of the surge at SBH, some pertinent questions arose that solidify some of the key lessons that were, and need to be, learned from a healthcare crisis of this magnitude and nature.

What is unique about an infectious, possibly viral health crisis? There are many characteristics unique to an infectious crisis versus other crisis, such as a hurricane, an earthquake, or a mass casualty event. An infectious crisis has an accumulative rapidly escalating surge with an acute burden on healthcare systems. Furthermore, an infectious crisis can affect the healthcare workers themselves, thus threatening hospitals' ability to cope with the crisis and deliver care to patients.

Can a hospital count on presetting a maximal capacity and executing a diversion to other hospitals in case of high demand during a surge of a crisis? Yes and No! Depending on the magnitude of the surge and the availability of other receptive hospitals, a hospital may or may not be able to divert to other hospitals. In the case of an extraordinary surge, maximal capacity may frequently have to be "stretched."

Can the triage of the various acuity of patient conditions and the designation of levels of care be preset prior to an infectious health crisis? While it is very important to include, in crisis preparedness plans, criteria for triage and designation of levels of care, such practices should be subject to frequent review and dynamic adjustment during a crisis, in order to achieve practical flexibility, maximal efficiency, and prompt response to a continuously changing situation.

The reflections on these questions and the key features of the SBH Health System response to the surge can provide lessons to develop a culture of preparedness in healthcare settings to lessen the impact on hospital services and workers, and hopefully mitigate the devastating impact on patient lives health crises can bring.

References

1. Frenk J, Gómez-Dantés O, Knaul FM. Globalization and infectious diseases. Infect Dis Clin N Am. 2011;25(3):593–9, viii. https://doi.org/10.1016/j.idc.2011.05.003. Epub 2011 Jul 2. PMID: 21896360; PMCID: PMC7135545.
2. Bloom DE, Cadarette D. Infectious disease threats in the twenty-first century: strengthening the global response. Front Immunol. 2019;10:549. https://doi.org/10.3389/fimmu.2019.00549. PMID: 30984169; PMCID: PMC6447676.
3. Zhou P, Yang XL, Wang XG, Hu B, Zhang W, et al. A pneumonia outbreak associated with a new coronavirus of probable bat origin. Nature. 2020;579:270–3. https://doi.org/10.1038/s41586-020-2012-7.
4. Wu F, Zhao S, Yu B, Chen Y, Wang W, Song Z, et al. A new coronavirus associated with human respiratory disease in China. Nature. 2020;579:265–9. https://doi.org/10.1038/s41586-020-2008-3.
5. Andersen KG, Rambaut A, Lipkin WI, Holmes EC, Garry RF. The proximal origin of SARS-CoV-2. Nat Med. 2020;26:450–2. https://doi.org/10.1038/s41591-020-0820-9.
6. Zou X, Chen K, Zou J, Han P, Hao J, Han Z. Single-cell RNA-seq data analysis on the receptor ACE2 expression reveals the potential risk of different human organs vulnerable to 2019-nCoV infection. Front Med. 2020;14(2):185–92. https://doi.org/10.1007/s11684-020-0754-0. Epub 2020 Mar 12. PMID: 32170560; PMCID: PMC7088738.
7. Wrapp D, Wang N, Corbett KS, Goldsmith JA, Hsieh CL, Abiona O, et al. Cryo-EM structure of the 2019-nCoV spike in the prefusion conformation. Science. 2020;367(6483):1260–3. https://doi.org/10.1126/science.abb2507. Epub 2020 Feb 19. PMID: 32075877; PMCID: PMC7164637.
8. Ghebreyesus TA. WHO Director-General's opening remarks at the media briefing on COVID-19-2020. https://www.who.int/director-general/speeches/detail/who-director-generals-opening-remarks-at-the-media-briefing-on-covid-19%2D%2D-11-march-2020.
9. Horton R. Offline: COVID-19 is not a pandemic. Lancet. 2020;396:874.

Chapter 3
Preparation, Planning, and the Command Center

Eric C. Appelbaum, Daniel P. Lombardi, Manisha Kulshreshtha, Mary M. Bolbrock, Zane S. Last, and Morena Lasso

Preparation and Planning for Health Crisis Management

A crisis in a healthcare system can arise from multiple different sources: political, socioeconomic, environmental, and/or infectious disease. Changes in political regulations or healthcare laws can result in a short-term subacute crisis, which is often met with changes in health system policy and procedures. Socioeconomic crises affect a given population and can result in a chronic long-term or subacute crisis within a healthcare system or within a given patient population. Environmental and infectious sources can cause an immediate and exponential crisis in the healthcare system. Another cause of a health crisis can be war or collapse in public order; during and immediately after war, health crises can arise resulting in massive illness and death.

Environmental crises such as hurricanes and earthquakes can result in a catastrophic loss of healthcare function and can affect operations for an extended period. Examples of such environmental crises include Hurricane Katrina (New Orleans/Gulf coast) and Hurricane Sandy (New York/East Coast). These environmental crises can also reveal vulnerabilities in a healthcare system, which are often

---

E. C. Appelbaum (✉) · D. P. Lombardi · M. Lasso
SBH Health System, Bronx, NY, USA
e-mail: eappelbaum@sbhny.org

M. Kulshreshtha
SBH Health System, Bronx, NY, USA

CUNY School of Medicine, New York, NY, USA

M. M. Bolbrock
Quality and Risk Management, SBH Health System, Bronx, NY, USA

Z. S. Last
Healthcare Analytics and Business Intelligence, SBH Health System, New York, NY, USA

© The Author(s), under exclusive license to Springer Nature Switzerland AG 2022
R. Shabsigh (ed.), *Health Crisis Management in Acute Care Hospitals*, https://doi.org/10.1007/978-3-030-95806-0_3

long-standing and complex to fix. Hurricane Katrina not only resulted in long-term operational disruption but it also revealed inequities affecting vulnerable populations [1]. On the other hand, Hurricane Sandy revealed both strengths and weakness in the coordination of emergency operations [2].

Infectious crises, as seen in an epidemic or pandemic, can also result in long-term operational changes. These long-term operational changes must be managed to continue effective and safe healthcare operations. Such a crisis was experienced during the historic Flu Pandemic of 1918, a global health catastrophe determining one of the highest mortality rates due to an infectious disease [3]. Similar to the 1918 pandemic, the COVID-19 pandemic has created similar challenges. Infectious crises are different from environmental crisis in that infectious crises threaten the healthcare workforce, thus endangering the existence of the healthcare system.

Planning for a health crisis is paramount in order to maintain effective continuous health system operations. Key components – staff, supplies, and space – to the delivery of care must be identified, considered, and monitored in order to continue to function in any given crisis. Additionally, triggers or benchmarks must also be considered and planned for so that a given system can adjust overall operations in accordance with a well-developed plan.

The Hospital Incident Command System

The hospital incident command system (HICS) is an established and defined process in the USA, which incorporates emergency plans, policies, and procedures necessary to achieve a state of ongoing readiness and preparation in response to an emergency. It also includes mitigation strategies to address system recovery in response to an emergency. When an emergency situation arises which impacts and affects the functionality of a healthcare system, the emergency preparedness coordinator/safety officer will collaborate with internal and external resources to determine the need for activation of HICS to manage the situation. If and when HICS is activated, it is necessary to report this activation to the state regulatory body. In New York State, HICS activation is reported through the New York occurrence reporting and tracking system (NYPORTS).

HICS Command Center and Communication During a Healthcare Crisis/Pandemic

When a healthcare crisis develops and is deemed a pandemic, it is necessary for the healthcare system to maintain continuous communication with both internal and external resources at the state, local, and federal government levels. Through the HICS process, a command center is established with representation from assigned administrators to address the issues that evolve as a result of the pandemic. In responding to a pandemic, the healthcare system must take action to address policies and regulations which have been formulated to address the pandemic and develop strategies to mitigate and limit the spread of disease. The healthcare system must be forthcoming in addressing new challenges that develop in response to the pandemic and incorporate information, received from the state and the federal government, into healthcare delivery for the management of a pandemic. Daily communication circulating ongoing updates with the state regulatory agency is imperative and it is necessary to assign administrative staff as designated representatives specifically responsible for the coordination of this ongoing communication. Establishing contact persons within the healthcare system is also needed to facilitate direct and rapid access of communication with the state and federal regulatory agencies. In addition, communication with the state agency is necessary to address any complaints that they may receive in response to the pandemic crisis.

Expanding the Role of the Command Center During a Health Crisis

The command center in a hospital is a designated location – physical, virtual, or hybrid – where a command team convenes to direct the response to a complex incident or a crisis, including the coordination of activities, resources, and information. The command center's main goal is to aid patient care and hospital operations and improve patient outcomes through centralization of activities during an emergency. The command center also supports staff to ensure safety of staff and patient care activities. Under the direction of the incident commander, leaders and directors/department heads collect information within the hospital and off-site, these activities often being aided by local, state, and federal regulatory agencies. Additionally, the command center aids in the coordination of care, focusing on maximizing bed capacity, and helps improve efficient and safe movement of patients within the healthcare system. Like a good umpire in baseball, the majority of the command center's function may go unnoticed by most of the frontline staff and patients, that is, when the command center is functioning well for both staff and patients.

HICS is part of the larger command center and consists of the following principles: emergency management planning, response (continuation of patient care activities), and recovery. The command system is subdivided into five major areas: command, operations, planning, logistics, and finance. Each of these five major areas ensures that all necessary patient care needs are met and that resources are available and used efficiently without duplication.

In the face of a healthcare crisis, HICS will be set up immediately and at the discretion of the senior management, nursing supervisor and/or administrator on call (AOC). An identified leader will then act as the incident commander. The incident ccommander's role will be determined by the order of authority; however, a senior authority can delegate to most qualified or available individual(s): chief operating officer, senior administrator, senior vice president or vice president, chief medical officer, and nursing supervisor in consultation with the AOC (during off-hours, weekends, and holidays).

One of the biggest responsibilities for the command center team is the action taken to return to a normal and even safer situation after the emergency or crisis.

Recovering can take weeks, months, and sometimes years. During a pandemic caused by an infectious disease, special infection prevention considerations must be considered and infection control practices followed in order to protect the command center team and command center operations. This should, at minimum, include creation of a smaller in-person team that practices social distancing, hand hygiene, and mask wearing. Development and utilization of a virtual command center offer even greater protection to the staff and operations, and relevant technology can then be utilized to effectively communicate with team members and healthcare staff.

The shift from an in-person command center team to a virtual team requires careful planning and practice in the form of pre-pandemic drills. These drills must focus on communication and, in particular, chain of command communication. A small, physically present command center team acts as the central hub of communication where phone calls are answered and command center activities documented. Electronic mail is also useful for communication; a group "command center" e-mail address can be created to assist in communication. The group e-mail can help expand the center response and improve communication. Figure 3.1 illustrates the command center functions, relationships, and communications.

Communication

Communication during any disaster is critical. All levels of an organization must be well-informed during the rapid changes that are inherit in a disaster response. A thoughtful communication plan must consider effective ways to communicate to leaders, managers/directors, and frontline staff/workers of an organization.

A senior leadership team is necessary to help allocate resources in an efficient and concise manner during a prolonged disaster. The formation of a senior leadership daily communication call can help in the execution of both long- and short-term plans and needs and should be tasked with making quick and effective

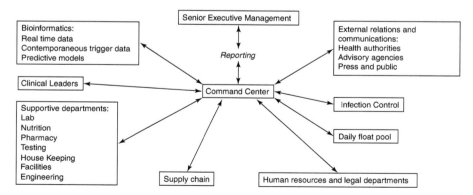

Fig. 3.1 Command center functions, relationships, and communications

decisions. The team should be small to increase effectiveness, though stakeholders should be present when critical decisions are made. Many of the agenda items for the senior leadership daily call emerge from the experiences and needs of the department heads of the organization, since many of these key department heads are involved in the disaster planning and prep team (see Box 3.1).

> **Box 3.1: The Plan, Do, Study, Act Process**
> Rapid cycle performance improvement with the process of plan, do, study, and act (PDSA) for the improvement of the functioning of data acquisition and presentation on a daily basis.
>
> - PLAN: Review requirements and collect data from the SQL databases and update table every day.
> - DO: Link the Tableau dashboards with EMR and update the dashboards.
> - STUDY: Validate and analyze the data.
> - ACT: Present the dashboards depending on the periodical update of the data. Get feedback from the end user for any future changes needed in the dashboards.

Departmental communication is essential not only to disseminate communication in a top-down approach but also to allow feedback from the bottom-up to higher levels of the organization. Frontline staff are not only essential in providing care during peaceful, regular times, but their experience and feedback during a crisis are even more essential. They experience firsthand the processes and structures put into place during a crisis and can therefore provide highly valuable feedback as to which processes work well and which do not. Additionally, frontline staff also provide valuable insight into needed processes, supplies, and support, some of which may be overlooked during the planning and execution of a crisis response, since each crisis presents its own individual challenges.

The Daily Safety Call

A 15-minute daily safety call, which serves as a weekday operational and safety organizational huddle during peaceful regular times, can be utilized to communicate updates to managers and directors during crisis times. This weekday daily call is extended during a crisis to include weekends. The call utilizes a roll call format to allow different operational and clinical departments to provide updates and communicate any safety or operational events. This format lends itself to rapid escalation and resolution of issues or events. This typical daily call includes reports from all inpatient clinical units as well as ambulatory clinics, infection prevention and control, clinical engineering, patient access, security, facilities, environmental services, and clinical support services, such as radiology, lab, and pharmacy. The report also includes any communication that has been escalated to the AOC.

Float Pool: Supporting the Care Teams

During a health crisis, many non-essential clinics and services are shut down and the employees from those services can be placed in a daily float pool. The command center team receives lists of daily available float pool healthcare workers and allocates them to needed functions and locations.

Creating a Team to Coordinate Transfers to Alternative Care Sites and Partnering with Other Health Systems

Setting up such a team should be a vital part of any crisis preparedness planning, especially in small- and medium-sized hospitals where transfers may be anticipated once capacity is overwhelmed. When the COVID-19 pandemic surged in New York City in March, April, and May of 2020, the federal and state governments developed alternate care sites (ACS) where acute care hospitals transfer patients due to patient capacity/space issues. At SBH Health System, a team was developed to help identify and aid in the transfer process. The team acted as a subgroup of the command center and consisted of medical staff, patient access, and pharmacy personnel. The group was under the leadership of a hospital senior vice president.

Emergency Operations Plan

Due to the significant impact emergencies can have on the operations of a healthcare system, it is necessary for a healthcare system to have a process for continuous readiness to manage and recover from any emergencies they may encounter; this is addressed in the emergency operations plan. The plan encompasses a comprehensive "all hazards" command structure which addresses six critical areas:

1. Communications
2. Resources and assets
3. Safety and security
4. Staffing
5. Utilities
6. Clinical activities

The response procedures within these six areas are established to address any and all emergencies which can adversely impact healthcare systems operational processes, as well as patient safety and the ability to provide care, treatment, and services for an extended length of time. In response to an emergency, this plan utilizes HICS to assist in addressing emergency situations that develop from both internal and external resources and it also establishes policies, action plans, and processes in preparation to address any possible emergency that may impact the healthcare system, as well as the community.

The Dashboard

When it comes to bioinformatics, the underlying data is a pure representation of the raw facts; the raw truth of a health crisis. It is the solemn task of the data analytics department to take the raw data and present it to the management, the command center, and decision-maker in a structured and organized manner that represents those facts truthfully and in context. Data visualization tools are used to convert the underlying data to graphical presentations of that data providing accurate, clear, and fast understandings of information gathered. Using data visualization tools allow data analytics to provide the audience with valid and robust information, showing the true direction, trends, or facts buried within the dataset. These tools are also used to convert data to information using visual elements like charts, graphs, and maps. The dashboard is mentioned in this chapter in the context of the command center and the role it plays for the command center functioning. More details on the dashboard can be found in the chapter on information technology, healthcare data, and analytics.

Case Study 1: Meaningful and Actionable Presentation of Data to Decision-Makers During a Crisis: The Case of SBH Health System During the 2020 COVID-19 Pandemic

Data Visualization Tools Tableau, a visual analytics engine, was leveraged at SBH Health System during the COVID-19 pandemic to create interactive visual analytics in the form of dashboards. Dashboards were easier for non-technical analysts and end users to convert data into an understandable format with the use of interactive graphics. Tableau facilitated the use of data from multiple sources in combination with proprietary data, empowering new and beneficial insights. With this engine, it was also possible to pull data from the electronic medical record (EMR), creating own views – a simple process to connect datasets to make dashboards.

Daily Meetings (Teleconference) Frequent meetings allowed the teams to utilize a rapid iterative process linking clinical, financial, and analytical teams together to review, discuss, and provide feedback to the developers. Rapid implementation of timelines and updates to developed dashboards were possible because of this team approach. Meetings would look to validate underlying data provided as well as the visualization dashboards created, allowing for stakeholder objectives to be fulfilled, quickly identifying next steps and subsequent actions required.

Timely Actions As the pandemic progressed, it was clearly apparent that not only was the underlying data evolving but the data elements themselves were developing, changing, and maturing. For example, new tests on-boarded frequently and new inpatient locations were created. This required constant review of existing data extractions and dashboards which subsequently required frequent updates to bring in new datasets and revise existing visualizations.

With the ever-changing nature of the pandemic, stakeholders needed to be continually updated with ever increasing needs to incorporate new data elements. Frequent working sessions were an invaluable resource to allow for discussion and review of clinical, operational, and financial reporting needs, as well as to solidify the feasibility of developing and/or delivering any data-related reports and dashboards in a timely fashion. Timely follow-through with any and all urgent and non-urgent updates and/or bug fixes were prioritized due to stakeholder's requests or the nature of the data. The rapid cycle performance improvement method of PDSA was used to improve the functioning of data acquisition and presentation on a daily basis (see Box 3.2).

Transparency All aspects of this dashboard creation process were open and transparent to the stakeholders for validation of the data. Ultimately, it was clear that SBH needed to be cognizant of eliminating or avoiding any inherent "garbage in, garbage out" scenarios. Transparency allowed for the rapid identification of any incorrect, inappropriate, or misleading data from propagating and diminishing the value of our dashboards. End-user requirements were obtained, analyzed, and reviewed with the team for appropriateness of the following:

- Types of data available and required
- Sources of the data
  - EMR
- Validation of the data
  - Data pulled following organizational rules was validated, not to become degraded due to inconsistencies in type or context. The ultimate goal was to create data that was consistent, accurate, and complete so to avoid any errors during a move.
- Extraction of the data
- Required data conversions
- Creation of visualization utilizing powerful business intelligence tools

3 Preparation, Planning, and the Command Center

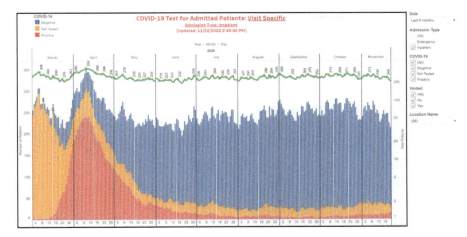

Fig. 3.2 COVID-19 test for admitted patients: visit specific

Dashboard as a Tool to Aid in Employee Morale The creation of a cumulative discharge dashboard was made available on multiple monitors throughout the SBH Health System for employees and visitors to see, as a way of increasing morale. Those who were found to be focused or locked within their own world view of the pandemic were afforded a broader picture of the efforts of the larger team. It was possible to provide near real-time data tabulating the successful discharge of the COVID-19 patients, as well as the discharge of those patients previously intubated. The acknowledgment of our successes was a welcome distraction by the entire organization.

Example of Dashboards for Crisis Management The following dashboard (Fig. 3.2) conveys each day's total number of admitted patients (green line) along with the total number of COVID-19's tests performed (negative and positive), providing an extremely useful visualization of outcomes. The viewer can leverage the use of provided filters to manipulate multiple aspects of the visualization such as admission date, admission type, COVID-19 results status (positive, negative, etc.), ventilation status, and admitted locations.

Leading Leaders and Creation of the Leadership Team

Leadership is an essential element to any crisis response. Effective leadership in managing crises and emergencies can minimize the damage inflicted by an event while lack of successful leadership can exacerbate the impact [4]. Leadership has two very essential roles in crisis response; the first is to manage the response and the second is to communicate the management of that response throughout the organization.

However, before any of this, leaders need to first anticipate and plan for a crisis. Emergency management systems and drills are essential to help frame and structure crisis planning, and these drills can help expose weaknesses in a disaster response. Crisis management involves significant changes compared to management of the "everyday". The Kotter's 3 tenets of change management are extremely relevant in a state of health crisis; leaders must consciously create a climate for implementing and sustaining change, alongside engaging and enabling the whole organization.

Supporting the Clinical Leadership and Frontline Healthcare Workers

Supporting the clinical leadership and frontline teams is a 24/7 core function of the command center during a health crisis. Crises are, by definition, met with many stressors such as changes in workflows, assignments, overwork, sleep deprivation, suboptimal work conditions, staff shortages, high patient mortality, grieving families, and others. Material, logistical, and psychological support is necessary to maintain the workforce and sustain fulfilling the mission during a health crisis. Supporting healthcare workers may include larger items such as rotating work schedules, leadership rounding, and providing adequate call rooms and facilities. However, small items may also go a long way to alleviate healthcare workers' stress such as the provision of free parking, meals, snacks, refreshments, and others (Box 3.2).

> **Box 3.2: Examples of Support Provided to Clinical Leaders and Frontline Healthcare Workers**
> - Support for difficult decision-making – team approach, senior leadership and management, end-of-life support
> - Bereavement support
> - Rotating work schedule with fairness and transparency
> - Townhalls
> - Regular and frequent leadership rounding
> - Adequate, clean, and comfortable call rooms, bathrooms, and showers with daily fresh sheets and towels
> - Free parking
> - Free meals, snacks, and refreshments
> - Napping arrangements
> - Calm lounge
> - Employee support hotline
> - Counseling and psychological services
> - PPE

Managing Clinical Volunteers – Medical Reserve Corps

Volunteerism can be great during a time of crisis due to the innate human trait to want to help each other. This trait extends to doctors, nurses, and other healthcare professionals. A crisis can also bring out less desirable traits in people, but more often, the kindness and generosity of people shine. When healthcare systems and staffing are overstretched, working with volunteers and voluntary groups to provide community services has the potential to fill acute gaps and prevent public agencies from being overwhelmed during crisis events [5].

Case Study 2: The COVID-19 Pandemic, Expansion of Clinical Services, and Crisis Surge Management

In the very early stages of our COVID-19 response, the planning team consisted of the chief medical officer and two associate medical directors. The team recruited frequent input from the chief nursing officer and director of infection control. Once the pandemic further developed, was more clearly understood, and the likelihood of a surge established, additional stakeholders were quickly recruited and the command center was set up. Table 3.1 shows a tool that was used during the surge of the COVID-19 pandemic for the management of expansion of services.

Surge Planning and Management During the stages of the initial epidemic, the COVID-19 surge plan was created. Many of the triggers and phases were developed from the collective experiences during the 2009 H1NI pandemic [6]. An infectious viral crisis typically involves an initial small number of cases followed by a rapid increase, creating a surge which quickly reaches a peak and then slowly declines. A good understanding of this pandemic crisis flow by the senior leadership and command center can result in the development of a surge plan early in a crisis. Table 3.2 shows a sample surge plan that was produced by the SBH senior management and command center early in the COVID-19 pandemic in 2020. The plan contains

Table 3.1 Sample of tool for inventory and expansion of critical care areas, regular medical/surgical areas, and surge plan (the numbers are for example purpose)

Bed categories	Total beds in service	Surge capacity (# of beds) beyond beds in service	Estimated number of days until surge beds could be in service	How many surge beds can you staff with internal staff?	Bed(s)	Ventilator(s)
Total	234	117	21	67	85	24
ICU	16	23	5	23	0	10
Isolation	10	0	0	0	0	0
Med/Surg	184	90	21	40		10
NICU	12	4	7	4	0	4
Pediatrics	12	0	0	0	0	0

triggers for the different phases of a surge indicating the severity of the surge, with phased responses for the various departments and teams of the hospital. The triggers deserve a special discussion; scientifically, there are 2 types of triggers: contemporaneous triggers and predictive models (Box 3.3). Contemporaneous triggers use "cross sectional in time" events and data such as census data on numbers of patients in the ED, number of admissions, bed occupancy, ICU bed occupancy, available and remaining human and material resources, available and remaining disposables, rate-limiting factors, and others. Predictive models use "rates and trends over recent time" such as rate of arrivals to the ED in the past 3 days, rate of admissions, rates of admissions to the ICU, rate of ventilator utilization, probability of recruitment of additional healthcare workers, rate of consumption of equipment, supplies and disposables, probability of replenishment of supplies and disposables, and others. Contemporaneous data is relatively simple and can be acquired easily from hospital data sources. However, predictive models are more complex and require a significant data infrastructure, statistical analysis, and special information technology applications. Finally, while producing a well-designed surge plan is very important before or at the early beginnings of a crisis, the senior management and command center should exercise, in real practice, utmost flexibility and agility in timely responding to the unfolding events of a surge of a crisis, in accordance with the "dynamic decision-making" principles. While surge planning may be a science, surge management is a science and an art! More on dynamic decision-making can be found in the chapter on dynamic decision-making and effective communications.

Box 3.3: Types of Triggers
There are 2 types of triggers: contemporaneous triggers and predictive models

1. *Contemporaneous triggers*
   - Cross-sectional in time events and data such as census data on numbers of patients in the ED, number of admissions, bed occupancy, ICU bed occupancy
   - Available and remaining human and material resources
   - Available and remaining disposables
   - Rate-limiting factors such as ventilators and ICU staff

2. *Predictive models*
   - Rates and trends over recent time such as rates in the past 3 days including arrivals to the ED, admissions, admissions to the ICU, ventilator utilization, consumption of equipment, supplies, and disposables
   - Probabilities of recruitment of additional healthcare workers, replenishment of supplies and disposables, and others

Table 3.2 COVID-19 surge plan

Levels	Triggers	Actions in different departments										
		Expansion of COVID-19 in-patient beds	Out-patient clinics	Peri-operative services	Visitors	Tent	Meetings	Infection control isolation	Staffing	Residents	Rapid discharge process	Employee screening
A or phase 1	ED volume and/or confirmed cases	Status quo	Status quo	Status quo	Status quo, ill visitors not permitted	Drills and training	Status quo	Status quo	Status quo	Status quo	Not applicable	Per CDC guidelines
B or phase 2	<275 ppd for 3 days; <5 COVID-19 cases	Conversions of detox and pediatric units	Status quo	Status quo	Status quo, ill visitors not permitted	Assembly and preparation	Virtual as much as possible	Modification of rules to balance isolation and need for expansion	Additional staffing	Redeployment to other duties and departments as needed	Initiation of rapid discharge process	Per CDC guidelines
C or phase 3	275–325 ppd for 3 days; >5 COVID-19 cases	Ambulatory surgery center, PACU	Partial reduction	Elective canceled, urgent and emergent only	Limited visitors with case by case approval	Launch tent operations	Virtual as much as possible	Modification of rules to balance isolation and need for expansion	Additional staffing	Redeployment to other duties and departments as needed	Continuation of rapid discharge process	Per CDC guidelines
D or phase 4	>325 ppd for 3 days; widespread COVID-19 cases	Obstetrics, cardiac cath lab, NICU	Urgent care mode	Elective canceled, urgent and emergent only	Not permitted	Launch tent operations	Virtual as much as possible	Modification of rules to balance isolation and need for expansion	Additional staffing	Redeployment to other duties and departments as needed	Emphasis on rapid discharge process	Per CDC guidelines

Please note – triggers/surge plans may change if a specific service line(s) is/are affected by COVID-19

Summary and Conclusions

The occurrence of unexpected incidents around the globe can cause health crises which impact world economies and result in mass fatalities. Having procedures and plans in place to manage and mitigate such crises is critical, especially for a healthcare center that has a significant role in disaster management. A management system playing a prevalent role in empowering healthcare centers is the hospital incident command system, a system incorporating emergency plans, policies, and procedures in order to tackle a crisis situation, and also one which attempts to build a coordination between hospitals and other involved institutions through using a rational and integrated management structure [7]. Departmental communications are essential not only to disseminate communication in a top-down approach but also allow a bottom-up feedback communication to the senior management and command center. Supporting the clinical leadership and the frontline teams is a 24/7 core function of the command center.

References

1. Quinn SC. Hurricane Katrina: a social and public health disaster. Am J Public Health. 2006;96(2):204. https://doi.org/10.2105/AJPH.2005.080119.
2. Shipp Hilts A, Mack S, Eidson M, Nguyen T, Birkhead GS. New York state public health system response to Hurricane Sandy: lessons from the field. Disaster Med Public Health Prep. 2016;10(3):443–53. https://doi.org/10.1017/dmp.2016.69.
3. Martini M, Gazzaniga V, Bragazzi NL, Barberis I. The Spanish Influenza Pandemic: a lesson from history 100 years after 1918. J Prev Med Hyg. 2019;60(1):E64–7. https://doi.org/10.15167/2421-4248/jpmh2019.60.1.1205.
4. Demiroz F, Kapucu N. The role of leadership in managing emergencies and disasters. Eur J Econ Pol Stud. 2012;5(1):91–101.
5. Miao Q, Schwarz S, Schwarz G. Responding to COVID-19: community volunteerism and coproduction in China. World Dev. 2021;137:105128. https://doi.org/10.1016/j.worlddev.2020.105128.
6. 2009 H1N1 Pandemic (H1N1pdm09 virus). 2019. Retrieved 29 Dec 2020, from https://www.cdc.gov/flu/pandemic-resources/2009-h1n1-pandemic.html.
7. Bahrami P, Ardalan A, Nejati A, Ostadtaghizadeh A, Yari A. Factors affecting the effectiveness of hospital incident command system; findings from a systematic review. Bull Emerg Trauma. 2020;8(2):62–76. https://doi.org/10.30476/BEAT.2020.46445.

Chapter 4
Internal Medicine, Infection Control, and Occupational Health Services

Edward E. Telzak and Judith Berger

Internal Medicine and the Usual Role of the Internal Medicine Department

Internal Medicine is a branch of medicine that deals with non-surgical prevention, diagnosis, and treatment of diseases in adults. There are numerous services within the department including but not limited to the following: General Internal Medicine, Cardiology, Infectious Diseases, Gastroenterology, Geriatrics, Nephrology, Neurology, Dermatology, Addiction Medicine, Rheumatology, Endocrinology, Hematology/Oncology, and Pulmonary and Critical Care Medicine. At SBH, General Internal Medicine is divided into the Hospitalist Division and the Division of Primary Care.

The Hospitalist Service is responsible for overseeing the care for patients who are admitted to the hospital with an acute medical illness and was an essential component of SBH Health System's response to the COVID-19 surge. During normal times, there are 7 teams, each one responsible for between 15 and 20 patients with a variety of illnesses. Each team consists of an experienced attending physician who is board-certified in Internal Medicine and one second-or third-year resident in

E. E. Telzak (✉)
Department of Medicine, SBH Health System, Bronx, NY, USA

Department of Medicine, CUNY School of Medicine, New York, NY, USA

Albert Einstein College of Medicine, Bronx, NY, USA
e-mail: etelzak@sbhny.org

J. Berger
CUNY School of Medicine, New York, NY, USA

Infection Control, Division of Infectious Disease, Department of Medicine, Occupational Health Services, SBH Health System, Bronx, NY, USA

© The Author(s), under exclusive license to Springer Nature Switzerland AG 2022
R. Shabsigh (ed.), *Health Crisis Management in Acute Care Hospitals*,
https://doi.org/10.1007/978-3-030-95806-0_4

training, two first-year residents, and generally two third-year medical students. Each patient is seen every day by the entire team together during morning rounds, and often seen numerous times a day by one or more members of the team to discuss clinical status and updates, scheduled tests, results of tests already completed, and discharge planning with particular attention to follow-up. Typically, one member of the team also makes afternoon rounds to review the day's events with the patient and speak with family members if available. Each morning, there is a scheduled 30-minute "group" meeting called White Board Rounds where the entire medical team, or two teams on one floor, assemble with the nursing staff, physical therapists, hospital-to-home navigators, and case management and social work staff to discuss the progress of every patient, potential or actual delays in treatment and discharge, and how to best arrange a safe discharge. As a substantial proportion of patients discharged have housing and food insecurity, are homeless, and/or have coexisting substance use and mental health disorders, a "safe" discharge can often be challenging and time-consuming. Fidelity to this process, and these practices and procedures, are very high during normal times.

Expanding the Role of Internal Medicine During the COVID-19 Crisis

Beds

Enormous preparation, starting in mid-late February, went into expanding the ability of the Department of Medicine to care for large numbers of patients who were expected beginning in mid-March. SBH Health System followed the initial Chinese epidemic and response, and subsequently the Italian experience, extremely closely. Those who worked in hospitals saw what was happening to their colleagues and patients in China and Italy, and there was profound concern and fear that SBH Health System, too, was soon to experience something comparable. As is now well known, it was only 1 week before the onslaught of patients arrived into most New York City's (NYC) emergency rooms that there was a lockdown and schools closed, crowds were limited in both number and a broad range of activities, and people were strongly encouraged to work from home and wear masks. Of course, one week was far too short a time frame to significantly impact the curve for hospitalizations and ultimately it took a month or longer of lockdown and associated decrease in viral transmission to significantly impact the flow of patients into hospitals and into SBH.

With the expectation that SBH Health System would need to care for an extreme number of extremely sick patients infected with SARS Co-V2, extensive preparations were made to expand SBH Health System bed capacity for patients who would require oxygen but not critical care interventions such as mechanical ventilation and cardiac monitoring. A separate committee was tasked with expanding those critical services. A team consisting of the Chair of Medicine, an Associate Medical Director, the Chief Nursing Officer, and others, met frequently and began thinking broadly about required preparations to expand medical services during the subsequent weeks to 1 month. With the expansion of beds, a comparable expansion in the number of physicians, nurses, respiratory therapists, and support staff was also required. In contrast to numerous other exercises to prepare for emergencies, it was felt that the likelihood of SBH confronting a very significant challenge from COVID-19 was far more likely to happen than not, and this provided the impetus and dedication to commit fully to make changes to prepare for this likely impending near-term pandemic.

The Department of Medicine worked with the senior administration to identify areas that could be converted into additional bed capacity for sick patients likely to require oxygen. The second floor of the hospital was divided into 2North, a ward of 30 beds largely made up of double rooms, and 2South, a former hospital ward that had been converted into office space housing the Risk Management Department, the Patient Experience Department, two Associate Medical Directors, a large Hospitalist office with 7 work stations, and other offices. Given the pandemic on the horizon, within a relatively short period of time in late February, all of these functions and personnel were relocated and the 2South ward was converted, with considerable effort, back to 13 double-bed rooms able to care for 26 patients. Similar additional efforts went into reconverting 23 beds that had been converted, many years ago, from hospital rooms into administrative space (12 beds on one general medical floor and 11 beds from Physical Therapy). With the canceling of elective surgery, most of the 28 surgical beds were repurposed to primarily care for patients with COVID-19. When it became apparent that this was not sufficient and that additional beds would be required, it was possible to make arrangements with a Children's Hospital in the Bronx to care for the pediatric patients requiring hospitalization who came to the Emergency Department; this allowed the utilization of the 22- bed Pediatric Floor to care for the relatively small proportion of patients who were COVID-19 negative and to separate them from the large number of COVID-19 positive patients. This separation was crucial to minimize disease transmission within SBH patients. Lastly, all of the patients from the Addiction Medicine floor were discharged; and over the course of 2 weeks, SBH was able to repurpose these 24 beds to be capable of caring for patients diagnosed with COVID-19. In all, it was possible to create >100 additional beds that were potentially capable of managing patients with COVID-19, who did not require critical care, and to establish a 22-bed COVID-19-negative floor for the relatively small proportion of patients requiring acute care who tested negative for SARS Co-V2 and had a low clinical suspicion for COVID-19.

Floors opened up very quickly during the surge of late March 2020. Very soon the importance of a very detailed checklist prior to the opening of each new COVID-19 unit became obvious, as the first repurposed area opened without fully appreciating the range of equipment that would be required. One notable example was the opening of a unit on a weekend day when far too many patients were being cared for in the emergency department (ED). A new team was assembled of residents and a subspecialty attending, a cardiologist, which admitted a large number of patients to the unit from the ED, most of whom required supplemental oxygen. As these patients came to the floor, it became apparent that not all of the rooms had the ability to provide oxygen to the patients. It was made certain that oxygen could be effectively delivered to each of the 26 beds and that we had adequate numbers of nasal canulae and ventimasks. However, what was lacking was an adapter to take the oxygen being piped in to connect to the nasal canula or Ventimask. When this was realized, it also was recognized that there was not sufficient numbers of adapters in stock and this had initially been neglected on the "checklist." Patients were provided with oxygen through tanks while the adapters were being acquired. Obtaining adaptors took time because every other hospital in New York, and many hospitals elsewhere, were also ordering this equipment.

Physician Staff

During the beginning of the preparation for the COVID-19 surge, it became apparent that the full-time hospitalist staff of 7 was not adequate, given the numbers of expected COVID-19 patients and their acuity. Of course, in addition to the hospitalists, as a teaching hospital, there were internal medicine residents. Although residents are physicians in training, they are an important part of the healthcare workforce. At times of crisis, their presence is even more significant. The hospitalists at SBH Health System work 5 days (M–F)/week and cover one weekend/month when they are required to complete rounds on their entire floor, seeing each patient and writing progress notes for both Saturday and Sunday. Under ordinary circumstances, this is a substantial amount of important and hard work, and it became apparent after their first weekend on call during the beginning of the surge that it was not reasonable to have hospitalists working so many consecutive days, let alone 12 days in a row. The Department of Medicine leadership requested ideas from the hospitals, one of which was ultimately enacted.

The hospitalist schedule became 12-hour days – 7 days on followed by 7 days off. Night call was via telephone with complete home access to the electronic medical record. For this one-week period, they managed approximately 25 patients each with a full complement of residents, covering both day and night. Though the week was very challenging, it provided for continuity of care for the patients and one senior experienced physician who knew the patients when residents contacted them at night. In order to operationalize this schedule, a more than doubling of the hospitalist service was required to cover the greatly expanded seven medical services. To cover these units, medical chief residents, who having graduated would normally function as attending physicians, were utilized with appropriate supervision and one volunteer hospitalist who was an SBH Health System graduate overseeing a unit. In addition, two interventional cardiologists covered one unit in alternating weeks; two gastroenterologists covered a second unit; two oncologists covered a third unit, and four primary care physicians were responsible for two units. In total, there were eighteen attending physicians covering the seven COVID-19-positive units and the one COVID-19-negative unit. Given the high needs, it was expected to make hospitalist coverage mandatory for specific physicians; however, the primary care physicians and medical subspecialists who ultimately became hospitalists all volunteered for this important responsibility. Our full-time hospitalists each covered the largest number of patients, approximately 25 each, followed by primary care physicians who covered 15–18 patients each and the subspecialists generally covered the smaller new units of <15 patients. This group functioned as the hospitalist team from the end of March 2020 until early June when it was possible to return to pre-COVID-19 surge schedule. It was possible to repurpose the primary care physicians, cardiologists, gastroenterologists, and oncologists because, in part, of the dramatic decrease in their respective workloads during the surge. In fact, interventional cardiology closed, the endoscopy suite became an ICU, and only emergent endoscopies were performed during this period and most patients stopped coming to clinics which greatly decreased the workload for oncologists and primary care physicians. Though intensivists, surgeons, and anesthesiologists, in addition to full staff of ED physicians, were on the premises during the night to assist the residents with any emergencies, the addition of at least one "nocturnalist" was strongly considered to cover the hospitalist service and admit patients during the night.

Each day every hospitalist met with the Department of Medicine Chair to assess needs, review patient medical conditions, and communicate particular challenges. Based on these daily rounds, numerous real-time changes took place that significantly improved and influenced care. Though many examples could be cited, two very important changes that took place relatively early in the surge are worth emphasizing as learning points. Given the rapidity with which respiratory deterioration took place on the general medical floors, *widespread distribution of pulse oximeters* to all of the residents and hospitalists was initiated. Subsequent to this, a program to *teach patients self-proning* was also started. Both of these are described in greater detail below.

Role of the Residents

Internal Medicine residents at SBH Health System play a very important role and, under close supervision, help diagnose and manage the majority of admitted patients to the hospital. With the onset of COVID-19, their role in dealing with this pandemic at SBH Health System, and, similarly in the teaching hospitals throughout the New York area, became critical. Though the most pressing concern was how to optimally staff the units in preparation for the impending surge, numerous other activities were initiated well before the first patient with COVID-19 was admitted on March 3, 2020.

One week before the first COVID-19 patient was admitted, all teaching conferences, including Medical Grand Rounds, became virtual. Soon after COVID-19 patients began to be admitted, virtual conferences were also canceled and residents were given a list of pre-recorded COVID-19-related lectures to be viewed weekly. Nightly remote meetings by the chief residents were initiated to keep the residents informed of all changes. In addition, the Residency Program Director had, as frequently as needed, remote meetings to update residents on the number of patients with COVID-19 in the hospital, expansion of the floors and ICU to accommodate these patients, scheduling changes, updates on the ever changing proven and unproven treatment modalities, and especially to determine how the residents were coping and ensuring that they were getting adequate rest and mental health support. In addition to these formal meetings, the Chair of Medicine and the Program Director made daily rounds on each of the medical floors to provide these updates in real times, assess issues and problems related to patient care and speak with all staff, especially the residents, and determine how they were coping with the enormous stress of the pandemic.

Numerous discussions within the department involving the residents occurred focusing on creating resident schedules that would allow for flexibility to staff the opening of more medical and ICU units as well as to give residents time to decompress and rest. After several schedule "optimizations," the situations settled on 12 hour shifts with a team of one post-graduate year (PGY) 1, one PGY2, and one PGY3. The schedule which was voted on by a majority of residents had an 8-day cycle: 4 days on service followed by another 4 days that included 3 full days off and 1 day as a floater (the floater allowed us to cover residents who were sick as well as units that would open from one day to the next). Residents were relieved of all ambulatory responsibilities including primary care and subspecialty clinics. Medically high-risk residents worked from home to help with remote outpatient visits, renal consults (the number of renal consults increased substantially due to COVID-19's impact on kidney function and need for hemodialysis), and ongoing COVID-19 studies for expanded access of remdesivir and convalescent plasma. Medical students were pulled from all rotations. All vacations were postponed and residents were strongly requested not to travel.

Many residents from other departments such as surgery, dentistry, psychiatry, and osteopathic manipulative medicine (OMM) worked in tandem with the Internal Medicine residents to serve a diverse group of needs for patients and the institution. Perhaps one example is most noteworthy. It became almost immediately apparent that close monitoring of the patients' respiratory status was critical. It was evident that patients, although appearing stable, could, and often did, decompensate rapidly from a respiratory point of view. The medical teams requested additional pulse oximeters to more closely monitor patients' oxygenation status. The hospital purchased several hundred pulse oximeters and residents from other specialties, including dental, podiatry, and psychiatry, were tasked with obtaining regular and frequent monitoring of patients' respiratory status and oxygenation status. As proning for non-intubated patients also was thought to be beneficial, other residents, including OMM, began to teach patients to "self-prone" and would check on them regularly. A geriatric physician who was also a former pulmonologist from the Department of Medicine met with the team regularly to discuss problems and issues as they arose. Another example was the role that anesthesiology played for patients who were acutely decompensating. Residents, under hospitalist guidance based on predetermined criteria, were able to call anesthesiologists directly to intubate patients bypassing the need to have the overly stressed ICU physicians approve the request. During this intensive period, residents acquired strong skills in managing patients' respiratory status and understanding different modalities of oxygen delivery.

Residents continued to be responsible for writing admitting notes. However, in order to decrease the work load for residents, abbreviated progress notes were being written by the attending staff. Residents would write a brief note for any new information that would occur during their shift. Toward the end of the surge, residents were writing COVID-19-template progress notes that were brief but that captured the relevant information on each patient.

During the COVID-19 surge, residents had to assume new roles. For example, they received training to start IV drips on newly intubated patients. They were also taught to manage "smart" pumps – pumps with libraries that included programmable infusion rates for a wide variety of drugs. Despite the increasing number of patients and the thinning of all staff on units, the residents devoted many hours calling family to keep them appraised of the patient's status. Residents were often using their phones to allow patients face time with their family. Before intubation, if time allowed, the residents would make it a point to give the patient and the family a moment to see/talk with one another.

By the end of May, the patient census began to normalize: 2–3 auxiliary ICUs closed; some expanded units closed; other units reverted to pre-pandemic functions. However, clinics remained closed. Residents were now able to take their scheduled vacation time and eventually revert to their original schedules, rotations, and conferences that remained primarily virtual.

Critical Shortages of Specific Physicians

Despite the ability and moderate success in redeploying numerous full-time primary care physicians and subspecialists to a hospitalist role, there were physician areas where critical shortages continued. Perhaps most noteworthy were the challenges in providing hemodialysis services to the many patients already on hemodialysis who were admitted to the hospital with severe COVID-19 and patients admitted with COVID-19 who subsequently developed acute kidney injury and required hemodialysis for the first time while in the hospital.

As with all safety-net hospitals with limited budgets, recruitment of physicians and other healthcare workers is a challenge; at the baseline, the nephrology division was very "lean." There was one full-time nephrologist on the verge of retirement who stayed until the COVID-19 surge was manageable, a full-time hospitalist who was an experienced board-certified nephrologist and was always available to cover the inpatient nephrology consultation service and see a portion of the chronic hemodialysis patients, and a part-time nephrologist who covered weekends, staffed clinics, and contributed to the overall nephrology effort.

Very aggressive attempts at recruitment of volunteer physicians from around the country were made by contacting physicians who voluntarily enlisted in the Medical

Reserve Corporation (MRC) and sending e-mails to graduates of the SBH residency program. The MRC is a national network of volunteers, organized locally and generally deployed locally to improve the health and safety of their communities. These volunteers include medical and public health professionals. The MRC became available during the surge to provide medical support for NYC hospitals. One individual in clinical leadership received lists of potentially available volunteers several times per week, including ICU physicians, hospitalists, and nephrologists.

A very high proportion of physicians from around the country who were contacted expressed considerable interest in coming to New York to assist SBH Health System during this crisis. There was great empathy for the patients and healthcare workers. However, most could not commit to work at SBH Health System until they had administrative permission from their respective clinical Chairs and hospital administrations. Though most physicians called and provided follow-up information, the overwhelming majority could not get administrative permission to work at SBH Health System for a multiplicity of reasons. Most commonly, there was concern that they would become infected with SARS Co-V2 and would not be available to work at their home institutions if the pandemic spread to their communities. Also of great concern was the potential liability of their home institutions. In all, 4 ICU physicians received emergency credentialing and worked in the ICUs of SBH. Despite considerable efforts, it was not possible to bring an additional nephrologist. Lastly, 3 Locum Tenants critical care medicine physicians were hired for various periods of time. Military physicians and physicians from the 5 large medical centers in the Bronx and Manhattan, including emergency room and ICU physicians, who were redeployed to many of the overwhelmed community hospitals in New York City, unfortunately were not available to SBH Health System.

Treatment Protocols

It was significantly after the peak of the surge that remdesivir was documented to shorten hospital stay [1, 2] and that dexamethasone was shown to have a mortality benefit in the treatment of COVID-19 [3]. Given the very high mortality rates seen during the surge and the lack of documented beneficial therapeutic modalities, numerous treatments were implemented based on very limited clinical information. Most notable were the almost routine use of hydroxychloroquine and azithromycin [4]. Treatment algorithms were implemented including names of medications, dosing and duration, route of administration, indications, contraindications, and adjustments for renal function. These were developed and disseminated with input from the pharmacy and infectious disease team.

The importance of participating in clinical trials was clearly understood. It proved very challenging to conduct research at SBH Health System as all local institutions were extremely stressed battling the pandemic and consequently could not provide help. When expanded access for remdesivir became available, overseen by pharmacy and infectious disease physicians, eligible patients at various stages of illness were enrolled expeditiously. Residents from various departments, including pharmacy, psychiatry, and medicine, were instrumental in enrolling and following patients in the expanded access trials. A "Treatment Guidelines Committee" made up of pharmacy, clinicians from the Department of Medicine – infectious diseases, pulmonary and critical care medicine, hematology, and others – and the Emergency Department was constituted and played, and continues to play, a critical role in guiding treatment throughout the institution well beyond the surge.

Discharging Patients with COVID-19

Each of the units and areas that were repurposed for COVID-19 patients, and the one unit that was meant for COVID-19-negative patients, became filled with the exception of one unit, the 24-bed unit for patients who were admitted for alcohol and opiate detoxification, i.e., the Detox Ward. By the time all of these other units were open and filled, the staff were stressed well beyond their maximum capacity. This was staff at all levels – from doctors and nurses, to respiratory therapists, to environmental services personnel, pharmacy services, and the transport department. Attempts were made to not have to open this last unit, given the very significant shortage of staff at all levels. As a result, the sufficient numbers of discharges each day became critically important to be able to accommodate the large number of patients being admitted.

One very significant obstacle in discharging relatively "stable" patients was the availability of home oxygen. Though the capability of home health agencies to obtain home oxygen during the surge was apparently very compromised, this was particularly true for both patients on Medicaid and almost impossible for uninsured patients. Thus, patients often spent as long as an additional week or more being weaned off oxygen which, if not for the lack of availability of home oxygen, could likely have been done in a home environment. An important alternative to home oxygen for many of our patients became transfer to the Jacob Javitz Center (JJC) where the oxygen could be administered in a hospital-like setting.

The federal government, working with the New York State Department of Health (NYSDOH), established two off site facilities for patients to be transferred to, when hospitals were at their limits of capacity: The JJC, which functions as the Convention Center for New York City in ordinary times, and the USS Comfort, a naval medical ship capable of providing care to very ill patients, including those requiring mechanical ventilation. Originally their mandate was to accept only COVID-19-negative patients and free up space for the hospitals to care for COVID-19-positive patients. However, there were very few COVID-19-negative patients coming to, and being admitted to NYC Hospitals, so both the JJC and the USS Comfort remained initially empty. After a great deal of discussion, they began to allow patients with COVID-19. Ultimately, fewer than five patients were transferred to the USS Comfort from SBH Health System. The USS Comfort was docked on the west side of Manhattan. Quarters were extremely cramped, the rooms had no windows, and beds were stacked. Though the USS Comfort was capable of caring for very ill patients, there was very little interest on the part of the patients, or their families, to be transferred from their community hospital to a ship. In fact, some people asked if the ship was going to take them, or their loved one, away given the hostilities that had been expressed toward immigrants. The experience with the JJC was very different. The JJC had very strict parameters in accepting patients. The patients needed to be ambulatory because of a lack of nursing personnel and needed to be clinically stable with only minimal supplemental oxygen requirements. A long list of comorbidities made patients ineligible and perhaps most noteworthy was the inability to provide methadone maintenance. Nevertheless, a process was established at SBH Health System. The hospitalists and residents were educated about these alternative care sites. Though many patients refused to be transferred and would not give the required consent, ultimately almost 40 patients over several weeks were discharged to the JJC. These additional discharges were sufficient to not have to open the 24-bed detox unit which was extraordinarily helpful, given the impact opening this additional unit would have had on further diluting the limited available medical, nursing, respiratory therapy, and other support staff.

Infection Control and Occupational Health Service

Infection control (IC) played a critical role in the initial response to the pandemic and was instrumental in the hospital's evolving adaptation to the pandemic. As in prior emerging infectious disease outbreaks, the infectious disease and infection control team, and many others, needed to educate themselves on the manifestations, incubation period, and modes of transmission of the emerging pathogen, and review guidance if available from the Centers for Disease Control and Prevention (CDC). Early on, IC and the Department of Medicine took leadership roles in educating staff throughout the institution about this newly emerging pathogen and integrating guidelines from the CDC, the New York State Department of Health (NYSDOH), and the New York City Department of Health and Mental Hygiene (NYCDOHMH) into hospital policy. Given the rapidly changing guidelines and recommended practices as the pandemic evolved and as the approach to the pandemic matured, IC became responsible for keeping the hospital policies and IC practices and procedures up to date and both internally and externally consistent.

From the very onset, identifying and isolating persons potentially with COVID-19 – persons under investigation (PUI) – became a priority and urgent concern. Efforts to identify the infection at the various entry points of the hospital, i.e., stopping the infection at the door, several weeks before the first case, were instituted so that appropriate infection control practices and effective isolation could be implemented. Screening and triaging all persons at presentation to the emergency department, the multiplicity of ambulatory practices, Occupational Health Service (OHS), and other entry points to the institution were prioritized.

At triage, patients and staff were questioned about any of the symptoms and/or signs of the infection, exposure to someone who was either known or suspected of having the infection, and travel to an area where the infection was known to be prevalent. Identifying PUIs at presentation allowed isolation of the individual and containing the infection to prevent spread to others. The triage questions became part of the Electronic Medical Record (EMR) and were part of all initial evaluations. Alerts/posters were prominently displayed at all entrances to the hospital and patients and staff were notified to inform the Concierge on entry if they answered yes to any items of concern.

Protocols and algorithms for triage, isolation, laboratory and radiologic workup, consultation with relevant clinical services including Pulmonary and Critical Care Medicine, the Emergency Department and Infectious Diseases, and treatment and administrative escalation were widely disseminated to appropriate staff. These were updated regularly as more information became available from federal, state, and city public health authorities and a better understanding of the pathogen emerged. Performing tracers to walk through the actual steps in the emergency department from patient presentation, identification, the path to the isolation room(s) on the medical floors or the ICUs, and appropriate clinical interventions were practiced before a case ever came to SBH.

Clearly, diagnosis of the emerging pathogen in a timely manner was critical. The hospital was greatly impacted early on by our lack of on-site rapid testing. The testing algorithm, approval for testing, the EMR testing order, testing kits, laboratory preparation of the specimen, transportation of specimens to the NYCDOHMH and resulting of the test in the EMR and to the responsible healthcare worker were implemented within a short period of time. Concurrently, a focus for IC and many others became the obtaining of in-house testing for the emerging infection. This took many weeks and was not fully implemented until well into the peak of the surge.

Very early on and within several days after our first confirmed COVID-19 case, when a patient presented to the hospital with any signs/symptoms of COVID-19 or with any risk factors (e.g., travel to Wuhan, China), the patient was taken directly to the highly infectious pathogen patient room in the emergency department. These PUIs were evaluated and testing was completed upon approval from the NYC Department of Health. PUIs with pending test results and requiring admission to the hospital were placed in a single patient room when available or, far more commonly, in a double patient room necessitating blocking a bed. As the number of patients positive for COVID-19 increased, two groups of patients were cohorted: confirmed COVID-19-positive patients and those with pneumonia with negative COVID-19 test results.

Soon thereafter, the number of COVID-19 patients increased exponentially. As the ED became full of patients with pneumonia and at high suspicion for COVID-19, a transition was instituted, very reluctantly, into cohorting PUIs based solely on clinical criteria when the COVID-19 test results were still pending. However, over the first few weeks, well in excess of 90% of PUIs who were cohorted were found to be positive for the COVID-19 virus. Once the rapid test became available at SBH Health System, it became possible to obtain COVID-19 status within an hour and base a decision regarding cohorting on both clinical presentation and test results.

Institution-wide education around personal protective equipment (PPE) was among the critical roles performed by the IC team. Appropriate use of PPE when readily available, and when in short supply, was especially important with the goal of keeping healthcare workers safe while taking care of patients with a highly infectious respiratory pathogen. Initial guidelines recommended "full PPE" to include N95 masks, and gowns and gloves to be used once and then discarded. With shortages, additional local and federal guidelines encouraged reuse of N95 masks until soiled or damaged with a goal of each N95 lasting for 1 week for each healthcare workers. Gowns and eye protection, also traditionally used once and then discarded, were recommended to be reused and reworn between patients with the goal of keeping a healthy workforce and preventing nosocomial transmission. Ongoing PPE education and oversight were critical to all members of the hospital community but especially to the clinical staff.

The Occupational Health Service (OHS) also played an important role in the overall management of the pandemic. Testing healthcare workers for the emerging infection, investigating exposures, advising isolation and quarantine at home procedures, and providing return to work clearance were all guided by the OHS. As was the case with many areas of this pandemic, guidelines changed and evolved as our knowledge increased. Guidelines for healthcare workers were different from those of the general population, given the necessity of these essential workers to continue to care for patients (Box 4.1). Having adequate staff remained a major challenge during the surge, given the exposures that took place in the hospital as well as in their homes and community. Most importantly, guidelines for return to work after an exposure differed between healthcare workers and the general population.

Box 4.1 Healthcare Worker (HCW)-Specific Guidelines (July 2021)
- *Universal masking for all HCWs throughout the facility at all times unless alone in a room by themselves*
- *N95 masking AND full PPE (gown, eye protection, and gloves) for all COVID-19 Person Under Investigation (PUI) or proven COVID-19 positive patients*
- *Preferred N95 masking though droplet mask acceptable AND eye protection for care of all COVID-19 negative and not PUI patients*
- *Occupational Health Service (OHS)-driven testing for symptomatic or COVID-19-exposed HCWS*
- *OHS COVID-19 specific e-mails for HCWS who are symptomatic, exposed, or traveling*
- *To maintain an adequate workforce for the overwhelming number of patients, guidelines allowed for symptomatic masked HCWS to return to work and evolved as fewer HCWS were sick and the surge decreased to isolating at home till cleared by OHS updated guidelines with 14 days post-COVID-19 evolving into 10 days.*
- *Present guidelines: Symptomatic HCWs stay home or go home for any COVID-19 symptoms and isolation till cleared by OHS*
- *COVID-19 vaccines available for all HCWS and strongly encouraged*

OHS and IC needed to be informed about any and all healthcare workers or patient exposures to COVID-19 or potential healthcare worker COVID-19 symptoms in order to control transmission of COVID-19 within the hospital. A COVID-19 e-mail was set up which allowed communication between supervisors and OHS and between exposed and/or sick healthcare workers and OHS. It facilitated healthcare workers notifying the OHS about their ongoing health status and facilitated the ability of the OHS to provide emotional and medical support as well as communicating return-to-work requirements to the healthcare worker.

Ready availability for COVID-19 testing of healthcare workers was essential to the "health" of the hospital. Rapid testing for staff in a separate area than for patients was implemented early on in the pandemic. An outdoor tent was set up on hospital grounds. Dental residents, medical assistants, and other staff whose clinics were closed were utilized during the pandemic surge to perform COVID-19 testing.

Conclusion

This chapter summarizes the enormous work and effort involved by the Department of Medicine, Infection Control, and the OHS in preparing for the COVID-19 pandemic and its initial surge in a community-teaching hospital in the Bronx, the epicenter of COVID-19 in the spring of 2020 in the United States. To care for the large number of very sick patients who suddenly required hospitalization, this preparation was necessary but unfortunately was not sufficient. Interventions such as opening and transforming units, greatly expanding the number of available beds to care for patients with COVID-19, repurposing physicians within the Department of Medicine to focus on the specific issues essential to caring for patients sick from this new pathogen, and developing new policies and procedures and educational programs related to infection control and the importance of the OHS all collectively undoubtedly saved lives. But if we were to honestly speak to the physicians in the Department of Medicine, as hard as they worked, there was a sense that their best was not good enough. No one was nearly as prepared as one needed to be; no one in recent memory has lived through a crisis of this intensity. An enormous amount was learned in the process, and now, with a more modest second surge and third surge, the performance is definitely much better. Those key lessons learned can also be carried forward to help prepare and mitigate future crises (Box 4.2). It is hoped that this chapter provides a framework for all, the next time a crisis of this type and this magnitude must be confronted.

Box 4.2 Key Lessons Learned from the Initial COVID-19 Surge in the Internal Medicine Department at SBH Health Services

- *For the preparation and management of a health crisis, expansion of internal medicine capacity can be achieved in a relatively short period of time by implementing the following measures:*
  - *Doubling beds in single bed rooms*
  - *Repurposing certain areas*
  - *Creating integrated teams of physicians, nurses, and others to increase efficiency and maximize sustainability*
  - *Converting non-clinical space to clinical space*

- *In an infectious disease health crisis with a transmissible agent, hospital planning and preparation should include large areas for infected patients and a separate area for non-infected patients. This is important because during a health crisis, a hospital will have to continue to care for patients with "routine" illnesses and emergencies.*

- *In an infectious disease health crisis related to a respiratory pathogen, rapid deterioration of respiratory function should be anticipated. Given the rapidity with which respiratory deterioration may take place on the general medical floors, widespread distribution of pulse oximeters to all of the residents and hospitalists should be initiated. In addition, a program to teach patients self-proning can be very effective in certain circumstances.*

- *Ongoing training of all personnel, including attending physicians, residents, and fellows is an immensely valuable resource for the successful management of a health crisis. Furthermore, empowerment and support of medical residents can highlight their leadership qualities during a crisis. As frontline healthcare workers, residents can provide highly effective dynamic suggestions and creative solutions for the inevitable challenges as they arise.*

- *During the COVID-19 surge, residents assume numerous new roles after appropriate training. These included the following:*
  - *Starting IV drips on newly intubated patients*
  - *Management of "smart" pumps; pumps with libraries that included programmable infusion rates for a wide variety of drugs*
  - *Calling families to keep them appraised of the patients' status, often using their phones to allow patients face time with their family*
  - *Before intubation, if time allowed, allowing the patient and the family a moment to see and speak with one another*

- *In a health crisis, multiorgan failure can be a common occurrence in a large number of patients. The department of internal medicine should plan contingency staffing for such specialties as nephrology (for hemodialysis), pulmonary medicine, and palliative care as the needs during crisis times will vastly exceed "lean" staffing during peaceful regular times.*

- In a health crisis, it is very important to have a significant focus on timely, expeditious, effective, and safe discharge of recovered patients. This will allow the hospital to continue to serve the incoming patients and reduce the strain on its limited resources.
- Treatment protocols must be implemented and disseminated as soon as available. The treatment team must research the availability of treatments and, if necessary, advocate obtaining these from pharmaceutical companies, especially those treatments only available on expanded access or in investigational studies.
- Safety of healthcare workers is of utmost importance. OHS protocols for identification of symptomatic healthcare workers, infectious agent testing availability for healthcare workers, isolation, and return-to-work protocols need to be implemented and updated regularly.

Infection Control Specific Key Lessons

- In a health crisis, given the rapidly changing guidelines and practice recommendations, infection control should be responsible for keeping the hospital policies and infection control and prevention practices and procedures up to date, both internally and externally.
- Infection control, with guidance from infectious disease experts, should produce and keep up-to-date protocols and algorithms for triage, isolation, and laboratory diagnostic evaluations for the infectious agent.
- In-house testing capability for the new infectious agent is critical to acquire as soon as possible to manage isolation and treatment.
- In preparing for an infectious disease health crisis, tracers should be practiced by walking through the actual steps in the Emergency Department from patient presentation, identification, the path to the isolation room(s) on the medical floors or the ICUs, and appropriate infection control interventions.
- Tracer simulations should teach lessons on the prevention of spread of infection, patient safety, and protection of the healthcare workers and other hospital staff.

Acknowledgments Susan Singh, MPH Director of Infection Control
Victoria Bengualid, MD, Director of Graduate Medical Education
Anita Soni, MD, Director of Hospitalist Service.

References

1. Beigel JH, Tomashek KM, Dodd L, Mehta AK, Zingman BS, Kalil AC, et al. Remdesivir for the treatment of Covid-19. N Engl J Med. 2020;383(19):1813–26. https://doi.org/10.1056/NEJMoa2007764.

2. Wang Y, Zhang D, Du G, Du R, Zhao J, Jin Y, et al. Remdesivir in adults with severe COVID-19: a randomised, double-blind, placebo-controlled, multicentre trial. Lancet. 2020;395(10236):1569–78. https://doi.org/10.1016/S0140-6736(20)31022-9.
3. Tomazini BM, Maia IS, Cavalcanti AB, Berwanger O, Rosa RG, Veiga VC, et al. Effect of dexamethasone on days alive and ventilator-free in patients with moderate or severe acute respiratory distress syndrome and COVID-19: the CoDEX randomized clinical trial. JAMA. 2020;324(13):1307–16. https://doi.org/10.1001/jama.2020.17021.
4. Kalil AC. Treating COVID-19—off-label drug use, compassionate use, and randomized clinical trials during pandemics. JAMA. 2020;323(19):1897–8. https://doi.org/10.1001/jama.2020.4742.

Chapter 5
Critical Care

Christopher A. Grantham, Dmitriy Karev, Robert D. Karpinos, Rocco J. Lafaro, Edward E. Telzak, Ralph Rahme, and Ridwan Shabsigh

---

C. A. Grantham
Medical Intensive Care Unit, Department of Medicine, SBH Health System, Bronx, NY, USA

CUNY School of Medicine, New York, NY, USA

D. Karev
CUNY School of Medicine, New York, NY, USA

Division of Trauma and Surgical Critical Care, Department of Surgery, SBH Health System, Bronx, NY, USA

R. D. Karpinos
Perioperative Services and Department of Anesthesiology, SBH Health System, Bronx, NY, USA

CUNY School of Medicine, New York, NY, USA

R. J. Lafaro
CUNY School of Medicine, New York, NY, USA

Division of Cardiothoracic Surgery, Department of Surgery, SBH Health System, Bronx, NY, USA

E. E. Telzak
Department of Medicine, SBH Health System, Bronx, NY, USA

Department of Medicine, CUNY School of Medicine, Bronx, NY, USA

Albert Einstein College of Medicine, Bronx, NY, USA

R. Rahme
CUNY School of Medicine, New York, NY, USA

Division of Neurosurgery, Department of Surgery, SBH Health System, Bronx, NY, USA

R. Shabsigh (✉)
Department of Surgery, SBH Health System, Bronx, NY, USA

Department of Urology, Weill Cornell Medical College of Cornell University, New York, NY, USA

CUNY School of Medicine, New York, NY, USA
e-mail: rshabsigh@sbhny.org

© The Author(s), under exclusive license to Springer Nature Switzerland AG 2022
R. Shabsigh (ed.), *Health Crisis Management in Acute Care Hospitals*,
https://doi.org/10.1007/978-3-030-95806-0_5

Introduction: Critical Care as a Crucial Pillar in Health Crisis Management

Health crises may produce patients and illnesses at various levels of acuity and severity which can result in large numbers of patients being admitted to a hospital. In addition to requiring regular care, patients may also require intermediate care and/or admission to the intensive care unit (ICU). The result is that hospital resources are severely impacted during a crisis. Preparation and delivery of critical care are vital in order for a hospital system to successfully respond to a health crisis. This is reflected in the lessons learned from the 2020 COVID-19 pandemic at its USA epicenter in New York City.

What Is Critical Care?

Critical care is the practice of delivering comprehensive optimal care to patients who are either severely ill and unstable or who have the potential to become so. Critical care patients are those who not only require but will benefit from the highest level of care delivered in a setting that is optimized for observation, multimodal monitoring, intervention, treatment, and life-supportive care. Critical care may prevent patients from decompensating by optimizing the treatment and support of various organ systems. Optimizing care provides patients with the necessary time for stabilization and healing. These patients are on continuous cardiac monitoring both at bedside and at central stations for arrhythmia analysis. Blood pressure monitoring can be done both noninvasively and invasively, with arterial lines for real-time assessment. Central lines allow for infusion of pressors, concentrated solutions, rapid volume infusion, and assessment of oxygen utilization. Advanced/complex hemodynamic monitoring including Swan-Ganz catheters can be used to assess cardiac index, systemic vascular resistance, right-sided heart, and pulmonary artery pressures. Transesophageal echocardiography (TEE) and transthoracic echocardiography (TTE) can also be utilized as minimally invasive tools to obtain "snap shots" to further assess interventions and their impact on anatomy and physiology. Pulmonary dynamics can be monitored directly at the ventilator allowing for acute adjustments/interventions in airway pressure: peak and plateau, air flow, and the pressure gradients created under specific conditions of ventilation. Pulse oximetry and end-tidal CO_2 ($ETCO_2$) can and should be monitored on a continuous basis, providing ongoing feedback from interventions as well as alerting staff if there is a need for additional intervention. Respiratory monitoring is done with continuous pulse oximetry and end-tidal CO_2 analysis, as needed. Ventilatory support of intubated patients is done with various ventilator modes, utilizing both volume-cycled and pressure-cycled ventilation. Some patients require various levels of both inspiratory and expiratory pressures to optimize oxygenation. Patients who have inadequate ventilation, despite appropriate optimized support, may be candidates for extracorporeal membrane oxygenation (ECMO). Dialysis capabilities include intermittent hemodialysis (HD), continuous renal replacement therapy (CRRT), and peritoneal dialysis (PD). Nutrition support is a very important function of critical care since many patients are at risk of nutritional depletion and its deleterious consequences. Many patients require various forms of parenteral nutrition whereas others may need gastrointestinal tube nutrition.

Numerous patients in intensive care units suffer from multi-organ failure. Critical care provides diagnostics and therapeutic support to multiple vital organs. Such support requires the involvement of multiple specialties and subspecialties in addition to the critical care team.

Components of Critical Care

In order to achieve the primary goals of diagnosing and treating critically ill patients, the range of functions encompassed by critical care is broad. These functions include the following:

- Monitoring of vital signs, heart rhythm, oxygen saturation, $ETCO_2$, fluid input and output, and laboratory tests
- Specialized monitoring as needed for cardiac output, either noninvasively or invasively
- Intracranial pressure (ICP) monitoring
- Intravenous (IV) access capable of safely delivering necessary medications, fluids, and blood products
- Mechanical ventilation
- Ventilator support capabilities
- Noninvasive ventilation alternatives: continuous positive airway pressure (CPAP), bilevel positive airway pressure (BIPAP), and high-flow nasal cannula (HFNC)
- Respiratory therapy by trained specialists
- Nursing care at a level adequate for patients' severity of illness, with nurse/patient ratio of 1/2 or 1/1 registered nurse (RN) according to severity of illness
- Physician care by physicians specialized in critical care

Critical care is a general specialty that provides services to diverse types of acute severe illness. There are also sub-specialties in critical care, including medical, surgical, neuro, trauma, cardiac, pediatric, and neonatal critical care. Such sub-specialties have different scopes of work, separate training, and certification processes. In large medical centers, especially large university medical centers and tertiary hospitals, such diverse critical care sub-specialties exist in separate ICUs, creating the medical ICU (MICU), surgical ICU (SICU), pediatric ICU (PICU), neonatal ICU (NICU), cardiac care unit (CCU), and neuro ICU (neuro ICU), among others. However, in small- and medium-sized hospitals, not all such sub-specialized ICUs exist. In planning and preparing for a health crisis, accounting for all possible critical care capacity is important. Cross-coverage of critical care should be possible among the various subspecialties, with some preparation and cross-training.

In most hospitals, ICUs are so-called "closed units." The closed unit model of care means that the critical care physician team is exclusively responsible for the care of all patients in the ICU, regardless of the initial admitting physician-of-record or prior physicians caring for a given patient. The critical care team responsible for the ICU usually directs patient care, writes orders, and consults with other physicians and specialists, as appropriate for each patient. This model of care assures that each critically ill patient can receive the specialized services, treatments, and procedures specific to critical care, with continuity of care and a clear definition of responsibility.

The Patients

ICU patients are critically ill and unstable or at risk of becoming so. They may have a variety of medical problems requiring the highest level of monitoring available. These conditions may include respiratory failure, cardiac failure, ST-elevated myocardial infarction (STEMI), renal failure, liver failure, multi-organ failure (MOF), traumatic brain injury (TBI), central nervous system (CNS) events, strokes, shock, sepsis, pneumonia, acute respiratory distress syndrome (ARDS), bleeding, metabolic derangements, malnutrition, coagulopathy, medication side effects and overdoses, and toxidromes, and they may require peri-operative care.

Critical Care Health Workers

Physicians caring for critically ill patients are intensivists, trained specifically in critical care through fellowship programs. Intensivists are commonly also trained in pulmonary medicine. Specialists trained in critical care may include surgeons, neurosurgeons, anesthesiologists, pediatricians, nephrologists, cardiologists, and neurologists, among others. These specialists have the knowledge, skills, and experience to perform and deliver all the functions of critical care mentioned above.

Multidisciplinary critical care teams also incorporate clinical pharmacists, registered nurses, nurse practitioners, physician assistants and others. Registered nurses working in the ICU are specialty-trained and certified to care for critically ill patients. This is necessary in order to deliver the high level of care that is required in the ICU. Respiratory therapists (RTs) are an integral part of the critical care team as many patients are on ventilators or require noninvasive ventilator support with frequent bedside assessment and treatment by the RTs.

The facilities necessary for ICU care require rooms with multiple life support systems and essential capabilities, bedside and central station monitoring, oxygen therapy, suctioning, dialysis capability, and optimally negative pressure isolation rooms. Equipment for the ICU needs to be readily available for emergent care such as airway support, intubation, chest tubes, bronchoscopy, central line access, arterial lines, defibrillation, and ICP monitors. Medications needed for emergent use must also be readily available such as those for sedation-analgesia, paralysis, BP control, arrhythmia treatment, and thrombolytics.

Levels of Critical Care

In most arrangements, there are generally two levels of critical care: intensive care and intermediate care (although in some settings, sublevels of intensive and intermediate care may exist). It is vital to at least have these two levels available when planning and preparing a hospital for a health crisis. Since well-defined admission criteria to either level of care are highly important factors for the effective and efficient delivery of critical care, the resulting impact on efficient utilization of tight human and material resources will be significant.

Admission criteria to intensive care includes patients with ventilators, respiratory distress, hemodynamic instability, shock, arrhythmias, requirements for frequent neurologic assessment and invasive lines, patients needing frequent or high-level nursing care or respiratory monitoring. A variety of medications may only be administered in a highly monitored ICU setting such as pressors and thrombolytics. The nursing care requirements are high with a staffing ratio of 1:1 or 1:2 nurse: patient.

Admission criteria to intermediate care include patients requiring cardiac and respiratory noninvasive monitoring. These patients have noninvasive blood pressure and heart rate monitoring, pulse oximetry, and end-tidal CO_2 monitoring, as needed. The nursing care requirements are less and allow for a staffing ratio of approximately 1:5 nurse: patient.

Expanding Critical Care During a Health Crisis

During a health crisis, the need for critical care may escalate rapidly and far exceed available capabilities at the facility. In order to prepare for a potentially quickly evolving situation, initiatives can be put in place.

Planning

Planning for these situations is crucial to allow time to escalate ICU patient care and volume. An inability to provide critical care when indicated will result in unsafe and suboptimal care.

Once the ICU is full, placement of patients may be logistically difficult. Finding adequate appropriate ICU bed space for an escalating unknown quantity of patients then becomes one of the primary institutional needs. The danger of inadequate ICU bed capacity may cascade to impact care in multiple ways:

- Patients waiting in the emergency department will overwhelm the emergency department capabilities.
- Infectious patients, with inadequate infection control, will put staff and others at risk.
- Patients with worsening conditions on the regular floor awaiting ICU transfer will have suboptimal monitoring.
- Staffing outside of the ICU will likely be inadequate for the severity of illness and patient needs, leading to higher morbidity and mortality.

Building a new ICU rapidly during a crisis is generally not a feasible solution. Mobile Army Surgical Hospital (MASH) units and temporary ICU-capable tents or trailers require financial capabilities beyond those of independent small safety net hospitals, such as the SBH Health System. This can usually only be accomplished by a governmental organization or the military medical services.

Requirements for newly added ICU beds include the following:

- Available space
- ICU equipment
- Monitoring capability
- Adequate ventilator and noninvasive ventilator alternatives
- Infection control and isolation capability
- Dialysis capability
- Personal protective equipment (PPE) supplies
- Staffing trained for ICU-level patient care
- Pharmacy supplies and other supplies for critical care

If available ICU bed capacity has been exhausted faster than expected, rapid decisions and contingency plans must be made and new areas allocated for critically ill patients as effectively as possible (Box 5.1).

Box 5.1. Summary of Steps on How to Improvise Regular Care Areas for Critical Care
- Optimize visualization of patients in room (e.g., convert solid doors to paneled see-through/consider camera options).
- Portable bedside monitor if no remote central monitoring capability is available.
- Pulse oximetry with alarms.
- Optimize alarm audibility.
- Optimize infection control: Negative pressure room conversion (if possible), mobile HEPA filters in rooms and on devices, demistifier tents, helmet noninvasive ventilation with high-flow nasal O_2.
- Maintain adequate PPE for all personnel (gowns, masks N-95, face shields, goggles, PAPRs for intubations).
- In case ICU nurses are not available, staff new critical care areas with nurses who have experience with ventilators and in caring for unstable patients (e.g., ED or PACU nurses). Also consider accessing the retired experienced ICU nursing pool.
- If medical intensivists are unavailable, utilize physicians with most experience in caring for unstable ICU patients (i.e., surgeons, anesthesiologists, hospitalists with additional critical care training).
- Utilize telemedicine with experienced physicians to optimize rounding and specialized care delivery.
- Incorporate palliative care team into decisions regarding goals of care and identifying patients who are not candidates for ongoing ICU care.

Minimum requirements include the following:

- Cardiac monitoring/pulse oximetry/alarm capabilities
- Medical air and oxygen capabilities for ventilators and noninvasive ventilator alternatives
- Dialysis capabilities
- Electronic medical record (EMR) capabilities for ordering and documentation
- Access to ICU medications with rapid deployment

ICU-Ready Areas

Because critical care is one of the pillars enabling the successful response of a hospital system to a health crisis, preparation for expansion should be done during normal times. Such preparation includes ICU-ready areas equipped with the capabilities of central monitoring, ventilator connections, hemodialysis, isolation, and other physical requirements. These ICU-ready areas can be used as needed during normal times for regular-level care, intermediate-level care, telemetry, and others. However, during crisis times, these areas can quickly be converted to ICUs. In addition to ICU-ready physical space, preparation must also include supplies, medications, staffing, etc. It is important to note that when new ICU bed locations are created, there may be specific care limitations in these areas. For example, some new locations may lack dialysis capability. This obstacle then affects staffing, transport stability, and infection control logistics if transportation to dialysis facilities outside the ICU is required.

Location Considerations: Advantages and Disadvantages

- Large open areas: greater bed capacity, greater efficiency in monitoring and utilization of staff especially at times of shortage, but less infection control.
- Closed rooms: better infection control but higher staffing utilization.
- Specialty areas (post-anesthesia care unit (PACU), cardiac cath recovery): full monitoring but loss of specialty service and reduction of infection control.
- Medical floor beds: can isolate patients but may have no negative pressure and no central monitoring.
- ED holding area: has all advanced monitoring capabilities but potential infection control issues in open areas and overburdened ED staff capabilities means real-time monitoring may be overlooked.

Critical Care Crisis Team Building

Integrated Tiered Critical Care Teams

The concept of an "integrated tiered critical care team" relates to the integration of the specialties of medical and surgical critical care and anesthesiology. It, in turn, includes the downstream integration of physicians, residents, fellows, nurses, respiratory therapists, and many others. The result is a layered tiered team that is able to maximize utilization of limited resources and therefore broaden the ability of coverage of expanded areas (see Fig. 5.1).

Cross-Training of Non-critical Care Physicians in Critical Care

The COVID-19 pandemic resulted in a critical care crisis, the immediate concern being the availability – or lack – of medical resources required to meet both the challenges posed by and the number of critically ill patients. Advanced critical care skills including ventilator management, hemodynamic monitoring, use of invasive technologies, and advanced therapeutics, require hospital personnel capable of critical care training and skills.

For example, in order to meet the challenges of the COVID-19 pandemic, the SBH Health System expanded critical care resources and personnel by cross-training. Building critical care teams was a priority.

One strategy employed to meet the challenges created by the pandemic was to create a reserve critical care physician workforce by cross-training non-critical care physicians (surgeons of all specialties, anesthesiologists, medical doctors, podiatrists, and dental specialists). The aim was to ensure that an additional layer of support was available to care for rapidly increasing numbers of patients, should critical

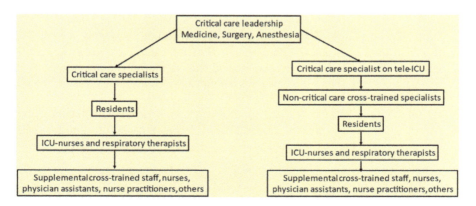

Fig. 5.1 Example of a critical care integrated tiered team (SBH experience)

care specialists become unavailable due to COVID-19-related isolation, illness, or simply overwhelmed by fatigue and burnout.

The first step in the program was to provide education, both didactic and practical, in order to prepare non-critical care physicians to care for critically ill patients at the intensive care and intermediate care levels. The program provided safe and effective systems under the direct supervision of senior critical care staff.

The program is a self-study educational course on *Critical Care for Non-ICU clinicians* of education, training, credentialing, indemnification, deployment, and support. It is instituted, free of charge and offered by the Society of Critical Care Medicine (SCCM): https://www.sccm.org/Clinical-Resources/Disaster/COVID19/COVID19-ResourceResponseCenter.

Didactic sessions include clinical case presentations, detailed discussion of cases, review of pathophysiology, respiratory failure, shock, sepsis, care of the older patient, nutrition, utilization of therapeutics, and other critical care illnesses (Box 5.2). Participants are required to reason through clinical cases, engage in discussion with the group, and answer quiz-type questions. The sessions are led by a senior critical care specialist, who remains available to the group throughout the training for additional review and discussion.

The didactic sessions are followed by practical training. Each non-critical care physician attends a training session on the use of the ventilator, including modes of ventilation and settings. This session is a hands-on use of a ventilator taught by a senior anesthesiologist and critical care physician.

The practical training includes the non-critical care physicians rounding with critical care physicians in the ICU setting. The participants actively participate in-patient care and management under the supervision of a senior critical care specialist.

On completion of the didactic and practical training, the non-critical care physicians can be deployed to critical care areas including ICU, telemetry, and ventilator units. The physician becomes part of a team which includes residents and nurses under the supervision and guidance of a critical care physician. The supervising critical care physician can guide the team for 24 hours at a time and remain available throughout via remote (tele-ICU) technology. This model allows the critical care

Box 5.2. The Didactic Training Sessions Include the Following
- Assessment of the seriously ill patient
- Airway management I
- Airway assessment and management
- Critical care for older adults
- Diagnosis and management of acute respiratory failure
- Nutrition of critically ill patients
- Mechanical ventilation I
- Mechanical ventilation II
- Diagnosis and management of shock and sepsis
- Use of therapeutics, including antibiotics, vasopressors, and inotropes.

team leader full access to the patient with all available data, imaging, and view of the patient for 24 hours.

The follow-up program includes didactic sessions, with an emphasis on simulated cases and ventilator review. The program will be provided as a timely ongoing maintenance. This program will include ongoing review of up-to-date COVID-19 guidelines, including ventilator modes, new technologies, and therapeutics. All services will discuss their response and management during the crisis.

Cross-training of non-critical care physicians is a feasible, effective, and safe program with the aim of creating a replacement and supplementary workforce in areas facing challenges due to a critical care crisis, such as the current pandemic. The concept of non-critical care trained physicians and the integrated tiered team will hopefully remain an ongoing tool for crisis management in hospitals. The success of the integrated team is built on a system of supervision and guidance of a critical care physician, who remains available to the team throughout. Timely review of the program will ensure that up-to-date knowledge and skills are available, and this in turn will reflect upon the readiness of physicians when faced with prolonged current and future health crises.

Multidisciplinary Critical Care Committee

A carefully planned, designed, and operated critical care committee is an absolutely essential part of a hospital's critical care response. Such a committee should form a core part of advanced planning for hospital crisis preparedness.

Mission, Goals, and Composition

The mission of this committee is planning, information exchange, providing leadership, allocating resources, coordination, dynamic response to rapidly changing conditions, and assurance of effective communications. The goal is for the committee to become an efficient platform in order to achieve its mission.

It is also equally important to understand that critical care, especially in crisis times, is a true multidisciplinary endeavor. This should be fully reflected in the membership and conduct of the critical care committee. The composition of the committee should be represented by all departments and stakeholders of critical care. Table 5.1 explains the recommended membership in a critical care committee and their roles. Figure 5.2 illustrates the relationship of the critical care committee with the command center, other departments, and entities.

5 Critical Care

Table 5.1 Recommended membership in the health crisis critical care committee with representation and roles

Department or discipline	Division	Representative	Role(s)	Comments
Internal medicine	Medical Intensive Care Unit (MICU)	Director of MICU	Joint leadership of overall critical care services	The 3 leaders of medical critical care, surgical critical care, and anesthesiology can provide strong joint leadership of overall critical care in time of crisis by uniting their departments into one large hospital-wide critical care service. In addition, the 3 leaders coordinate the continuity of care from the ED to the ICU and other floors in alignment with treatment plans and ongoing interventions
Surgery	Surgical Intensive Care Unit (SICU)	Director of SICU	Joint leadership of overall critical care services	
Anesthesiology		Chair of anesthesiology	Joint leadership of overall critical care services	
Surgery	All surgical services including trauma and acute care surgery	Chair of surgery	Multilateral coordination	Chair of surgery may modify surgical services and reallocate resources to support critical care during a crisis
Internal medicine	General internal medicine	Chair of medicine	Multilateral coordination	Chair of internal medicine may modify internal medical services and re-allocate resources to support critical care during a crisis
Other clinical departments	If available: neuro, cardiac, trauma, pediatric intensive care units (all ICUs)	Directors of other ICUs if available	Provision of additional services for expansion of critical care	Other ICUs may all be combined and converted to provide critical care services specific to the current crisis
Emergency medicine		Representative of chair of emergency medicine	Coordination of emergency medicine and critical care	
Nursing	General nursing	Chief nursing officer or director of nursing	Coordination of critical care services	

(continued)

Table 5.1 (continued)

Department or discipline	Division	Representative	Role(s)	Comments
Nursing	Critical care nursing	Director of critical care nursing	Coordination of critical care nursing services	
Respiratory therapy		Directory of respiratory therapy	Coordination of critical care respiratory care services	
Nutritional medicine		Director of nutritional medicine	Coordination of critical care nutritional services	
Pharmacy		Director of pharmacy or director of intensive care pharmacy	Coordination of critical care pharmaceutical services	
Rehabilitation and physical therapy		Director of rehab and physical therapy	Coordination of rehabilitation of survivors after critical care	
Information technology and medical informatics		Director of medical informatics	Coordination of medical informatics and IT needs for critical care	
Facilities and engineering		Director of facilities and engineering	Coordination of facilities and engineering needs for critical care	
Infection control		Director of infection control	Infection control oversight and coordination of services	
Supply chain		Director of supply chain	Assurance of equipment and supplies for critical care	

Meetings

The frequency of meetings of the critical care committee is based on the contemporary needs and the intensity of the healthcare crisis. In the preparedness planning phase, weekly meetings may be appropriate. During the escalation phase and the peak phase of a crisis, daily meetings are necessary. At such times, daily meetings of the entire committee are necessary on all days, including weekends and holidays.

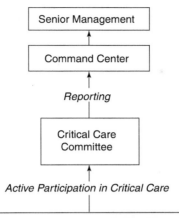

Fig. 5.2 Relationships of the critical care committee with the command center and other departments in the hospital during a crisis

Box 5.3. Frequency of Meetings of Critical Care Committee

Planning phase:	weekly
Escalation phase of crisis:	daily
Peak of surge of crisis:	daily or twice daily
De-escalation phase of crisis:	daily or less frequently
Immediate post-crisis phase for reflection and learning:	weekly
Normal times:	monthly

In addition to the regular meetings, the leadership of the committee may meet any time and as much as needed. A master list of mobile numbers and e-mails of all committee members should be distributed and updated. In the de-escalation phase of the crisis, the frequency of meetings may be adjusted to the needs of the current status. It is strongly recommended that critical care committee meetings are conducted virtually for many reasons, including efficiency, infection control, and assurance of attendance. Availability of the digital infrastructure for efficient virtual meetings and communications is indispensable. The meetings should be formal, each with an agenda and minutes. It is the duty of the leaders of the committee to assure timely and effective communications both inside and outside the committee (see Box 5.3 for the suggested frequency of critical care committee meetings).

Agenda

The agenda should reflect the long-term goals, short-term goals, resources, operations, tasks, updates, trouble-shooting, and representation of all stake holders.

Minutes

The minutes should be a live document that is updated regularly. The minutes should include action items clearly assigned to the various committee members (see Box 5.4 for a sample agenda that can also be followed for the minutes).

> **Box 5.4. Example of Agenda/Minutes of a Critical Care Committee Meeting**
> Critical Care Committee Meeting
>   Agenda/Minutes
>   Date
> *Section 1: Baseline Information*:
>
> - Introduction:
> - Goals:
> - Assumptions:
> - Resources:
> - Human resources: physicians, nurses, respiratory therapists, pharmacists, laboratory technicians, etc.
> - Patient care teams: Integrated teams
> - Training:
> - Critical care committee:
> - Physical space/beds:
> - Escalation/expansion plan:
> - De-escalation:
> - Ventilators:
> - Ventilator alternatives:
> - Proning:
> - Medical informatics and telemedicine:
> - Supplies and disposables:
> - Supplies conservation guidelines, education and enforcement:
> - Pharmacy:
> - Infectious disease and infection control:
> - Environmental services:
> - Medical students' involvement:
> - Guidelines for rationing and bioethics:
> - Coordination of care and practice between critical care and Emergency Medicine:

Section 2: Implementation, Gap Analysis, and Updates as of "Date":

- Status:
- Critical care teams:
- Lessons learned:
- Emergency medicine:
- Nursing:
- Pharmacy:
- Respiratory therapy:
- Proning:
- Ventilators:
- Ventilator alternatives:
- Supplies:
- Infectious disease:
- PPE:
- Renal failure and dialysis:
- Clinical guidelines:
- Participation in clinical trials:
- HCW morale and emotional status:
- New literature watch:
- New problems:

Section 3: Summary of Action Items:

- What, how, who, when, where?

Timely Actions

Since critical care deals with the most ill patients, timely decision-making, communication, and execution are of the highest importance. This is especially the case during a crisis. The critical care committee must assure timely actions with effective communications and effective follow-up. The leaders of the critical care committee should foster the necessary culture of accountability and collaboration.

Transparency

During a healthcare crisis, managing critical care cannot afford misinformation or missing information. Regardless of how bad the news is, all news and all information related to critical care should be brought up to the critical care committee with transparency and timeliness. Transparency fosters confidence, trust, and engagement. This can be reflected not only in the deliberations of the committee but also in its minutes and communications. An important element to promote transparency is for the hospital to provide full legal and liability coverage during a crisis to all ranks of its healthcare workers, especially the decision-makers. It is inevitable during a crisis, especially at its highest intensity and peak, that incorrect decisions will be made, complications will occur, and unsatisfactory outcomes might be reached. Such is the nature of a crisis! To assure that all healthcare workers give their strongest effort and rise to their highest performance, it is necessary to provide legal and liability coverage with transparency and clarity. However, such coverage should not be misunderstood as absolving from accountability in case of gross egregious negligence.

Bottle Necks and Service-Limiting Factors

Critical care could be understood as a "veto system." A "veto system" is one which has many essential components so that any or many of its components could be rate-limiting, creating a bottle neck. Such is critical care! For example, any of the following factors could limit a hospital's critical care capacity: number of rooms with necessary equipment, number of ventilators, critical care supplies, number of specialized critical care physicians, number of specialized nurses, number of respiratory therapists, dialysis capability, and monitoring capability. Understanding this point should guide critical care planning for health crisis. A checklist with gap analysis can assure that all service-limiting factors are addressed. Table 5.2 shows an example of a checklist with gap analysis, actions, and tasks. Such a checklist can be used by the hospital senior management and the critical care committee to prepare critical care for a health crisis.

Creativity and Improvisation

This chapter would not be complete without mentioning creativity and improvisation. Regardless of detailed careful planning and meticulous preparedness, a severe crisis will challenge and expose previously implausible situations, unexpected deficiencies, and difficult problems. With the support of the hospital senior management, critical care leadership should be empowered to make dynamic decisions and use creative solutions to tackle unprecedented challenges and unexpected problems. Such creative solutions may include a broad range of unconventional practices, on-the-spot improvisations, cross-training, multi-tasking, re-assignments of resources, and others (see Box 5.5).

Table 5.2 Critical care crisis planning checklist with gap analysis, actions, tasks, and timelines

Type of item	Item	Max target capacity during crisis	Current capacity	Gap	Task/action	Assigned person/department	Timeline	Additional comments
Human resources	Physicians							
	Residents/fellows							
	Nurses							
	Respiratory therapists							
	Other workers							
Physical facilities	Critical care rooms							
	Isolation rooms (negative pressure)							
Equipment	Central monitoring							
	Dialysis capability							
	Ventilators							
	Ventilator alternatives							
Supplies	Oxygen							
	IV pumps							
	Specialized beds							
	Protective equipment							
Supportive services	Laboratory							
	Pharmacy							
	Nutrition							

(continued)

Table 5.2 (continued)

Type of item	Item	Max target capacity during crisis	Current capacity	Gap	Task/ action	Assigned person/ department	Timeline	Additional comments
Systems	Electronic medical record system with critical care templates and care pathways							
	Medical informatics							
	Tele-medicine, Tele-ICU							
	Virtual communications and virtual meetings							
Additional support	Patient relations and family support							
	Mortality management							
	Rehabilitation after ICU							
	Ethics committee							
	Practice guidelines							
	Emerging literature updates							
	Physical, emotional, and moral support of healthcare workers							
The bottom line	Finance							
Other	Other							

> **Box 5.5. Examples of Creative Solutions and Improvisations**
> - Cross-training of non-critical care physicians in critical care
> - Utilizing dental staff in medical care
> - Utilizing orthopedic staff in proning of ventilated patients with acute respiratory distress syndrome (ARDS)
> - Utilizing medical students for virtual ICU rounding and subsequent communication with patients' families
> - Utilization of medical students and medical school librarians for frequent summaries of rapidly emergent literature on the current crisis
> - Placing IV pumps and ventilator monitors and controls in hallways outside ICU rooms to reduce entry
> - Ventilator sharing

Utilization of Anesthesiologists in Critical Care

Anesthesiologists generally receive critical care training during residency. Some anesthesiologists choose critical care as a specialty and complete an additional fellowship that expands the role of the critical care anesthesiologist beyond the acute perioperative phase, with emphasis on longer-term critical care functions. Anesthesiologists who choose the perioperative arena may electively confine their practice to preoperative optimization, operating room (OR) anesthetic care, the post anesthesia care unit (PACU), and acute pain management. Largely, the intraoperative management of the acutely ill or trauma patient requires the most acute levels of critical care. In many institutions, the PACU has the same requirements and is considered an intensive care location. While systems and protocols may vary, the biggest difference in care delivered in a typical ICU setting and that delivered in the OR and/or the PACU is predominantly related to volume, focus, and duration. Adapting in order to provide complete ICU care for critically ill patients is actually a steep relearning curve and can be anxiety provoking and somewhat overwhelming, especially when time has elapsed after training. For this reason, while the anesthesiologist may seem well suited to jump into a full-service critical care setting, the support of the tiered system along with the educational reinforcement described above is essential.

Utilizing Dental Staff in Clinical Care

In the crisis condition, where the volume of care providers can easily be outpaced by need, it is essential to identify and create roles that may not be traditional but where additional manpower can ease the stress on the system. Many dental providers have combined DDS and MD degrees and a number have rotated in anesthesiology and surgical departments during training. Many dentists have an extensive background and experience in clinical fields, and this can prove extremely valuable in the pharmacy or the laboratory. The ability to interface with people, develop clinical relationships, and earn patients trust quickly makes these providers ideal candidates to perform testing for potential patients and to provide an interface with patient families, explaining medical conditions and providing comfort to families. Dental providers suited for and interested in direct patient care can adapt to, and be included, in the tiered delivery of critical care. Where dental anesthesiology is practiced, providers can contribute at the highest level to respiratory care and ventilator management, if not directly to ICU care and emergency airway management.

Utilizing Other Staff

Orthopedic staff can be used for proning of ventilated patients with acute respiratory distress syndrome. Medical students can aid virtual ICU rounding and subsequent communication with patients' families. Medical students and medical school librarians can help with frequent summaries of rapidly emergent literature on the current crisis.

Ventilator Sharing or Splitting

Due to the rapid onset of the pandemic, out-of-the-box solutions become a necessity, and one of these solutions is ventilator sharing. For example, since many COVID-19 patients had an acute need for ventilator therapy not only was bed availability and manpower rapidly overwhelmed, but in many cases, ventilators became in short supply as well. Every effort to provide each patient with an individual ventilator was made, and in many cases, ventilators that were not typically used for ICU patients, including anesthesia machines, bilevel positive airway pressure (BIPAP), and other non-traditional mechanical ventilation devices, were safely used outside of their general indications. At the same time, as the market was being flooded with new and novel adaptations for traditional ventilation devices, the concept of ventilator sharing became a firm reality as the supply and production of ventilators was rapidly outpaced by demand. Without this concept in place, the alternative was to ration care and objectively identify which patients should get a ventilator and which should not, and therefore be left to die. In the absence of objective data, initiating this sharing concept could be a daunting prospect but it might lead some systems to begin sharing ventilators between matched patients [1].

The Department of Emergency Medicine at St. John's Hospital in Detroit, MI, demonstrated that in theory, as many as four patients could be adequately ventilated for a limited time on a single ventilator with routine and commonly available equipment [2]. Using the same model, Lorenzo et al. demonstrated that four adult human-sized sheep could successfully be maintained on a single ventilator for up to 12 hours [3]. This solution was operationalized and successfully used in the immediate response to the 2017 mass causality Las Vegas shooting and reportedly also in Italy by Dr. Marco Garrone during the pandemic, with success.

The practice of "splitting" ventilators between patients was almost immediately condemned in a joint consensus statement of the Society of Critical Care Medicine, the American Association for Respiratory Care, the American Society of Anesthesiologists, the Anesthesia patient Safety Foundation, the American Association of Critical-Care Nurses, and the American College of Chest Physicians [4]. This position paper was looking specifically at the practice of splitting ventilators between patients with significant evolving pulmonary disease, where the limitation was the constant change of clinical conditions, making the modality near impossible. If the practice of ventilator sharing had been applied to chronic, stable patients who were well matched and remained sedated and relaxed, it could be an achievable though high-risk proposition, freeing up resources for the more unstable patients.

Sharing a ventilator between patients is a high-risk procedure that does require extensive evaluation for all involved patients. An in-depth review of the patients for adequate matching of ventilatory parameters is required prior to initiating the procedure and includes checking the following: tidal volume, driving pressure (plateau pressure – PEEP), respiratory rate, peak pressures, positive end expiratory pressure (PEEP), FiO_2, pH (>7.35), SpO_2, consistent ventilator settings with no anticipated changes necessary, no contraindication to quinolone or steroid NDMR, absence of infection or laboratory confirmation of identical pathogen, absence of asthma, or COPD. Both patients should also be hemodynamically stable and not requiring vasopressor.

Neuromuscular relaxation is required to ensure passive ventilation and pressure-controlled ventilation is recommended to prevent pulmonary dynamics in one patient from impacting the other. Infection control is a critical part of this procedure, and cross-contamination, while possible (if valves are incompetent), must be mitigated with additional filters. If patients do not meet all of the above criteria or are unable to tolerate PCV, pairing them on a single ventilator is NOT recommended.

The practice of ventilator sharing requires continuous monitoring, for each individual patient, of heart rate and blood pressure, end-tidal carbon dioxide, PCO_2, pH, and PO_2, in addition to the maintenance of the matched ventilatory parameters. In the presence of any new condition, the practice should be curtailed. This is labor intensive and does require a critical care physician who has an intimate knowledge of the ventilator to be immediately available at all times where the practice is being conducted.

Prior to vent changes:

- Ensure both patients are adequately sedated: RASS<-4.
- Ensure both patients are adequately relaxed: train of 4 = 0–1.
- Document baseline driving pressures (plateau PEEP), tidal volume, and respiratory rate for both patients.

Switch both patients to PCV:

- Adjust inspiratory time for each patient such that tidal volume is equal to base line and set to match between patients.
- PEEP is titrated to match in both patients optimizing oxygenation: ensure that tidal volume (TV) has not increased, which may indicate air trapping, or TV has not decreased, which may indicate de-recruitment.
- FiO_2 is expected to be the same for both patients with a resultant $SpO_2 > 96\%$.
- Confirm that all parameters are still matching, including minute volume.
- Verify that both patients tolerate the new PCV settings and that PCO_2 is acceptable in both.
- Set up single ventilator to ventilate both patients simultaneously.
- Set up of two patients sharing one ventilator:
- Color coding the inspiratory and expiratory limbs of the new multiport circuit is recommended to avoid confusion. By default, the expiratory limbs will be white and the inspiratory limbs will be blue.

It is recognized that ventilator sharing is not a standard of care and would be conducted only in the most extreme emergency conditions, where insufficient ventilators are available to support necessary use. In the case of the COVID-19 pandemic surge in Spring 2020, the practice had been approved by the Governor of New York. To proceed with ventilator sharing under other unforeseen circumstances such as this, it is recommended that the adopted protocol be supported by the hospital administration and that, in order to initiate sharing, the directors of the critical care committee all agree that the candidates are acceptable.

Creative Solutions

Staffing

In a healthcare crisis condition, hospital resources, including human resources, can rapidly become overwhelmed (Fig. 5.3). There are often members of the community who are willing and able to help, and reaching out to alumni residents who may be in practice locally or remotely where crisis conditions may not exist can provide an opportunity to bolster clinical staff. Administrative authority can allow for rapid emergency credentialing, and familiarity with community physicians or previously trained residents may allow the process to be expedited. Once granted privileges, volunteers can be added to the clinical staff and provide backup staff to allow much needed down time, in addition to filling in for staff that may have fallen ill.

Even if a service is well staffed and appears to be functioning well, having the added benefit of volunteers is a perfect opportunity to find new or additional roles, no matter how large or small, allowing people to participate and feel like they are contributing to the greater good. In many cases, people with fringe training or experience can provide additional support to services that are struggling.

5 Critical Care

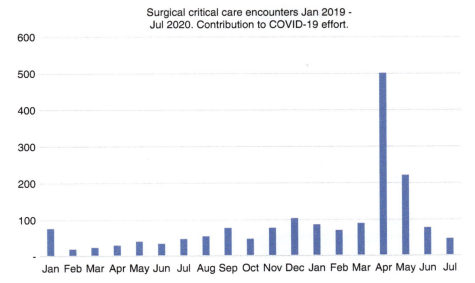

Fig. 5.3 Contribution of surgical critical care during the COVID-19 health crisis surge in April 2020

One example from SBH Health System is that of an alumnus dental anesthesiologist (DA) who had been practicing in an office-based setting in North Carolina. This DA alumnus came to NYC during the pandemic to "help out". Although there was not much need in the OR proper and bed-side critical care was well beyond this provider's comfort level and present scope of practice, a true hero, this provider took up a role as a respiratory therapist. His knowledge of ventilators was rapidly expanded and his ability to manage patients on ventilators proved incredibly valuable. This provider was able to help support the RT team and thus the critical care, ICU, and ED teams. This provider came from out of state with no local family and no place to stay. The need for creativity was not identified until the end of the first clinical day. Where to house this incredibly generous soul? Clearly, he should not sleep in his car as he had planned to do, and while many would have opened their homes under normal conditions, understandably these offers were rare during COVID-19. When presented with the request to assist with housing for volunteer staff, the team responsible for managing clinical spaces exercised some creative energy and identified that the general medical and surgical outpatient clinic spaces were also on pause. When supplied with available stretchers, sleep lab beds, and exam tables, these spaces became instant overnight dormitories for visiting volunteer staff.

Crisis Management of Critical Care Facilities and Physical Spaces

Ventilator-sharing protocols were established for the absolute extreme conditions that would make this practice necessary. However, prior to reaching this level of urgency, several other types of equipment were shared. Infection control precautions during the pandemic mandated conditions where additional space was created in-between patients in the COVID-19 and non-COVID-19 areas to avoid the potential for cross-contamination. In the COVID-19-negative PACU, every other patient bay was left empty. Half of the monitors, pumps, and other materials that were normally available for use in every PACU bay were now available and could be removed and repurposed in the expansion areas. In cases where there were no monitors, available transport monitors and battery dependent devices were used. Frequently, there were not enough monitors for each patient to have their own and central monitoring was not available, so screen splitting and multiple transducers on a single monitors system were set up. These systems are however not ideal and do require attention and verification to be sure that the correct patient's information is being addressed. Protocols were used to ensure uniformity and minimize confusion, i.e., where there are two arterial traces on a single shared monitor, the patient on the physical left (when standing at the foot of the beds) would be the top trace and the patient on the physical right would be the second or bottom trace.

Clinical Practice Adaptation

The original guidance for ventilator management in the COVID-19 patient was to keep tidal volume low and provide respiratory rate to create minute volume. PEEP would be added, consistent with ARDSNET protocols, to ensure oxygenation. Unfortunately, despite low tidal volume settings, high airway pressures were not uncommon in the atypical ARDS of COVID-19, and in this population, multiple patient attributes contributed to an incidence of ventilator-induced pneumothorax. In the adult population, volume-cycled ventilation with various subprotocols is much more common than the pressure-cycled ventilation that is most frequently used in the newborn and pediatric populations. Exercising clinical creativity, some of the units chose to initiate ventilator therapy for COVID-19 patients with pressure-cycled ventilation, which allowed for a wider distribution of air flow and improved tidal volumes with a greater delivery of volume at lower pressures. Limiting pressure while still following ARDS NET protocols had the advantage of avoiding both volume trauma and barotrauma and therefore lowered the inadvertent incidence of pneumothorax.

Supporting the Frontline Healthcare Workers

Frontline workers are an indispensable part of the workforce, especially in the realm of critical care. The success of a hospital system in responding to a health crisis is dependent to a large degree on the optimal functioning and well-being of the frontline workers. Supporting these workers should therefore be a high priority and a daily ambition and should be functional on several levels: the role of team leaders, management of overwork, long hours, intense situations, support for difficult decision-making, emotional and psychological support, material support, and daily rounds (see Box 5.6).

Team Leadership

In a healthcare crisis, the role of the team leader takes on several additional facets. The team leader must rapidly establish the guiding principles that will serve as a foundation. The goal is to create a highly functioning team able to tolerate long hours and incredibly intense situations, confounded by various supply limitations and often with less-than-ideal outcomes expected. Recognizing the significant stress levels associated with crisis is vital as it will contribute to continuous variability in the rational and relational makeup of the team. The team leader's goal is to develop each member of the team, recognizing and capitalizing on complementary skill sets and uniting the team with a common purpose and a common approach. The objective is also to develop autonomy and encourage individual accountability, without losing sight of the daily struggles and emotional health of each team member. As performance readiness develops, greater attention can be focused on the necessary emotional support of the team.

To create a strong and cohesive care team, the leader must motivate each member of the team to *want* to respond to the situation. The leader has a responsibility to ensure that each member of the team feels they are an integral and vital part of the unit and are ultimately key to its success. The leader can encourage this by stating

---

Box 5.6. Quick Daily Checklist of Status of Frontline Healthcare Workers
- Roll call of team members
- Attention to any absent member of the team, reason of absence, and any immediate needs
- Inquiry into any incidents, shortages, and problems since last meeting
- Addressing individual and team reaction to major events, such as patient death, colleague illness, and colleague death
- Inquiry into any immediate needs
- Inquiry into emotional status and morale
- Attention to any member who may need extra help immediately

clear goals and expectations with clear instruction, teaching and coaching, and providing leadership by example, thereby setting the standard by performing high-level tasks alongside the team. Shared decision-making facilitates task performance and builds the motivation to perform, and this will eventually allow the delegation to build trust, confidence, and autonomy.

The team leader will then settle into a supervisory role, adopting different leadership styles to address the strengths and challenges of each member of the team. Some will require focus on task management or task completion, while others will require relational support encouragement and a forum to express opinions and concerns. In the supervisory role, the team leader must listen and hear the team's concerns and ensure that the team is well rested and coping with the unfamiliar conditions of a very high failure or unavoidable mortality rate. When behaviors regress, and they inevitably will in these highly stressful conditions, it is essential that the team leader reverts and provides the appropriate task and emotional support to build back autonomy. The team will outperform expectation when they believe the leader has their best interests at heart and mind.

Overwork, Long Hours, Intense Situations

As the crisis persists, it is important to redistribute work and allow for a rotating-day or half-day away from the bedside. An option would also be to mix things up and have a junior member of the team conduct the rounds. Paying attention to where their focus is concentrated provides an opportunity for informal evaluation of the team leaders leadership success.

Support for Difficult Decision-Making

During a crisis, frontline teams as well as leaders and senior management are frequently confronted with difficult situations requiring rapid and difficult decision-making. Prevalent in such situations is "gray" decision-making, the outcome of which often has substantial consequences on patients' outcomes, morbidity, mortality, access to resources, taking risks, and others. Examples of these situations include triaging critically ill patients to overcrowded intensive care or intermediate care units, assigning limited resources to overwhelming numbers of patients, and making end-of-life decisions. In order to support frontline workers with difficult decision-making, there should be clear policies and rules, transparency, empowerment, availability of ethics and triage committees, palliative care, and rapid-cycle performance improvement cycles.

Emotional and Psychological Support

There is nothing harder in medicine than losing a patient. Although many coping mechanisms exist and some people are more skilled at employing them, no one was prepared for the overwhelming impact that COVID-19 would bring, including the devastating mortality rate. It is essential to take a moment at some routine time during the day or week to acknowledge that sometimes, despite our best and most complete efforts, we are going to lose patients. It is equally important to find some small success of each member of the team and celebrate at regular intervals (see Box 5.7).

Material Support

During a health crisis, healthcare workers need material support, not only in materials that support patient care but also in materials to support themselves. Basic items of support, however small, can go a long way in boosting morale and supporting teams. Such items may include free meals, all-day refreshments, short nap arrangements, quiet stations, laundry services, facilitation of transportation and parking, among others.

Daily Rounds

Daily rounds provide a perfect forum for the team leader to provide direction, manage tasks, distribute/redistribute, identify issues, and evaluate performance readiness which will foster growth, mutual trust, and respect. Conducted 2–3 times a day, the continuity of rounds not only provides the team with a formal expectation and forum to express concerns, but it also allows the less formal opportunity for the team leader to listen, understand, and assess the psychological and emotional health of the team. Particular attention should be focused on the team moral, and sources of frustration, and plans should be made and escalated to ensure rapid resolution of

---

Box 5.7. List of Emotional Support Resources
- Team leader counseling
- Colleague huddles
- Psychologist
- Psychiatrist
- Religious and spiritual services
- Virtual counseling

frustration and process impediments wherever possible. The team leader, or whomever is conducting the rounds, should keep an account of issues, both material and emotional, that are raised and a checklist for when each issue is addressed. The "punch list" format is not intended to be a list of gripes, rather a visible accounting of issue resolution. Starting rounds an hour late gives the team a bit of extra down time. Something as simple as decreasing the stress of the morning commute goes a long way. The work will get done and, in the crisis, no one is going home early so the extra hour in the morning can be a big bonus.

When more complex issues are afoot, it is important to acknowledge not only these issues but also the necessary complexity of a solution, so that appropriate expectations for resolution can be set. When a crisis such as COVID-19 persists, it is crucial to allow the human side of things to be present as well. Fatigue and burnout are real entities: recognize them, acknowledge them, and treat them aggressively. A crisis environment is the natural high-pressure setting for burnout and among the first symptoms to present itself is fatigue. At the same time, addressing human and emotional stress requires approachability. It is essential to be approachable so that your team feels comfortable bringing issues to your attention. Group discussion identifying stress, fatigue, and burnout may help us recognize these issues in ourselves and our colleagues. Bring councilors to the unit for a group discussion. Your team is your responsibility, and they cannot provide top level care if they are suffering.

The team will outperform expectation when they believe the leader has their best interests at heart and mind. Rounds are a great place for feedback and encouragement. This is where every small should be acknowledged and celebrated frequently.

Utilization of Critical Care Resources During an Overwhelming Health Crisis

Keeping track of all human resources (including support staff) is essential during a crisis. In case of a failure to arrive promptly at work, support teams should be triggered to ensure that the staff member is healthy and well. Back up staff should be sought, and staffing rotations should allow for people to be adequately rested.

Material resources should be made easily available at the local care unit. Materials should be maintained in a neat and orderly fashion and positioned so that everyone is aware when supplies are running low, and the appropriate requisitions for restocking can be completed.

Resource allocation and rationing should be the direct responsibility of the team leader. Daily rounds are a good time to take inventory of the necessary equipment and supply including essential PPE. No one should be allowed on the unit without the necessary protective gear. As supplies are depleted, this information should be escalated directly to supply chain management as well as the critical care committee. In a crisis, it is important to anticipate that material supply will run short, and frequent restocking is essential. Communication between unit leadership can ensure appropriate sharing and utilization of material. Unit security is important, and although supplies cannot be diverted, sharing among units is possible and may become necessary.

Managing the Flow of Critical Care Information, New Knowledge, and Clinical Practice Guidelines During a Crisis

As mentioned earlier, the tiered approach to critical care allows the local team leaders frequent opportunities to discuss clinical interventions that work, do not work, and in need of modification. This is a short loop that allows rapid cycle adjustment and dissemination of clinically relevant information. With good inter-unit communication, clinical pearls discovered in one unit can be implemented in real time throughout the institution.

Local information sharing between units is essential for system-wide success. However, equally as important and distinctly different from locally derived and discovered pearls is the management of the vast amount of information that floods the web pages of specialty societies and the popular press outside the critical care units. It is essential that newly emerging critical specialty information reaches providers rapidly and accurately. This includes practice guideline modifications, new standards, and precautions among many other forms of guidance. It is vital that emerging information be screened and accepted on an institutional level before it is implemented. Once accepted, modifications to current practice and new practice guidelines can be posted on an institutional electronic bulletin board in real time.

The amount of information that becomes available in the community during a crisis may be overwhelming and may vary in accuracy, integrity, and validity. Medical students and nonclinical and non-essential staff working from home can function as a resource to gather, collate, and present new information as it becomes available. Often information of a technical nature requires discrete levels of interpretation before it can be implemented. The critical care committee can also function as a vetting forum to identify which information is credible and in need of implementation.

To maintain the accuracy and validity of the information arriving at the clinical provider level, all new information should be presented, interpreted, and agreed upon by the institution, prior to implementation. When information is equivocal or further vetting is required, the institution can assign a subject matter expert such as the critical care committee or one of the critical care team leaders to attend a conference, read a report, or participate in a forum and then report back, so that the institution can decide whether to implement the new information or not. Once accepted by the institution, information can then be disseminated through the tiers at regular intervals until it ultimately reaches the clinical interface. When this happens on a regular and predictable basis, the teams will anticipate new, accurate, and validated updates and be eager to implement the latest advances and guidelines.

Continuation of Emergent and Urgent Services

While a hospital system prepares and plans for a health crisis, emergencies unrelated to the current health crisis will continue. A good example of this is the continuation of trauma admissions at our SBH Health System even during the peak of COVID-19 pandemic surge in April 2020. In fact, trauma admissions even increased after the peak of the pandemic (see Fig. 5.4).

Stopping elective surgery and deferring it until after the health crisis are relatively straight forward. However, assuring continuation of care for emergent and urgent cases during a crisis can be very difficult. This requires careful planning and attentive management of all resources, physical space, healthcare workers, equipment, supplies, etc. Not only are effective diagnosis and treatment needed, but safety is also of utmost importance in order to avoid contagious infection from spreading to the patients coming for trauma, acute surgery, myocardial infarction, stroke, and any other emergent and urgent illnesses.

Neurocritical Care During a Health Crisis

Ralph Rahme, Sahar Sorek and Aaron Miller

With the overwhelming crisis of the COVID-19 pandemic, significant disruptions in the care of non-COVID-19 patients were inevitable. Particularly significant is the impact of the pandemic on the care of neurosurgical patients. Neurosurgery is a high-acuity surgical discipline that commonly deals with life-threatening and permanently disabling conditions, and the COVID-19 pandemic posed a significant challenge to the care of neurosurgical patients.

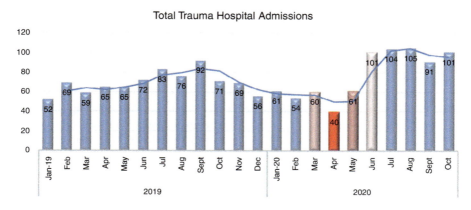

Fig. 5.4 Continuation of trauma admissions at the trauma center of SBH Health System during the surge of the COVID-19 pandemic in March, April, May 2020

Given its location in the South Bronx New York City, an underserved community with limited resources and one that has been disproportionately hard-hit by COVID-19, SBH Health System stood at the forefront of the challenges caused by the pandemic. Our neurosurgery division, a very active clinical service which is heavily geared toward high-acuity neurotrauma and stroke care, suddenly had to face and manage a whole new reality; one of confusion and chaos through which the care of neurosurgical patients could potentially slip through the cracks. In this section, the difficulties encountered and lessons learned during this pandemic are summarized.

Stroke Care

The relationship between COVID-19 and stroke has been the subject of extensive debate [5–8]. Although definite causality between the SARS-CoV-2 virus and stroke has not been well established, it is generally accepted that a subset of critically ill patients with COVID-19 may develop ischemic or hemorrhagic strokes during the course of their illness [5]. Notwithstanding this association, the impact of the pandemic on stroke care in general, affecting both patients with COVID-19 and those without, represented the biggest challenge for stroke patients and their healthcare providers during this crisis.

In fact, during the pandemic, a substantial reduction in hospitalizations for acute cardiovascular conditions, including acute coronary syndrome, ischemic stroke, and heart failure, has been observed worldwide [9–11]. Furthermore, global reductions in the rates of IV thrombolysis and interfacility stroke transfers were recently uncovered [11]. In the United States, delays in IV thrombolysis were reported, as was a 39% nationwide reduction in neuroimaging for acute stroke, a surrogate measure of endovascular thrombectomy for large-vessel occlusion [12, 13]. Likewise, a 38% nationwide drop in ST-elevation myocardial infarction catheterization lab activations was documented during the same period [10]. Very similar trends in stroke care were reported across France [14]. Our center has had a similar experience, including a 25–30% reduction in stroke case volume during the first few months of the pandemic (March–June 2020).

It is likely that a combination of patient-related and healthcare system-related factors accounted for those observations. Given the novelty, contagiousness, and severity of the disease, anxiety and widespread fear among the public have understandably dominated the first few months of the pandemic. The widespread fear of contracting COVID-19 was likely a catalyst for the delayed hospital presentation of stroke patients and self-selection of those with the most severe symptoms, a well-documented finding [9]. On the healthcare system side, a net redirection of resources from non-COVID-19 conditions including stroke, toward COVID-19, might have further contributed to stroke care disruption [11]. For instance, a rapid decline in stroke code activations, delays in obtaining brain imaging, and increased rates of stroke misdiagnosis were recently documented in a comprehensive stroke center [15].

In addition to resource redirection, other less quantifiable factors might have also contributed to the reduced quality of stroke care during the pandemic. One such example is the "tunnel vision of a pandemic." In the midst of the chaos generated by the pandemic, the constant pressure exerted by the surge of critically ill patients, and the inevitable state of physical and psychological burnout, a COVID-19-centered bias was likely to permeate the minds of healthcare professionals during these challenging times. As a result, non-COVID-19 diagnoses could be easily missed, potentially leading to suboptimal patient care and poor outcome. Sharp reductions in advanced stroke workup, including brain and cerebrovascular imaging, transthoracic and transesophageal echocardiography, and Holter monitoring, were observed during the pandemic.

Neurotrauma

During the COVID-19 pandemic, a significant reduction in neurotrauma case volume, ranging from 17% to 62%, has been recorded worldwide [16–20]. In one study, an 84% decrease in operative neurotrauma activity ensued [19]. Our trauma center had a very similar experience where a sharp reduction in neurotrauma activity and operative cases occurred during the 2 months of COVID-19 surge in NYC (March-April 2020), followed by a rapid rebound to normal pre-pandemic activity levels.

The nature of neurotrauma cases presenting to hospitals also changed significantly during the pandemic. In fact, mechanisms of traumatic injury were heavily impacted by the ubiquitous mandatory lockdowns and widespread public fear, both of which resulted in very limited social activity and road traffic. Moreover, home confinement and the accompanying high rates of unemployment and financial hardships brought about by the pandemic constituted a formidable psychological stressor for the population on a large scale. As a result, an increase in the rate of assaults, including gunshot wounds and abusive pediatric neurotrauma, was documented by several authors [17–19, 21–24]. In contrast, the impact of the pandemic on motor vehicle accidents was inconsistent, with some groups reporting an increase, possibly related to speeding on empty roads [16, 18, 19], while others reporting a decrease [17]. Falls, however, remained the most common mechanism of injury during the pandemic, with some reporting an increase in falls from a height, possibly due to the continued operation of construction businesses [19].

Similar to stroke, delays in hospital presentation have been observed in certain neurotrauma patient populations. For instance, statistically significant delays of up to 48 h have been documented in-patients with spinal cord injury during the pandemic, even after adjusting for injury severity. Likewise, elderly patients with chronic subdural hematomas tended to present less often and with worse symptoms, ultimately resulting in less favorable functional outcomes [16, 25].

Non-emergency Neurosurgery

In addition to its impact on neurosurgical emergencies such as stroke and neurotrauma, the COVID-19 pandemic took a tremendous toll on neurosurgical practices worldwide, most of whom had to cancel elective surgeries to help accommodate the growing public health needs [26]. This impact extended as well to non-emergency, yet urgent neurosurgical procedures, ultimately resulting in dramatic reductions in operative case volumes of previously busy neurosurgical services, reaching 60–70% in some cases [27, 28]. In line with those reports, neurosurgical case volume at SBH Health System dropped by about 70% during the NYC COVID-19 surge in March-April 2020.

Moreover, several challenges had to be overcome by neurosurgical services during the pandemic. First, the availability of operating room personnel was limited since many of those human resources had to be redirected to COVID-19 units across the hospital. Second, the surge of critically ill COVID-19 patients resulted in limited availability of intensive care unit beds and mechanical ventilators for postoperative neurosurgical care. Third, the risk of perioperative exposure to COVID-19 for neurosurgical patients without COVID-19 had to be incorporated in the surgical informed consent process, given its potential impact on the benefit-risk ratio of the procedure. For this reason, only true neurosurgical emergencies and time-sensitive urgent procedures (e.g., neuro-oncology) could be justifiable during the pandemic surge.

Neurosurgical Education

The pandemic constituted both a setback and an opportunity for neurosurgical mentors and trainees. Evidently, the training and hands-on experience of neurosurgical residents was negatively impacted by the transient but significant drop in case volume during the pandemic. In the United States, adjunct resident rotations (e.g., neuropathology, neuroradiology) were also postponed indefinitely. Notwithstanding, the availability of extra free time for neurosurgery residents and attendings provided a unique opportunity for increased participation in academic and scholarly activities, including conferences, mock board exams, and research. Moreover, social distancing guidelines led to the leveraging of previously available, yet not fully exploited communication technologies. Specifically, online communication platforms were used to maximize conference attendance and enhance education. In fact, the entire world of neurosurgery started connecting in unprecedented ways during the pandemic. Large organizations such as the Congress of Neurological Surgeons started offering virtual webinars, allowing the online dissemination of scientific information, ultimately improving communication and collaboration among neurosurgeons worldwide. Similarly, the potential power of telemedicine was fully unleashed during the pandemic, marrying the need for continued neurosurgical patient care with that of social distancing. The widespread use of online communication platforms and the continued development and refinement of telemedicine will likely be part of those added resources in the foreseeable future.

Lessons Learned

This pandemic may have granted neurosurgeons 7 pearls of wisdom for facing a public health crisis, summarized below:

1. *Recognize sober-mindedly the unique reality created by a public health crisis.* Recognize the looming chaos, resource shortage, exposure risks, public fear, healthcare provider burnout, and the disrupted nature of neurosurgical practice itself. In such instances, chance truly favors the prepared mind, preferably one that is open, flexible, and willing to learn and adapt.
2. *If you feel that you and your patients are on your own, then this is likely to be true.* A prepared neurosurgeon understands that whenever a non-neurosurgical public health crisis strikes, the care of neurosurgical patients may suffer. The limited resources, patient and healthcare system-related delays in care, tunnel vision of pandemic, and other factors beyond one's direct control are likely to prevail, potentially affecting the care of your patients. Being cognizant of this fact is key to protecting the interests of your patients and preserving their well-being.
3. *The efforts you used to invest in direct patient care may not be sufficient anymore. Double or triple your efforts, then double check and triple check them.* Missed diagnoses and delayed treatments are common features of public health crises. The onus is on you to fill the vacuum and protect your patients from easily slipping through the cracks. Luckily, given the slowing of your neurosurgical practice, you now have some extra free time to stay on top of things.
4. *Leverage your skills and help your struggling colleagues. You are a neurocritical care expert, after all.* Neurocritical care is a key component of neurosurgical training, particularly in North America, where residents in training are expected to demonstrate competency in the management of critically ill neurosurgical patients. Moreover, neurosurgeons in practice, especially those in stroke and trauma centers, often co-manage critically ill neurosurgical patients on a daily basis, alongside their colleague intensivists. Thus, among surgical specialists, neurosurgeons are uniquely positioned to help support their critical care colleagues in managing the growing demand of critically ill patients during a public health crisis. In fact, as the number of COVID-19 patients grew during the surge phase of the pandemic, overwhelming preexistent critical care services, many institutions redeployed their neurosurgeons to help manage the crisis [28, 29]. At SBH Health System, neurosurgeons and other surgical specialists underwent cross-training in critical care and were granted temporary privileges, allowing them to staff COVID-19 intensive care units during the pandemic surge.
5. *Remember that public health crises are generally limited in time. Stay ahead of the curve and prepare for the next phase: reopening and recovery.* While disruption can easily happen overnight, recovery is usually a much more deliberate, time-consuming, resource-intensive, and somewhat complex process, requiring careful planning, self-discipline, and a strong sense of organization. In order to stay ahead of the game, it is generally advisable to stay in touch regularly with your patients and keep your outpatient clinics running.
6. *Invest in your own education, grow your skills, catch up on your outstanding academic and scholarly work.* Invest in yourself and use technology to your advantage. This could include conferences and webinars, student and resident teaching, research projects and scientific papers; the sky is the limit.

7. *Most importantly, spend time with your family and those you love.* For once, you are temporarily relieved from the hustle of your busy and hectic daily schedule. Make the absolute best of this extra time bestowed upon you. Spend time with your family and reconnect with your spouse, kids, and those you love. Those are uniquely precious times in life. Also, use that time to care for yourself, catch your breath, and reflect. This will help you regain your much-needed physical stamina and psychological resilience. You will need that extra strength to help you manage the inevitable rebound in clinical activity after the crisis has passed.

Box 5.8. International Clinical Vignette: A Global Perspective on Health Crisis and Critical Care

Overall preparedness to crises has significant variations among countries and regions of the world. From the critical care point of view, middle- and low-income countries suffer from small numbers of ICU beds, consequently making them resource-limited and unable to deal with mass critical care (MCC). Figure 5.5, reported by Xiya Ma et al. [30], demonstrates the global availability of ICU beds.

Crisis standards of care (CSC) were developed by the US Institute of Medicine for the purpose of emergency crisis to ensure the best health care provided during disaster, recommended legal protection for healthcare workers, and recommended alternate models of care [31]. Crisis standards of care is defined as "a substantial change in usual healthcare operations and the level of care it is possible to deliver, which is made necessary by a pervasive (e.g., pandemic influenza) or catastrophic (e.g., earthquake, hurricane) disaster." CSC standards of care range from "conventional" to "contingency" to "crisis," in which risk of mortality and resource imbalance increases ascendingly. Conventional care is the usual care. Contingency is functionally equivalent to standards of conventional care, though with possible cancelation of elective surgery, utilization of all available critical care facilities (such as post-anesthesia care unit), and substitution of supplies. Crisis care is the inability to meet the usual standards and the existence of insufficient resources. CSC standards are mainly concerned with the 4 S's: Space, Supply, Staff, and System [30, 32]. The European Society of Intensive Care Medicine developed standard operating procedure (SOPs) as a recommendation for critical care management during disasters [33]. The American College of Chest Physicians (CHEST) task force published MCC recommendations known as CHEST consensus [34]. All such recommendations and guidelines are probably or at least partially outdated and in need for review and an update from lessons learned in reflections from the currently ongoing COVID-19 pandemic.

Mustafa Alwani, MD
Research Scholar, Men's Health,
Hamad Medical Corporation, Doha, Qatar

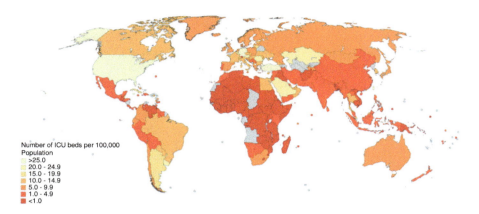

Fig. 5.5 The global availability of ICU beds per 100,000 population ranging from 0 to 21.3 per 100,000 in middle- and low-income countries, and from 0 to 59.5 per 100,000 in high-income countries. (Reprinted from Ma and Vervoort [30], with permission from Elsevier)

Case Study 1: Critical Care During a Health Crisis (SBH Health System in March, April, and May 2020)

Contingency Planning and Management

In order to quench ICU overflow, SBH Health System initially listed post-anesthesia care unit (PACU) and cardiac cath lab recovery as potential backup areas since they had all the necessary equipment and monitoring capabilities. The problems with these areas were the potential loss of services (operating rooms and interventional cardiology) and lack of infection control (isolation). Due to these limiting factors and the rapid need for ICU beds during the COVID-19 pandemic, the hospital ended up expanding the ICU by allocating all beds in the ambulatory surgery and post-endoscopy recovery room. These units had the necessary monitors and ventilator capabilities, but they were open units meaning that only COVID-19 patients could be placed and cohabitated and the staff had to be optimally protected with PPE at all times.

PPE guidelines may fluctuate during a new infectious outbreak until the science is clarified. PPE availability rapidly became limited at the beginning of the COVID-19 pandemic. The supply chain efforts to maintain adequate PPE supplies were enhanced by timely donations from a variety of groups and individuals. Although staff with direct COVID-19 patient contact had PPE priority, it was of paramount importance that all staff members have access to, and utilize, appropriate PPE for protection while working.

When planning for ICU expansion, the Critical Care Committee was represented by a diverse range of departments: nursing, medicine, surgery, anesthesia, respiratory, nephrology, engineering, supply chain, IT, infection control, and administration. Other departments were also brought into planning as needed. Having the stakeholders involved early saved time and allowed for rapid escalation of issues. One advantage that SBH Health System has, as a well-managed small hospital, is the capability for rapid dynamic decision-making and implementation to obtain effective operational goals in a timely manner. Some larger institutions may have administrative layers requiring more meeting time prior to actionable change.

Flexible and reliable staffing capabilities were a key component for maintaining safe delivery of ICU care. Plans for adequate staffing included nursing/intensivists/respiratory therapists and ancillary support staff. The importance of housekeeping and environmental services cannot be overemphasized enough. Delays in cleaning rooms and inadequate disinfection would slow patient flow and, if suboptimal, might cause infection control issues.

In the midst of the COVID-19 pandemic, multiple hospitals and care facilities were overburdened and the availability of critical care nursing sometimes led to lower nurse to patient ratios in the ICU at the peak surge times at SBH Health System and many other hospitals. While in crisis mode, this shortage was supplemented with other staff including cross-trained physicians, residents, dentists, physician assistants, nurse practitioners, therapists, and others, in order to assure proper attendance to critical care needs. The nursing and respiratory therapist shortages were difficult to fill on short notice when all per-diem and agency nurses were in high demand. Recruiting became difficult because of escalating financial offers from all staffing suppliers. Small safety net hospitals such as SBH Health System could not compete with larger endowed institutions for needed staff and this led to ongoing obstacles in staffing and in the delivery of ICU care. Overworked staff sometimes also succumbed to the stress of overwork and called in sick, exacerbating the problem.

Governmentally supported and coordinated staffing is crucial in a pandemic situation in order to maintain the delivery of ICU care for a given population. Load balancing between hospitals may attenuate the demand at any one facility. The load-balancing government mandates for hospital networks should be available for small independent hospitals as well to even the imbalance of critically ill patients and optimize safe care for a given population.

Effective bed utilization and patient flow is a continuous imperative when ICU beds are limited. Triage should be done by an intensivist with real-time knowledge of individual patient status and needs as well as total ICU bed status and patient flow. At SBH Health System, triage was done by an intensivist with ICU nurse managers, bed board personnel, and other physicians in order to effectively communicate and move patients. This position was known as a *quarterback/point person* (or pit boss) position and was found to be invaluable for multidisciplinary communication of information that requires action in a timely manner. With multiple moving parts, only people in this position could effectively triage patient flow to and from multiple ICUs.

Patient Scoring Systems

These may assist in triaging personnel with objective information predicting mortality for ICU patients. Sequential organ failure assessment (SOFA) is one of the common validated tools that can be used and trended (see Table 5.3).

Coordination of ICU care among subspecialty services had to be done in a timely manner to avoid unnecessary ICU bed utilization. Consultation done promptly allowed for downgrades to non-ICU beds resulting in an increase in ICU bed availability. Telemedicine capabilities also helped to avoid unnecessary decision-making delays (see Table 5.4).

Networking and Information Sharing

Networking and information sharing may facilitate rapid distribution of new information regarding disease understanding, treatment, and problem-solving. Resources include the internet, colleagues, societies such as the Society of Critical Care Medicine (www.SCCM.org) and relevant journal studies, among others. Improvisation and "out of the box" thinking may be needed for urgent

Table 5.3 SOFA score

Organ system	SOFA score				
Measurement	1	2	3	4	5
Respiration PaO_2/FiO_2, mmHg	Normal	<400	<300	<200 (with respiratory support)	<100 (with respiratory support)
Coagulation Platelets x1000/mm^3	Normal	<150	<100	<50	<20
Cardiovascular Hypotension	Normal	MAP<70 mmHg	Dopamine ≤5 or dobutamine any dose	Dopamine >5 or epinephrine ≤0.1 or norepinephrine ≤0.1	Dopamine >15 or epinephrine >0.1 or norepinephrine >0.1
Liver Bilirubin, mg/dL (micromole/L)	Normal	1.2–1.9 (20–32)	2.0–5.9 (33–101)	6.0–11.9 102–204	>12 (>204)
Central nervous system Glasgow Coma Score	Normal	13–14	10–12	6–9	<6
Renal Creatinine mg/dL (micromole/L or urine output)	Normal	1.2–1.9 (110–170)	2.0–3.4 171–299)	3.5–4.9 (300–440) or < 500 mL/day	>5.0 (>440) or < 200 mL/day

Table 5.4 Different specialties make various valuable contributions to critical care during a crisis

Specialty	Contribution to critical care during a crisis
Physicians of medical critical care, surgical critical care, anesthesia	Critical care in intensive care and intermediate care
Cross-trained non-critical care physicians	Critical care in intensive care and intermediate care with support by critical care specialists
Orthopedists	Proning and supining of patients with ARDS
Residents and fellows of various specialties	Critical care in intensive care and intermediate care under supervision by critical care specialists
Dentists, dental residents, podiatrists, podiatry residents	Supplemental staff as appropriate for competencies, skills, levels, and assignments under the supervision and support by critical care specialists
ICU-nurses, respiratory therapists	Critical care in intensive care and intermediate care
Nurses, nurse practitioners, physician assistants, medical assistants	Supplemental staff as appropriate for competencies, skills, levels, and assignments under the supervision and support by critical care specialists
Nutritionists, pharmacists	Provision of nutritional support and medications
Information technology and bio-engineering	Systems support and rapid engineering solutions for increased critical care demands and expansion of the ICU to new areas in the hospital
Supply chain	Assurance of equipment and supplies for the rapid expansion of critical care
Medical students	Virtual rounding in the ICU and communicating with patients' families on behalf of the teams

problem-solving. An example of where an urgent solution was needed during the COVID-19 surge was where IV pump tubing extensions ended up being used outside the room/room access portals for ventilator tubing and control panel cables. These techniques were rapidly adopted by multiple ICUs and allowed for decreased PPE usage and limited staff exposure to COVID-19 patients. Ventilator sharing/splitting techniques were rapidly disseminated by many and incorporated into treatment plans to conserve limited ventilator resources.

Overflow Planning (In the Hospital and Out)

In preparing for a health crisis in a hospital, it is important to set a plan for the case of overwhelming overflow of critically ill patients. Such plan should include patient workflow inside the hospital (expansion of ICU areas, ethics committee and ventilator triage, ventilator sharing, palliative care and management of hopeless cases), and strategies for management outside the hospital (pre-hospital triage, diversion, transfer).

Case Study 2: The COVID-19 Pandemic and Critical Care at SBH Health System

Repurposing Resources

Closing the elective surgery center – effectively the main engine of the hospital system – provided the perioperative leadership with an opportunity to reeducate and redeploy human resources to assist in frontline patient management. SBH increased its critical care capacity by over 500% in the initial days and weeks of COVID-19 (see Fig. 5.6 showing the rapid increase in the number of critically ill patients on mechanical ventilation during the COVID-19 health crisis in 2020 at SBH). The hospital acquired ventilators at a rapid pace to keep up with the accelerating surge of the COVID-19 pandemic. Prior to the pandemic, the number of available ventilators was always higher than the number of patients needing ventilation. However, during the pandemic surge, the number of admitted patients with respiratory distress twice came close to surpassing the number of available ventilators.

In addition to doubling the bed capacity in the ICU and expanding services in the step-down areas, critical care services would be provided in converted recovery rooms and ambulatory admissions suits. To accomplish this, the tiered team approach was adopted.

As described, the leaders of medical, surgical, and anesthesia intensive care units came together to create single critical care service. Governance of the service came from a newly created critical care committee that would meet frequently and function not only as a guidance committee, coordinating the multiple department interactions, but also as a sounding board and as the central repository for all clinical and administrative discussion and direction for the critical care service.

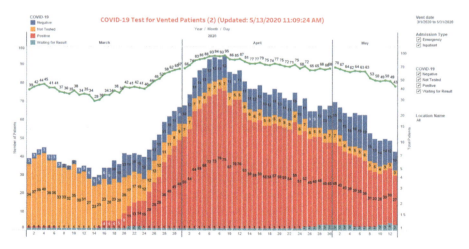

Fig. 5.6 Progression of COVID-19 and non-COVID-19 patients on mechanical ventilators during March, April, and May 2020 at SBH

The medical critical care team was the largest and most integrated with the other services in the hospital. The director of this team would function as the clinical "quarterback." As such, this director would maintain constant communication with each of the critical care locations and teams as well as with the ED. The quarterback would triage patients, manage the many dispositions, and assign beds as they opened in each unit. In addition, the quarterback would round several times a day to ensure that clinical needs were met in each of the locations.

Team leaders were not only direct care providers but would also build and support team morale, caring for the health and well-being of their teams, ensuring critical supplies were present, and providing effective guidance and direct support with dynamic decision-making in response to the ever-changing situations.

The second tier of providers would be the backbone of the teams and provide the daily care. Critical care refresher courses were conducted, giving the perioperative physicians the tools necessary to provide acute bedside critical care. This tier of providers was coached by the regular critical care teams as well as by the team leaders and were never truly alone. Each shift had identified providers, team leaders, and a quarterback.

Residents from all departments would be assigned and rotate through the units. The residents provided the largest physical group of providers with the most diversity of background and training. Rotating the residents through the units would add some variation within each unit but ultimately allowed for more uniformity between the units. This tiered approached allowed each unit to function both independently and interdependently with the other units and provided a fantastic forum for the integration of ideas and approaches to medical management from all the various backgrounds and specialties.

Expansion Units

The expansion of the ICU and step-down areas created a new and intense stress for the teams that normally cover a fraction of the patient volumes that these new areas would now be responsible for. In addition, the onslaught of patients into these expanded areas would all be incredibly sick. There were no historic treatment protocols and materials/supplies would rapidly become exhausted. While some of the critical care areas did have the benefit of staff and providers that were used to working in these locations, expansion brought new faces and new ideas. This was particularly true on the resident level, where neophytes were called upon for expertise within their respective fields. Under these conditions, team building was everyone's responsibility. The concept of exploiting the strengths and supporting the less strong was never more important and every team member had value, no matter background training or experience. Immediate gratification was achieved through early and frequent recognition and celebration of small wins.

Many of the critical care teams in the expanded units had worked together previously, and by comparison, the teams that would be called upon to provide critical care in the new areas were exactly that: NEW. Save for a few of the team leaders, these new teams largely lacked experience as individual critical care providers or as teams, yet they were asked to provide the highest level of care to the sickest of patients under incredibly stressful conditions. Relying on makeshift teams, with nursing support from various units throughout the institution, often with little or no critical care experience, as well as travelers or fill in services with variable degrees of experience, created an additional dimension of complexity (see Tables 5.5 and 5.6).

The notion that the new areas would care for less acute patients, or perhaps those with more easily treated conditions, was considered during the planning phase. This concept was however necessarily and rapidly abandoned as the volume of new and very sick patients needing the highest level of critical care rapidly outpaced bed availability in the expanded ICU and step-down areas.

Summary and Takeaway Messages from Critical Care

The COVID-19 epidemic revealed how susceptible and unprepared the healthcare system is in the face of a pandemic and how quickly overloading can happen when ICU bed and ventilator resources become overwhelmed (Box 5.8) [31]. Healthcare disaster planning has grown from its early place as an occasional consideration to become a rapidly evolving field [35]. As a fundamental pillar of the health crisis management system, reinforcing critical care capabilities and functionalities is

Table 5.5 Expansion of critical care areas: accounting of ICU areas and areas that could be converted into ICU for ventilated patients

Location	Current beds	Possible additions	Total potential	Comments
MICU	10	0	10	10 single rooms
SICU	6	6	12	6 rooms currently single; can be doubled
IMCU	22	0	22	22 rooms with telemetry; ventilators can be added
OR/PACU	7	0	7	Variable availability because of other emergencies
Chronic ventilation floor	14	14	28	Can be doubled
Cardiac cath lab	5	0	5	Variable availability because of other emergencies – open space
Endoscopy recovery room	5	0	5	Variable availability because of other emergencies – open space
Totals	69	20	89	

Table 5.6 Actual expansion of ICU areas for ventilated patients at the peak of the COVID-19 surge

Location	Current beds	Possible additions	ACTUAL	Comments
MICU			10	10 single rooms
SICU			11	6 double rooms
IMCU			22	11 double rooms
OR/PACU			0	Last resort
Chronic ventilation floor			11	Chronic non-COVID ventilated patients
Cardiac cath lab			0	
Endoscopy suite			5	Max capacity
ER			15	Open space with other patients
Amb surg			10	
Misc floor			9	COVID scatterd on several floors
Totals			93	

crucial, and the creation of an institution-wide unified critical care leadership, structure, and committee is paramount for the success of planning, preparation, and management of a crisis. Since the onset of the COVID-19 pandemic, predictive models have been developed to aid healthcare authorities in their planning of resources, personnel, ICU, and bed capacity. However, predictions can be challenging because known parameters of earlier epidemics are often not applicable [31]. Empowerment of the critical care leadership is absolutely necessary, especially during the surge of a crisis, to assure dynamic decision-making and effective responses to rapidly changing situations.

References

1. Beitler JR, Kallet R, Kacmarek R, Branson R, Brodie D, Mittel AM, et al. Ventilator sharing: dual-patient ventilation with a single mechanical ventilator for use during critical ventilator shortages. New York: Presbyterian Hospital; 2020. p. 20.
2. Neyman G, Irvin CB. A single ventilator for multiple simulated patients to meet disaster surge. Acad Emerg Med. 2006;13(11):1246–9. https://doi.org/10.1197/j.aem.2006.05.009.
3. Paladino L, Silverberg M, Charchaflieh JG, Eason JK, Wright BJ, Palamidessi N, et al. Increasing ventilator surge capacity in disasters: ventilation of four adult-human-sized sheep on a single ventilator with a modified circuit. Resuscitation. 2008;77(1):121–6. https://doi.org/10.1016/j.resuscitation.2007.10.016.

4. American Society of Anesthologists: COVID-19. http://www.ASAHQ.org/carona (2020). Accessed 1st Aug 2020.
5. Miller A, Segan S, Rehmani R, Shabsigh R, Rahme R. Letter: dismantling the apocalypse narrative: the myth of the COVID-19 stroke. Neurosurgery. 2020; https://doi.org/10.1093/neuros/nyaa419.
6. Oxley TJ, Mocco J, Majidi S, Kellner CP, Shoirah H, Singh IP, et al. Large-vessel stroke as a presenting feature of Covid-19 in the young. N Engl J Med. 2020;382(20):e60. https://doi.org/10.1056/NEJMc2009787.
7. Sweid A, Hammoud B, Weinberg JH, Oneissi M, Raz E, Shapiro M, et al. Letter: thrombotic neurovascular disease in COVID-19 patients. Neurosurgery. 2020;87(3):E400–E6. https://doi.org/10.1093/neuros/nyaa254.
8. Jabbour P, Sweid A, Tjoumakaris S, Brinjikji W, Bekelis K, Nimjee SM, et al. In reply: dismantling the apocalypse narrative: the myth of the COVID-19 stroke. Neurosurgery. 2021;88(3):E277–E80. https://doi.org/10.1093/neuros/nyaa522.
9. Seidu S, Kunutsor SK, Cos X, Khunti K. Indirect impact of the COVID-19 pandemic on hospitalisations for cardiometabolic conditions and their management: a systematic review. Prim Care Diabetes. 2021;15(4):653–81. https://doi.org/10.1016/j.pcd.2021.05.011.
10. Garcia S, Albaghdadi MS, Meraj PM, Schmidt C, Garberich R, Jaffer FA, et al. Reduction in ST-segment elevation cardiac catheterization laboratory activations in the United States during COVID-19 Pandemic. J Am Coll Cardiol. 2020;75(22):2871–2. https://doi.org/10.1016/j.jacc.2020.04.011.
11. Nogueira RG, Abdalkader M, Qureshi MM, Frankel MR, Mansour OY, Yamagami H, et al. Global impact of COVID-19 on stroke care. Int J Stroke. 2021;16(5):573–84. https://doi.org/10.1177/1747493021991652.
12. Kansagra AP, Goyal MS, Hamilton S, Albers GW. Collateral effect of Covid-19 on stroke evaluation in the United States. N Engl J Med. 2020;383(4):400–1. https://doi.org/10.1056/NEJMc2014816.
13. Siegler JE, Zha AM, Czap AL, Ortega-Gutierrez S, Farooqui M, Liebeskind DS, et al. Influence of the COVID-19 pandemic on treatment times for acute ischemic stroke: the Society of Vascular and Interventional Neurology Multicenter Collaboration. Stroke. 2021;52(1):40–7. https://doi.org/10.1161/STROKEAHA.120.032789.
14. Kerleroux B, Fabacher T, Bricout N, Moise M, Testud B, Vingadassalom S, et al. Mechanical thrombectomy for acute ischemic stroke amid the COVID-19 outbreak: decreased activity, and increased care delays. Stroke. 2020;51(7):2012–7. https://doi.org/10.1161/STROKEAHA.120.030373.
15. Velez FGS, Alvarado-Dyer R, Brutto VJD, Carrion-Penagos J, Bulwa Z, Prabhakaran S. Impact of Covid-19 on stroke code activations, process metrics, and diagnostic error. Neurohospitalist. 2021;11(3):197–203. https://doi.org/10.1177/1941874420976517.
16. Horan J, Duddy JC, Gilmartin B, Amoo M, Nolan D, Corr P, et al. The impact of COVID-19 on trauma referrals to a National Neurosurgical Centre. Ir J Med Sci. 2021; https://doi.org/10.1007/s11845-021-02504-7.
17. Algattas HN, McCarthy D, Kujawski B, Agarwal N, Brown J, Forsythe RM, et al. Impact of coronavirus disease 2019 shutdown on neurotrauma volume in Pennsylvania. World Neurosurg. 2021;151:e178–e84. https://doi.org/10.1016/j.wneu.2021.04.004.
18. Lara-Reyna J, Yaeger KA, Rossitto CP, Camara D, Wedderburn R, Ghatan S, et al. "Staying home"-early changes in patterns of neurotrauma in New York City during the COVID-19 pandemic. World Neurosurg. 2020;143:e344–e50. https://doi.org/10.1016/j.wneu.2020.07.155.
19. Figueroa JM, Boddu J, Kader M, Berry K, Kumar V, Ayala V, et al. The effects of lockdown during the severe acute respiratory syndrome coronavirus 2 (SARS-CoV-2) pandemic on neurotrauma-related hospital admissions. World Neurosurg. 2021;146:e1–5. https://doi.org/10.1016/j.wneu.2020.08.083.
20. Zhang M, Zhou J, Dirlikov B, Cage T, Lee M, Singh H. Impact on neurosurgical management in Level 1 trauma centers during COVID-19 shelter-in-place restrictions: the Santa Clara County experience. J Clin Neurosci. 2021;88:128–34. https://doi.org/10.1016/j.jocn.2021.03.017.

21. Sidpra J, Abomeli D, Hameed B, Baker J, Mankad K. Rise in the incidence of abusive head trauma during the COVID-19 pandemic. Arch Dis Child. 2021;106(3):e14. https://doi.org/10.1136/archdischild-2020-319872.
22. Sinha S, Toe KKZ, Wood E, George KJ. The impact of COVID-19 on neurosurgical head trauma referrals and admission at a tertiary neurosurgical centre. J Clin Neurosci. 2021;87:50–4. https://doi.org/10.1016/j.jocn.2021.02.021.
23. Andalib A, Sanders MI, Sinha S. Traumatic paediatric neurosurgical emergencies during the COVID-19 pandemic: experience in a single regional paediatric major trauma centre. Childs Nerv Syst. 2021;37(1):5–6. https://doi.org/10.1007/s00381-020-04902-1.
24. Dyson EW, Craven CL, Tisdall MM, James GA. The impact of social distancing on pediatric neurosurgical emergency referrals during the COVID-19 pandemic: a prospective observational cohort study. Childs Nerv Syst. 2020;36(9):1821–3. https://doi.org/10.1007/s00381-020-04783-4.
25. Hecht N, Wessels L, Werft FO, Schneider UC, Czabanka M, Vajkoczy P. Need for ensuring care for neuro-emergencies-lessons learned from the COVID-19 pandemic. Acta Neurochir. 2020;162(8):1795–801. https://doi.org/10.1007/s00701-020-04437-z.
26. Hanrahan JG, Burford C, Adegboyega G, Nicolaides M, Boyce L, Wong K, et al. Early responses of neurosurgical practice to the coronavirus disease 2019 (COVID-19) pandemic: a rapid review. World Neurosurg. 2020;141:e1017–e26. https://doi.org/10.1016/j.wneu.2020.06.167.
27. Deora H, Dange P, Patel K, Shashidhar A, Tyagi G, Pruthi N, et al. Management of neurosurgical cases in a tertiary care referral hospital during the COVID-19 pandemic: lessons from a middle-income country. World Neurosurg. 2021;148:e197–208. https://doi.org/10.1016/j.wneu.2020.12.111.
28. Khalafallah AM, Jimenez AE, Lee RP, Weingart JD, Theodore N, Cohen AR, et al. Impact of COVID-19 on an academic neurosurgery department: the Johns Hopkins experience. World Neurosurg. 2020;139:e877–e84. https://doi.org/10.1016/j.wneu.2020.05.167.
29. Caridi JM, Reynolds AS, Gilligan J, Bederson J, Dangayach NS. Letter: news from the COVID-19 front lines: how neurosurgeons are contributing. Neurosurgery. 2020;87(2):E248. https://doi.org/10.1093/neuros/nyaa205.
30. Ma X, Vervoort D. Critical care capacity during the COVID-19 pandemic: global availability of intensive care beds. J Crit Care. 2020;58:96–7. https://doi.org/10.1016/j.jcrc.2020.04.012.
31. Aziz S, Arabi YM, Alhazzani W, Evans L, Citerio G, Fischkoff K, et al. Managing ICU surge during the COVID-19 crisis: rapid guidelines. Intensive Care Med. 2020;46(7):1303–25. https://doi.org/10.1007/s00134-020-06092-5.
32. Crisis standards of care: summary of a workshop series. The national academies collection: reports funded by National Institutes of Health. Washington (DC); 2010.
33. Sprung CL, Zimmerman JL, Christian MD, Joynt GM, Hick JL, Taylor B, et al. Recommendations for intensive care unit and hospital preparations for an influenza epidemic or mass disaster: summary report of the European Society of Intensive Care Medicine's Task Force for intensive care unit triage during an influenza epidemic or mass disaster. Intensive Care Med. 2010;36(3):428–43. https://doi.org/10.1007/s00134-010-1759-y.
34. Christian MD, Devereaux AV, Dichter JR, Rubinson L, Kissoon N. Task Force for Mass Critical C, et al. Introduction and executive summary: care of the critically ill and injured during pandemics and disasters: CHEST consensus statement. Chest. 2014;146(4 Suppl):8S–34S. https://doi.org/10.1378/chest.14-0732.
35. Daugherty EL, Rubinson L. Preparing your intensive care unit to respond in crisis: considerations for critical care clinicians. Crit Care Med. 2011;39(11):2534–9. https://doi.org/10.1097/CCM.0b013e3182326440.

Chapter 6
Emergency Medicine

Daniel G. Murphy, Jeffrey D. Lazar, and Brian J. Dolan

The Emergence of a Global Crisis

On January 13, 2020, a routine department email update was sent out to the physician staff in the Department of Emergency Medicine at SBH Health System (consisting of approximately 30 attending physicians and 60 residents). The email was sent by the hospital's Director of Infectious Disease Division, Dr. Judith Berger; she wanted all Emergency Department (ED) staff to be aware of a newly identified respiratory virus in Wuhan, China. Given the daily battles fought against diseases and trauma endemic to the local community, it was difficult to fully internalize and appreciate her alert. So, when this message was sent to the staff, it was with a figurative 'roll of the eyes' and not very subtle facetiousness, that it acknowledged the existence of a virus halfway across the world and mentioned that we should be on the lookout for any patients who might have recently been shopping at the Huanan Seafood Wholesale Market. (Note: The local patient populations do not include many travellers to or from China.)

It was unlikely that such a brief email would have been remembered at all, except that at the height of the pandemic, when the ED was filled to capacity with air hungry and critically ill patients, two of our doctors were suddenly curious as to when COVID-19 was first mentioned in a departmental email. As one might expect, there were very many emails during the early days of the pandemic which corresponded with the spread of the disease around the globe. Alerts went out when COVID-19

D. G. Murphy (✉) · J. D. Lazar
Department of Emergency Medicine, SBH Health System, Bronx, NY, USA

CUNY School of Medicine, New York, NY, USA
e-mail: dmurphy@sbhny.org

B. J. Dolan
Department of Emergency Medicine and Department of Nursing, SBH Health System, Bronx, NY, USA

© The Author(s), under exclusive license to Springer Nature
Switzerland AG 2022
R. Shabsigh (ed.), *Health Crisis Management in Acute Care Hospitals*,
https://doi.org/10.1007/978-3-030-95806-0_6

was first identified in the Bronx County, New York State, and New York City. There were elaborate drills to prepare for the management of the first patient and the subsequent waves of texts and emails that went out when it was thought that there might be just a single positive patient. It is with a mixture of wonder and sadness that how truly unprepared New York hospitals were for what was ultimately experienced: thousands of patients and staff to care for during the pandemic.

On many levels, it is believed that the response of the SBH Health System, and particularly the Emergency Medicine Department, to the pandemic was remarkably successful: the department expanded its capacity, a patient was never turned away, and essential medical equipment and personal protective equipment (PPE) were always available. Spaces and staffing were flexed to meet the needs and demands as they evolved throughout the pandemic. Team members from all disciplines (respiratory, registration, environmental services, security, pastoral care just to name a few) came together to allow the department to function effectively and efficiently and to provide care throughout the surge that struck New York City, despite the hospital being an independent, resource-challenged safety net hospital in one of the city's hardest hit communities. This chapter chronicles the experience of the ED at SBH Health System during the COVID-19 pandemic surge in the Spring of 2020 with highlighted lessons learned.

Governance and Communication

The most important thing in communication is hearing what isn't said. Peter Drucker

As the hospital and ED staff closely followed the events unfold in Asia and Europe, preparation for the worst progressed, but the risk still remained abstract. Whilst the fear of what might be coming was on everyone's mind, what was actually experienced to that point was a steady stream of 'worried well' [1] and people who needed COVID-19 to be 'ruled out' in order to go back to work. They all looked and checked out just fine. But this was short-lived, and things changed over the weekend of March 14.

High acuity COVID-19 patients began to roll in by ambulances. Most had dyspnoea and abnormal vital signs, some had an altered mental status, and most had an unusually profound hypoxemia. Their chest imaging was consistent with 'ground-glass' patterns [2]. These sick patients tended to have similar risk profiles, including hypertension, renal disease, diabetes, and a high body mass index. Many were suffering thromboembolic complications. The emergency physicians were caught unawares; they discussed among themselves 'what does this bug do? How does it affect so many systems?'

As the first week progressed, staff concerns about a litany of issues arose. Sick calls were increasing, as were anxiety levels. ED leadership realized that an intervention was necessary to keep the team together. It was decided to implement the old-fashioned, tried-and-true, management technique of team huddles on a regular and reliable basis. At the end of every night shift (at 6:30 am) and the beginning of every day shift (at 7:30 am), the leadership team stood together at the back of the ED with all staff on duty in a group of 20–30. This was done every day for 31 consecutive days, and it was clearly the most important managerial intervention. All staff were invited, any job description. Early on, physicians stood in front, with the nurses, registrars, patient care technicians, radiology technicians, medical assistants, security, and environmental workers standing at the back.

The earliest meetings were emotional and stressful. The anxiety levels were high and understandably so, with some staff members having vulnerable adults or infants at home. Indeed, many were afraid to work. Each huddle would start with the same question posed by leadership to frontline staff: 'what had happened till now, and what do we need to fix today?' There was a myriad of responses, with some with broader implications, whilst others were very specific. By far, the most prominent and important issue of the staff at the beginning of the surge in cases was the availability and access to personal protective equipment (PPE) across all job descriptions. Although there had been a great deal of emergency management preparation in advance, there were some brief disruptions in the supply chain. This matter was addressed on a daily, if not hourly, basis, in those early days. But by the end of the first week, all staff were decked out in similar PPE. Success in addressing this issue efficiently built confidence in the staff, who felt that any issues raised by them at the huddles would be heard and acted upon.

In subsequent huddles, the contributions of 'alpha' physicians were soon drowned out by the technicians and environmental workers. Looks of anxiety or frustration were being replaced with confidence and determination. The huddle meetings that took place at the same time, every time, no matter the circumstance gave the staff a sense of reassurance. More and more of them attended with lists in hand. After the huddle each morning at about 8:30 am, ED leadership would take their notes and distribute a report with daily stats as well as complaints, issues, opportunities, and suggestions made during the meeting. In this manner, the entire hospital's management team, including the highest echelons of the hospital's leadership, were made aware of the specific concerns of the ED workforce. There was no filtering – except perhaps some added decorum. 'Straight talk' was encouraged at the huddles.

It is worth taking a moment to acknowledge what the staff were experiencing whilst on duty. The ED was taking care of more critically ill patients simultaneously than any one had ever experienced. An extraordinarily high ratio of patients required intubation, ventilation, central venous catheters, emergency dialysis, and vasoactive medications. Cardiopulmonary arrests were frequent and often simultaneous throughout the large unit. Visitors were not permitted, for their own sake and for the sake of the staff. Patients were dying in crowded rooms, without their loved ones. Ironically, during the darkest moments, morale was high. This was sad but important work; staff were saving lives and placing themselves at risk for others.

It is difficult to forget the staff huddle on Monday morning, April 6, at 6:30 am, at the peak of the surge. Started as usual 'What has happened and what do we need to get fixed today?'. After a list of more pedestrian observations and suggestions, a diminutive female patient care technician in the back of the group softly asked,

'Doctor, so many are dying and we are running out of stretchers. Last night, we had to put 2 bodies on one stretcher. Some of the patients are heavy. I need some help lifting and pushing the stretchers to the morgue'. She was not complaining. She was making a matter-of-fact operational observation. She was not emotional. The leadership of the department worked many shifts during the surge but stood and stared at her for some time, in awe, before, responding: 'I'll get you help. I'll help you push them myself if it comes to that'. Whilst aware of the impact of this disaster, there was a strong feeling of pride in the ED team.

On Tuesday, April 7, at about noon, the ambulances began to slow down, and they stopped rather precipitously. The next days and weeks were spent getting back to normal. Why did the surge wane so discretely and precipitously? As of this writing, it remains uncertain. What can be stated with confidence is that this inner city, stand-alone community hospital with an efficient, coordinated, and horizontal management team, did very well. It should also be emphasized that reliable face-to-face two-way communication among all job descriptions was the ED's most crucial strategy. This strategy of maintaining regular communication to deal effectively and decisively with the pandemic extended to include the leadership of the hospital. Indeed, the value of daily conversations with the leadership became evident very early on, and at the time, these calls were telephonic, as the institution was gradually becoming familiar with videoconferencing. ED leadership calls occurred at 10 am, late enough in the morning to have gathered significant data from the past 24 hours but early enough to intercede and affect the operations for the day. These conversations happened 7 days a week until a point where the surge had subsided, then reduced to business days, and ultimately eliminated.

Although the structure of these calls was unclear at the onset, it quickly evolved to include:

- ED chairman, who hosted the call and reported on issues from the morning leadership huddles
- ED medical director, who reported globally on ED operations and plan of action for the day
- ED nursing director, who reported on nursing operations and staffing
- Residency program director, who reported on resident scheduling and sicknesses
- ED volunteer logistics officer, who assisted with arranging receipt of donated supplies and delivery of items to staff out sick
- ED wellness director, who would discuss ongoing wellness activities
- ED pharmacist, who reported on any drug shortages, replacements, and recommendations
- ED administrator, who reported on attending sickness and sick call status/schedule

Lesson Getting all staff, of all levels, in a shared space twice a day, 7 days a week, to allow a space for asking questions, share feedback, and address the department's leaders is invaluable. Daily leadership calls critically facilitate sub-departments reporting and communicating key information. They promote a team approach at the leadership level, which then suffuse to the entire ED staff.

Departmental Reconfiguration of Space and Processes

> The art of life lies in a constant readjustment to our surroundings. Kakuzo Okakura

The ED at SBH Health System utilizes an open floor plan. With a few limited exceptions, all patients are located either on stretchers or chairs that may or may not be separated by a curtain.

The ED operates utilizing four zones, which are:

- High acuity (ED1): 46 patient stretcher spaces
- Low acuity (ED2): 38 patient stretcher/chair spaces
- Paediatric ED: 10 patient stretcher/chair spaces
- Behavioural health (ED4): 29 stretcher/chair spaces

Along with these four zones, there are zones for:

- Resuscitation/trauma: three patient stretcher spaces
- Geriatric ED: ten patient stretcher spaces
- Highly infectious patient (HIP) room: two patient stretcher/chair spaces

In the very early stage of the pandemic, a lot of time and energy went into preparing the HIP room for diagnosing and managing COVID patients. There were numerous monitored drills and simulations conducted prior to the department's first COVID patient, and these early simulations did indeed help iron out any glaring weak spots and shortcomings. However, no one could have anticipated the scale of the pandemic, and the single room was very quickly obsolescent as the department experienced an exponential increase in-patients. Very quickly the idea of isolating patients in the existing isolation areas was discarded, and by sheer necessity, COVID-19 patients were incorporated into ED1. Given the open floor plan, this did not allow for any sort of sequestration of infectious patients. As the numbers continued to rise, it was decided that the department's behavioural health zone (ED4) would be converted into a 'COVID-19' unit. There were many benefits to having an isolated zone, the most obvious one being improved infection control for both patients and staff (and by staff, it is important to recognize the multidisciplinary operations of an ED and how many different departments might 'touch' an ED patient during their visit). Having a separate zone for COVID-19 patients afforded the ED staff and others increased awareness of infection risks in that area, thus improved their use of PPE, and reinforced the need adhere to guidelines (Fig. 6.1).

One of the major drawbacks of having a dedicated COVID-19 zone was the occasional reluctance of a very small number of staff members, to enter the unit to provide necessary services. More often than not, this reluctance stemmed from unique concerns of the individual staff member, who may have been more vulnerable to infections or was at a higher risk, rather than sheer negligence or lack of professionalism. The respective department leadership usually handled such issues with generalized feedback, and individualized escalation of the matter was never warranted.

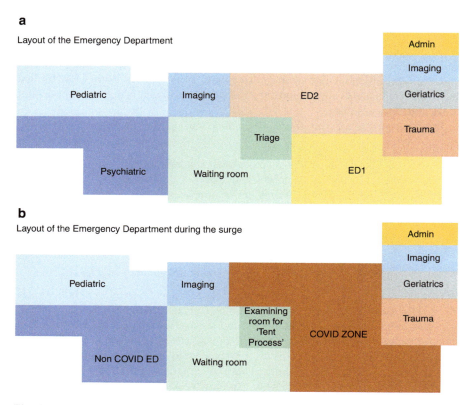

Fig. 6.1 (**a**) Schematic representation of the physical layout of the SBH ED prior to the Covid surge. (**b**) Reconfiguration of the layout of the ED at SBH Health System at the peak of the COVID-19 surge to manage the increase in-patient numbers

It also became quickly apparent that just because an available and/or dedicated floor space for care exists, that doesn't mean that that area necessarily conducive to focused patient care. In addition to physical space, staff and supporting supplies are as vital for providing optimal care and must be considered when such decisions are made. Whilst ED4 proved to be an ideal care zone for COVID-19 patients (a spacious unit with the monitors, medical gasses, a Pyxis machine capable of storing essential medications, and an existing and sustainable staffing model), other areas in our ED that often seemed appealing to staff external to our department, such as the geriatric zone, often had limitations that were recognized internally (i.e. no monitors, no existing/sustainable staffing model), or the paediatric zone which had limited supply of medical gases and where stretcher mobility was hindered.

Although ED4 had approximately 33% of the combined capacity of ED1 and ED2 and served its purpose for a number of days, it was fast becoming clear that a much larger space would be required to accommodate the increasing volumes of COVID-19 patients that were presenting requiring hospitalization. It was then decided to transpose units: ED1 and ED2 would become the 'COVID-19 zone', capable of housing close to 100 patients, and ED4 would become the 'regular' ED for patients presenting with non-COVID-19-related complaints. This was affected on an early Sunday morning, with the amazing participation of a large squad of environmental services workers, who, as soon ED4 was emptied of its COVID-19 patients, performed an aggressive terminal cleaning of the zone. Maintaining the operations of a 'regular' ED alongside a COVID-19 zone might have provided the staff some semblance of normality in a shift and a welcome break from the emotional toll of seeing patient after patient suffering from COVID-19. In addition to creating new care spaces for patients, the department also created new care spaces for staff. What had previously been a psychiatry consult office became an emergency medicine resident lounge where residents could store belongings and snacks and have a place to decompress; the department's Morning Report Conference Room, previously restricted to educational and administrative meetings, became a donation distribution/meal room that at points was utilized by all hospital staff.

During the surge, the paediatric patient volumes dropped precipitously in the ED. And given an almost complete absence of paediatric patients with COVID-19-like symptoms, the paediatric ED was utilized without any significant modifications with respect to patient triage/type.

Lesson Be dynamic. Be willing to reimagine a unit that serves one purpose to be renamed, resupplied, and re-staffed and serves a totally other purpose. And then, don't be afraid to switch back.

The 'Tent Process'

The scale of the pandemic meant that in addition to large numbers of patients with moderate or critical symptoms, the numbers of the 'worried well' were also increasing. An expeditious process to safely and effectively screen, treat, and discharge these patients was vital for the efficient functioning of the department. In a deviation from standard operating procedures, a 'tent' process was devised to deal with these 'worried well' patients. Under usual circumstances, a thorough and sophisticated but nevertheless inefficient electronic medical record (EMR) system is utilized for all patient encounters, beginning with a 'quick registration' process, through triage, full registration, exam and workup, results, and disposition. However, this wasn't best suited to deal with the exponential increase in the patients who were presenting to the ED and who needed to be moved through the system quickly, efficiently, and safely.

The 'tent' process, so named because of the 20′ × 40′ outdoor tent where it took place, involved the use of fit-for-purpose paper charts, in place of the EMR, and relied on senior residents who operated without what would otherwise be mandatory attending physician oversight for every case. A screening nurse served as the point of contact with the ambulance services or at the walk-in entrance who would refer the patients to the outdoor tent for registration, screening, evaluation, or discharge, based on bespoke criteria.

The tent was staffed with a medical assistant to triage vital signs (please note the patient had already encountered a nurse immediately upon arrival for triage to the tent) and a medical registrar who registered the patient demographics for eventual transfer to the EMR. Finally, a senior medical resident would evaluate the patient, documenting details on the paper chart, and release the patient unless the patient required a higher level of care (and if the patients did, they would be escorted by staff to the main ED for assignment inside).

The tent was utilized primarily during business hours when walk-in volumes were at peak. Although it was highly efficient from a patient workflow perspective, the 'tent process' put a strain on the resources, especially the staff who were split between the indoor ED and the outdoor tent. Eventually, to overcome this strain, the outdoor tent process was shifted indoors, though it kept the name 'tent process' for ease of use. The staff had all grown familiar with what this meant from a patient care perspective. A triage bay took the place of the tent as an examining room, which then allowed for routine processes to complete the triage and registration, and then shifted to the tent process for the final evaluation by a senior medical resident conducted independently. Being indoors, an attending physician was always proximal and available for supervision, with the option of transferring the patient to the main ED.

Lesson Don't be afraid to invent and refine. The tent process was set up without truly knowing how it might work and refined in real time. Don't allow 'perfection' be the enemy of 'good'. Allow for a process to capture suggestions in real time to aid refinement. However much you prepare an area for a new purpose, it isn't until the area goes live that the best is discovered about its particular needs. Having a clipboard in new areas for requests quickly identifies crucial needs to allow a unit to function more effectively.

Patient Transfers

A few weeks into the surge, a formalized transfer pathway was devised for moving ED patients who had been boarded but were waiting for a non-available inpatient bed into other departments of the hospital. This required a crosstalk between the ED and the remainder of the hospital for a seamless transfer of patient data. As one might expect, the process of transferring a critically ill patient involved a large amount of information and data exchange. It was realized that using a worksheet might assist and streamline the process, and though it started with a physical paper sheet, it later moved to an EMR document (Fig. 6.2).

The identification of patients suitable for transfer was dependent on the severity of their illness as well as the bed-type available in the receiving department. The process was facilitated by direct communication between the physician 'bed tzar' of hospital system and the medical director for ED.

Lesson A checklist/worksheet can facilitate efficient and safe transfer of patients with complex needs.

SAMPLE COVID Surge Transfer Document

1. CONFIRM ELIGIBILITY:

Patient IS stable for inter-hospital transfer (per general clinical assessment) **AND**
Patient has NOT had any clinically significant escalation of 02 needs in last 12 hours (ex. Being on nasal canula and now requiring NIPPV) and is NOT deemed at risk for acute decompensation

Please note: Intubated patient with stable 02 sat IS considered stable from respiratory status

☐ Yes, patient is eligible

2. IF PATIENT IS ELIGIBLE, PLEASE COMPLETE:

- Patient's current 02 source (please circle):

  ☐ NC at __ L   ☐ NRB   ☐ HFNC   ☐ Mechanical Ventilator

- How long the patient has been on current source: ____ Hours

- Patient's ambulation status (please circle):
  ☐ Ambulatory ☐ Bed ☐ Crib ☐ Stretcher   ☐ Transport Isolette   ☐ Wheelchair

- Is patient aware that he/she is being transferred, reason for transfer and consents?
  ☐ YES   ☐ NO
  If patient <u>UNABLE</u> to provide consent for transfer, does N.O.K provide consent?
  ☐ YES   ☐ NO

- Is the patient on dialysis? YES NO
  If <u>YES</u> what is the status: Date of last HD:
  ☐ No HD due today
  ☐ HD scheduled today
  ☐ HD completed today, OR
  ☐ HD due today but not schedule

- If the patient is on any drips/infusions, please list all:
  1.
  2.
  3.
  4.

- Sending Clinician Name & Contact Number:

Please make the unit clerk aware of transfer so that all appropriate lab work and imaging is transferred with the patient. Please email **XXX** to report the transfer with **XXX**.

Fig. 6.2 COVID-19 surge transfer document which acted as a checklist to facilitate the exchange of a large amount of information and data efficiently

Diversion Status

A diversion request to a different hospital or facility is triggered when there is an inadequate capacity in the ED to treat additional patient volume or if there are certain specific services lacking. During the first surge of COVID-19, diversion was never triggered nor requested due to inadequate capacity, and in any case, it was unlikely that such a request would have been granted.

Diversion for lack of specific services was determined by the healthcare system. During the surge, several hospital units were closed to facilitate creating bed space for increasing numbers of COVID-19 patients. The medically managed detox unit (MMDU), paediatrics, ambulatory surgery, and the catheterization laboratory were some of the units that were reassigned. The ED was therefore placed on diversion for paediatric and ST elevation myocardial infarction (STEMI) patients.

Lesson In a health crisis such as an infectious pandemic, discourage staff from believing that diversion might be a source of relief. Recognize and accept that the challenges will be unavoidable.

Visitation by Family

In response to the COVID-19 pandemic, most healthcare organizations implemented policies to restrict visitor access [3]. All visitations in the ED of SBH Health System were cancelled during the surge. At the time, there was also no formal mechanism to enable videoconferencing with family. However, the ED staff did facilitate telephonic communication between patients and families, and in some cases, patient or staff smartphones were used for videoconferencing. The hospital quickly moved to repurpose a team of non-clinical staff to facilitate patient-family communications and minimize isolation and separation.

Lesson Depriving patients of family and visitors is a difficult but necessary emergency measure to control transmission in an infectious (viral) health crisis.

Resources and Infrastructure

> The equilibrium between supply and demand is achieved only through a reaction against the upsetting of equilibrium. David Harvey

Personal Protective Equipment (PPE)

For effective control of COVID-19, a regular and consistent supply of PPE was vital. SBH Health System was able to supply necessary PPE throughout the pandemic and at a time when other hospitals nearby were making the news with staff reportedly wearing plastic trash bags and/or lacking for PPE [4].

A potential issue of contention could have been that the staff were bringing in self-purchased PPE, such as powered air purifying respirator (PAPR). Several hospitals in the vicinity found this unacceptable, and a nearby high-profile hospital made national news when a physician was sent home for wearing her own PPE which exceeded the requirements and level of protection offered by her hospital. Nevertheless, SBH Health System hospital chose not to prohibit personally provided PPEs but ensured that the staff knew that they always had access to PPE as per the guidelines recommended by the CDC. Furthermore, the ED leadership always only wore hospital-supplied PPE to demonstrate both its adequacy and equity. Some physician staff wore personal PAPR's during the surge. Additionally, SBH employed a PPE reuse initiative to ward off potential PPE shortages (Box 6.1).

Lesson Health institutions should prioritize the safety and welfare of their staff, especially during crisis. Leadership should consider the issues resulting from staff requesting to use personal PPE and potential resultant inequities.

Ventilators

The pandemic was leading to an unprecedented number of patients requiring critical care and a large proportion of them needing mechanical ventilation [5]. The ventilators for the ED came from a pool that was shared within the hospital, and initially the number of ventilators accessible by the ED was unclear.

A 'Ventilator Status Report' was devised and regularly distributed by the command centre for the hospital, which provided details regarding the availability of ventilators. This intervention helped alleviate some anxiety in ED physician staff, who were worried about the possibility of rationing care to the patients based on the availability of the ventilators.

Lesson A status report of critical equipment is a crucial intervention for better planning of care for patients; it builds confidence in staff to take care of the critically ill.

Lesson The use of different ventilator models almost caused a near miss safety incident in the ED. Consider having standard operating procedures, manuals, and troubleshooting guides available near all critical care equipment.

Box 6.1 The Reuse of PPE

The PPE had been handled largely very successfully by the SBH Health System's supply chain department. The availability and reliability of proper PPE was arguably a key determinant of morale. Whilst a shifting supply of brands and models was worked around, it was very obvious that the ability to make staff feel protected and cared for was a key factor in empowering and enabling them to be able to focus on the care of our patients. After a few weeks of very smooth sailing and perhaps in an attempt to be proactive and ward off potential PPE shortages, the hospital decided to embark on an N-95

> *sterilization/reuse initiative. Without formal communication to ED leadership, containers were placed at the hallway entrance of the ED to both collect and distribute N-95 s. Seemingly within minutes, information (and misinformation) spread among ED staff, raising concerns that supplies were out, that clean and dirty masks were being co-mingled, and that leadership had not communicated changes to PPE process and had lost control of a key ED safety process.*
>
> *As soon as the ED leadership team became aware of the initiative and the effect it was having on staff morale and confidence, they communicated with Hospital Leadership and obtained permission to immediately stop participating in the initiative. 'Damage control' was then done in the ED via thorough communication with staff.*
>
> **Takeaway: Emphasize that any new institutional initiatives that might affect your department be clearly communicated to your department before they begin.**

Pharmacy

Like with the ventilators, the availability and supply of drugs become a cause of concern early into the pandemic. Certain classes of drugs like antibiotics, sedatives, and those used for rapid sequence intubation (RSI) were in short and erratic supply. For the benefit of the clinical staff, who required up-to-date information or the availability of drugs and its option, our pharmacist created a 'Daily Medication Status Report' which included but was not limited to:

- Update on medications needed for RSI (given the large number of ED and hospital intubations, there was high utilization of RSI medications)
- Update on medications needed for post-intubation sedation
- Hemodynamic support medications
- COVID-19-specific medications
- Recommended substitutions/alternatives/non-traditional agents

Moreover, the medications were categorized as green (adequate supply), yellow (~7-day supply/of concern), orange (1–2-day supply/critical), and red (out of stock). This visual traffic light system provided a quick overview to the clinical staff on the availability of the drugs that they could use and informed purchasing priorities.

In the ED, the pharmacy staff included a clinical pharmacist and a pharmacy resident, who were typically scheduled to work together. However, during the pandemic, the working hours for the pharmacy resident were shifted to the evening shift to extend access to the pharmacy. Moreover, as the pharmacists were responsible for stocking and maintaining the supplies in the Pyxis machines, this allowed for tailoring supplies to the demands and to the zones in which the machines were located.

> **Lesson**
> A reliable, constantly updateable hospital pharmacy communication system is key to combating confusion, optimizing patient safety, and maintaining staff sanity. As a particular drug becomes short in supply, one can expect that its substitute or alternate will just as quickly become a supply challenge. Think proactively, not just for first-line substitutes but second and third lines as well. Encourage your hospital/institution to develop a standardized treatment regimen as soon as possible. Keep these resources handy and easily available to clinicians.

Staffing

> When you put people first and then surround them with processes and disciplines that recognize their efforts, performance will soar. David C. Novak

The pandemic brought with it unprecedented levels of challenges for healthcare staff in general and particularly for staff in the ED. This section will discuss some of the reconfigurations undertaken to increase capacity to manage the surge in-patients whilst providing a safe working environment for the staff.

Nursing Staff

The ED nursing team and ancillary staff, who although were preparing for the pandemic prior to the initial impact, were put under tremendous strain. Even at the start of the pandemic, the nursing staff was tenuous, with some full-time vacancies for registered nurses (RNs) and some full-time RNs on leaves of absences (LOA). This shortage in staff was compounded by some ED technicians on LOA and a vacancy.

The ED was searching, for a whilst, for supplemental staff with staffing agencies; however, the requests were late in comparison to other hospitals in the area, and at lower rates, which made it increasingly difficult to cover the shortfall. Furthermore, as the number of COVID-19 patients increased, there was also saw a rise in staff sick calls, with some cases of 'influenza-like illness' (ILI), which required a period of quarantine and extended absences. Every sick call was managed as a possible exposure to COVID-19 and was referred to the employee health service for evaluation and required quarantine. Some staff called in sick as a consequence of illness in their family or due to issues with day care.

Hospital staff from other departments would be reassigned to the ED to supplement the staff shortfall. The hospital was also able to emergently increase pay rates which helped increase staff recruitment and progress with staff on-boarding. Additional inpatient critical care units were opened that were able to take patients from the ED, decreasing their length of stay (LOS) in ED and ultimately making staffing more manageable. Another moderating force was the decrease in non-COVID-19 patient volumes as the pandemic progressed. This drop in non-COVID-19-related visits mitigated some of the nursing and ancillary staff shortages.

Lessons Anticipate workforce shortages early on, and have a plan to efficiently supplement staff. Implement agency contracts early for long-term staff recruitment, ensuring clauses for members leaving prior to completion of the contracted term.

Physician Staff

Prior to the pandemic, physician staff did not have a formal sick call schedule in place; if a physician was to call in sick, it was typically managed via volunteer moonlighters, shift swaps, administrative coverage, and/or cross coverage from other zones.

It was recognized early on that due to the likelihood of multiple physician sicknesses in the pandemic, the department would now clearly require a sick call schedule. Using Google Docs as the platform, a 2-month calendar allowed staff to sign up for a mandated number of shifts (weekday/overnight/weekend) in real time, in a process that allowed staff to assign themselves autonomously and remotely. Within hours of making the sick call calendar live, the majority of the staff had filled it in. The department's administrator subsequently managed the sick call process and was often able to avoid calling on sick call physicians, as other available staff, identified through the sick call calendar, were able to fill in.

Lesson Using a shared online platform allows for the self-assignment of sick calls. The knowledge that earliest responders would have the greatest flexibility in choosing shifts motivates staff to self-assign shifts as soon as possible.

Staff Wellness

Staff wellness was considered on two Maslowian levels [6]. Firstly, were basic needs of the staff being met, to foster a sense of physical and psychological safety so that they could feel secure and confident in coming to work? The daily leadership huddles described above were effective in monitoring staff wellness at this level and best suited to identify and address any concerns that might impede departmental functioning. Arguably, any failure to sufficiently address the most basic needs to feel safe and secure would have hampered any other higher-order goals.

Secondly, the aim was to bolster morale and team spirit. To do this, a 'Wellness Committee' was formed, which motivated the staff by showcasing the many letters and messages of gratitude that were received by the department. Members of the department were also given license to pursue outside donations, for example, one resident physician who had reached out to very well-recognized nutrition bar company ended up procuring dozens of donated boxes of bars for the department. The Committee also arranged the delivery of care packages to members of staff who tested positive and were quarantining. A volunteer supply officer, together with the departmental administrator, facilitated the picking up and delivery of donated items, which were often meals. Employee-driven fundraising initiatives were started to support staff but were quickly curtailed as potential threats to team unity arose (Box 6.2). On Sunday evening, virtual calls were arranged with a psychologist to discuss various topics of interest to the staff. Regular support meetings with the psychiatry and pastoral departments were arranged to provide an opportunity for the staff to discuss issues of non-clinical and more humanistic nature.

Lessons Prioritize staff wellness. Encourage and create opportunities for any staff to take leadership roles in wellness opportunities. Business, community, family, and friend donations and messages of gratitude to the ED can bring immense joy to the staff and a source of motivation.

> **Box 6.2 Fundraising: A Well-Intended Initiative That Had Negative Consequences**
> *Twice during the surge, two different groups of employees turned to social media fundraising platforms to seek donations. Whilst the genesis was well-intentioned, family and friends of one group had asked how they might make financial donations. This created the effect of a second group feeling left out, and so they then created their own fundraising initiative. Very quickly there were concerns about the veracity of some of the information included on one of the fundraising sites and an unwelcomed sense of competitiveness and a fracturing of what had been a very unified team approach within the department.*
>
> *Ultimately, the two initiatives were ended after consultation with the department and staff leaders. It did point out the need to stay ahead of staff-led initiatives and that well-intended projects that are not officially vetted can easily have negative consequences.*
>
> ***Takeaway: Prepare for what staff may wish to do personally in terms of seeking outside assistance and support. Have a pathway in place for staff to present ideas and requests before they go live with them.***

Risk Awareness in Staff

The ED is highly reliant on consultants and various admitting services, including medicine, surgery, and psychiatry, as well as clinical support services, such as radiology, respiratory therapy, and nutrition. Early on during the pandemic, reports were encountered of members of these teams being reluctant to enter the ED clinical areas housing COVID-19 patients. These events had multiple deleterious effects:

impacting the clinical care of patients, engendering a sense of abandonment among ED staff, and suggesting that they were more expendable and able to be exposed to risk.

As soon as such behaviour was reported, ED leadership reached out to the involved departments to emphasize on the unacceptability of such a conduct. It was also observed that different departments, and staff, had varying levels of knowledge of risks involved, use of PPE, and other guidelines associated with COVID-19 transmission. To address these, the ED worked tirelessly to communicate and educate the various service staff, to make them more aware and prepared to tackle the risks involved, and to make them feel a part of the team effort against COVID-19.

Lesson When thinking about your departmental staff, do not neglect the needs of the staff that support and serve your team.

Resident Staffing

The operation of any teaching/academic ED depends very heavily on a resident physician workforce. The ED at SBH Health System is home to a 4-year ACGME/AOA residency program with 60 residents. At any point in time, the ED can have as many as 18 resident physicians on duty. Ultimately a significant number of residents were infected by COVID-19, with most of those missing a few days of work and one requiring hospitalization. One occurrence that greatly assisted with resident staff was that a number of elective rotations were cancelled during COVID-19, providing the residency program with a reserve of residents that increased our coverage. A long-standing tradition of EM residency training is protected time for residency educational conferences. These were cancelled early on, both for infection control practices and to facilitate ED staffing needs. But as the rest of the world moved learning and teaching online and once the surge receded, these conferences also migrated to an online platform. A weekly clinical update and open-floor QA session with the medical director was incorporated into these conferences to keep the residents abreast with the rapid changes occurring during the pandemic (Box 6.3).

During COVID-19, it was also recognized that the residents were requesting a 'lounge', where they could store personal items, take breaks, and rest between long shifts. A decision was made to repurpose the office that had previously housed the department's emergency psychiatric consultation team, which had relocated out of the ED once the surge struck. Given the value of square footage in the department, this was a significant concession to the resident workforce, but one that was ultimately deserved and likely paid dividends in residents' performance and morale. It was also appreciated, post-surge, that the lounge could not easily, nor rightfully, be taken back and so eventually a new office was created for the psychiatry team.

Lesson In a crisis, consider pulling residents off non-essential rotations as soon as possible, and create a reserve body of resident physicians who could be called upon when staff are out sick. Be prepared to make administrative concessions to get buy-in and preserve morale among staff.

Box 6.3 A Resident's Perspective: Dr. Jackie Jian

As the COVID-19 pandemic slowly emerged, I was on my Fire Department New York (FDNY) Emergency Medical Services (EMS) rotation, listening in on 'FC' calls to the telecentre. Every call would contain the same dialogue. 'X year old M/F with fever and cough, with recent exposure to sick contacts, COVID-19 rule out'. Walking into the EDs of various hospitals of the Bronx, I noticed everyone was a bit more anxious as each day went by. Eventually, I returned to my own ED at SBH Health System and found that my own ED had become unfamiliar to me.

For a brief 2 months, it felt like no other pathology existed in the world. The only malady that came into our ED was acute respiratory failure due to COVID-19 infection. It was both an exciting and terrifying time to be in the frontlines battling an unknown disease. There was a strong sense of camaraderie among us. We became experts solely due to the fact that we were the primary contact for every patient presenting to the ED.

Patient after patient would come into our ED to the point where it all felt like a blur because every patient had the same disease and would end up on the same pathway: non-invasive ventilation leading to mechanical ventilation leading to vasopressors. It was horrifying to see patients decompensate despite everything we did. It was even more traumatizing to see both young and old patients die. We were forced to face our own mortality when members of our own residency program became sick as well. We became experienced in engaging our patients about goals of care early. Palliative care became another facet of our education.

Despite the stress and trauma, we felt overwhelming support that we never had before from our community. Support came from everywhere, from the local 7 am/7 pm applause to donated foods from local restaurants to our pediatric department answering calls from family to offload our work in updating our patient's loved ones. Our ED became a mini-ICU due to the overfilled ICU beds in the hospital, even though we had converted parts of our hospital into ICUs. We learned to manage all kinds of drips and even learned anachronistic forms of drip control such as old-school dial IV flow regulators. We became familiar with lesser-used medications for analog sedation as each day our pharmacist updated us to what medications we had access to.

As we face the surge of a second wave, reflecting on these memories has been bittersweet. If we can do it once, we can do it again. COVID-19 is no longer as mysterious as before, and we now have a better handle on how to manage it.

Staff Sickness

Once the surge was established, it was routine for a number of staff (nursing and physician) to be out ill with COVID-19 on any one day. A system was put in place to communicate with these staff, confirm their wellness and assess their needs, demonstrate the compassionate concern for their welfare, and keep them briefed on the status of the department and that their return, when appropriate, would be valuable.

The department was incredibly fortunate to not suffer any mortality among staff, though a significant number of staff did become unwell.

Lesson Daily check-ins with staff who are ill are not only deserved and courteous but likely contribute to their desire to return to duty as soon as possible.

> **Box 6.4 International Vignette: Health Crisis Management During the COVID-19 Pandemic in an Acute Care Hospital – The French Perspective**
>
> *Before reflecting on the overwhelming initial surge of COVID-19 patients in our acute care hospital in Paris, it is important to appreciate how the French Healthcare System functions and how the American Hospital of Paris is an integral part of this network. There are some key distinctions that set apart the healthcare landscape in France from other healthcare systems.*
>
> *First, when an emergency occurs, French citizens must choose between three different telephone numbers depending on what type of emergency they are experiencing. Rather than a single 911 number for any type of emergency as in the USA, a person in France must dial 17 to reach the Police, 18 to reach the Fire Department, and 15 for medical assistance. The central organizations that control these services are known as a SAMU, which stands for Service d'Aide Médicale Urgente. SAMU-Centre 15 is only dedicated to medical emergencies. Located in each 'Département' (equivalent to county in the USA), the 'SAMU-Centre 15' receives incoming calls, then provides rapid and appropriate answers to each caller, and dispatches help as needed. In cases where the caller does not have a life-threatening emergency, the SAMU-Centre 15 responses might include offering pertinent medical advice, sending a primary care physician for a house visit to consult with the patient (this could be a physician on duty or an emergency physician from 'SOS Médecins' a sort of 'doctor on wheels'), or sending adequate first aid assistance, such as a Fire Department Team or a basic ambulance like the French Red Cross, Civil Defense volunteers, or a private ambulance. In non-life-threatening situations, the call can be handled from the team in the SAMU-Centre 15. However, should the caller require urgent life-saving actions, the dispatcher would transfer the call to an emergency physician (regulateur) who would coordinate response efforts. This coordinator would send a Mobile*

Resuscitation Unit *(Service Mobile d'Urgence et de Réanimation (SMUR))*. This could be a red advanced cardiac life support (ACLS) ambulance from the Fire Department or a white ACLS ambulance from a public hospital. Either comes equipped with paramedics and an emergency physician or an anesthesiologist onboard. In other words, 'the hospital comes to you' and is able to initiate cardiopulmonary resuscitation (CPR), continuous positive airway pressure (C-PAP) ventilation, or tissue plasminogen activator (tPA) administration on site. Once stabilized, the patient would be transported directly to the intensive care unit (ICU), critical care unit (CCU), or catheterization lab/operating room (OR), therefore bypassing the emergency room (ER). This is probably a key difference between the French and the American emergency response systems. A very important thing to note is that the Fire Department and SAMU-SMUR are free of charge for the patient.

Second, the French Healthcare System is a dual system made up of both public and private hospitals. Public hospitals may be teaching or non-teaching hospitals. Physicians are paid monthly depending on their grade (from medical student to the head of the unit). On paper, these physicians work 35 hours/week. However, their work week is actually more like 50–60 hours/week for that same monthly salary. Private hospitals are either for profit or for non-profit. Physicians are usually paid on a fee-for-service basis. 'Les Cliniques' are not comprehensive care centers. They are specialized in general surgery, orthopedics, and/or obstetrics, but usually do not admit emergency cases.

Third, both public and private hospital care are 70% reimbursed by the basic French Social Security System. As 99% of people are covered with a complimentary insurance, even the remaining 30% of hospital fees are refunded to the individual. By hospital emergency services being effectively free of charge to French citizens, the French national budget suffers significantly. All these matters are important because the French Healthcare System was ranked number 1 in the world by the WHO in 2000 [7]. Over the past 20 years, the French Government has made desperate efforts to decrease the medical expenses of the healthcare system (close to 14% of the Gross National Product). To have better control, the government has exponentially increased the administrative management and administrative onus. For instance, every single action with a patient must be tracked through multiple software programs (which were not designed for use by the caregiver) as well as requiring the creation and maintenance of electronic health records. Health managers promise to deliver resources at low costs, yet unfortunately, it is not quite possible under these conditions. In developed countries around the world, we are witnessing a depletion of resources with patients unable to access services. The French Healthcare System has slipped to a ranking of 18 in the world today.

The COVID-19 Initial Surge in Paris

The duplication of processes, heavy workload, and the government regulations implemented to try to minimize costs had already led to the burnout of nurses and physicians. Without attractive work conditions, the public hospital is 'sick', and the private system is not much better. Strikes and protests in the streets by nurses and physicians had been common for some time. When COVID-19 struck, hospitals were supposed to be prepared to face this kind of crisis. Many studies and numerous reports for preparedness were previously published by distinguished professors in healthcare management, public health, and emergency and disaster medicine in the years running up to the COVID-19 pandemic. However, their messages were shelved rather than heeded. We were therefore left with an underprepared, tired workforce. Despite this, the healthcare workers and all members of the hospital systems who are involved in ensuring the provision of care for patients were persevering, selfless, and dedicated even under this great strain. In fact, at the beginning of the COVID-19 crisis, primary care physicians and private nurses gave care at great personal risk, without personal protective equipment (PPE), surgical masks, or N95 masks.

During the first wave of COVID-19, the French health agencies used only the public beds in hospitals. Clinics were almost always empty. Although they were prepared and ready to help, they were not considered or involved in the initial response. Instead, the lack of ICU beds in Paris caused the decision to evacuate patients via high-speed trains to hospitals in the southwest of France. In Alsace in the east of France, ICU patients were evacuated via helicopters to Germany as Germany has twice the French ICU bed capacity. Even in leading teaching hospitals, the workforce quickly became exhausted or ill. It became necessary to recruit nurses and medical students to lend a hand in COVID-19 units.

The American Hospital of Paris (AHP)

The American Hospital of Paris (AHP) is a very special member of the French Hospital Network. AHP is a non-profit hospital, but it charges the real cost of care. This means that patients who receive benefits from the French Social Security Program are not refunded 100% and the remaining bill could be substantial. For years, AHP has been the hospital of choice, preferred for visiting or native executives of international or French companies or VIPs from the entertainment industry.

APH Emergency Medicine in the COVID-19 Crisis

For the American Hospital of Paris, the COVID-19 crisis started on February 28, 2020. A COVID-19-infected patient was admitted through the ED. Immediately, the hospital administration and the president of the Medical Board set a taskforce to organize the way patients would be admitted and how COVID-19 units would be organized. During each daily meeting, the focus was on management and demand forecasts of intensive care capacity, hospitalizations in internal medicine, and operating rooms and ED resources. Due to the shortage of intensive care beds, hospitals in France functioned beyond capacity and were required to transfer stable patients as soon as possible to normal units in order to face the demand. At AHP, we turned recovery beds into ICU beds by equipping them with appropriate ventilators. Two different care pathways were set in the ED: one for possible/suspect COVID-19 patients and another for non-COVID patients. Nurses and emergency physicians received PPE. Information was communicated to ancillary services as well as transport services, CT scan technicians, and radiologists about COVID-19 suspicious case, to be sure to utilize PPE. The implementation of new protocols and the extra time needed to update staff and families were exhausting.

Infectious disease specialists, pulmonologists, and internists defined new units dedicated to both unconfirmed and confirmed COVID-19 patients. Of course, we postponed all elective, non-urgent services during the surge of the COVID-19 crisis. We experienced patients with long hospitalizations, especially in intensive care with unexpected high utilization of ICU pharmaceuticals, as did many other hospitals. However, AHP was not concerned with shortages in sedatives or curare drugs. We secured enough PPE and staffing to maintain our standard of care.

Physicians specialized in infectious diseases, and internists gave 'teleconsultations' on FaceTime and assured follow-up of discharged patients. To prevent COVID-19 transmission, the hospital limited the visitation of relatives, even for patients in critical condition. As a result, secretaries, nurses, and physicians spent a lot of time on the phone to keep families and relatives informed about their loved ones.

Remarkably, during the first surge of COVID-19 due to the lockdown, we experienced a marked reduction in all usual emergencies, no more ankle sprains or kidney stones! Even abdominal pains remained at home. One thing that puzzled us: 'What about chest pain or strokes?' No one came and no one knows!

As COVID-19 disease was a new disease, it was very labor-intensive to read all the abstracts published every day from around the world. Fortunately, hospital newsletters with summaries allowed us to remain updated, thanks to the tireless work of team members Prof. Anne-Claude Crémieux and Prof. Frederic Adnet. Also, we cannot overlook the crucial role of the social network (e.g. WhatsApp groups) to keep us informed about new drugs or new ventilation guidelines. Physicians never shared experiences so quickly and timely around the world.

Reflection

For the first time in decades, doctors once again became key people in the management of care in the hospital as a dynamic and reactive force on the frontline of patient care. Quicker and impactful decisions had to be made, and

lessons can be learned from this system of emergency management. Specifically, an emergency management system in healthcare should prevent and react to crises effectively, as well as avoid unpreparedness and miscommunication. It is important that political and public leaders listen to and read recommendations provided by professionals dedicated to disaster and crisis management. As we use a National Transportation Safety Board (NTSB) to investigate plane crashes and provide appropriate changes and adaptations to prevent them, the healthcare system should consider the need for a similar agency with equivalent power. Then these factors may help prepare healthcare systems for any future crises.
   Jerry Papon Benoit, MD, FACEP
   Title: Clinical Assistant Professor of Emergency Medicine
   Weil Cornell Medical College
   Former Head of the Emergency Department
   American Hospital of Paris, Paris, France
   Email: bjpapon@hotmail.com
   Phone number: +33 6 16 33 33 35

Easing of the Initial Crisis

As the patient volumes began to decrease, doing so rather dramatically, the department then deactivated and/or reversed the majority of the emergency procedures and processes that were instituted to cope with the surge (Box 6.4). Units were reopened and diversion ended. The department was able to end the tent process and return ED4 to being a behavioural health zone. And whilst COVID-19 patient numbers dropped off dramatically, there was not a concomitant return of routine patients which offered the staff a much-needed form of decompression. As the department moved forward, there was a sense that the lessons learned from this pandemic thus far would serve well the department and perhaps others. It is worth noting that whilst the department experienced a second wave in the late fall of 2020, the volumes never mandated any of the significant changes of the first the surge. The department's success energized the confidence in the ability to act quickly and decisively to handle any challenges this pandemic might throw at us in the future.

References

1. Chatterjee SS, Vora M, Malathesh BC, Bhattacharyya R. Worried well and Covid-19: re-emergence of an old quandary. Asian J Psychiatr. 2020;54:102247. https://doi.org/10.1016/j.ajp.2020.102247.
2. Cleverley J, Piper J, Jones MM. The role of chest radiography in confirming covid-19 pneumonia. BMJ. 2020;370:m2426. https://doi.org/10.1136/bmj.m2426.

3. Downar J, Kekewich M. Improving family access to dying patients during the COVID-19 pandemic. Lancet Respir Med. 2021;9(4):335–7. https://doi.org/10.1016/S2213-2600(21)00025-4.
4. Bowden E, Campanile C, Golding B. Worker at NYC hospital where nurses wear trash bags as protection dies from coronavirus. 2020. https://nypost.com/2020/03/25/worker-at-nyc-hospital-where-nurses-wear-trash-bags-as-protection-dies-from-coronavirus/?utm_source=url_sitebuttons&utm_medium=site%20buttons&utm_campaign=site%20buttons.
5. Wunsch H. Mechanical ventilation in COVID-19: interpreting the current epidemiology. Am J Respir Crit Care Med. 2020;202(1):1–4. https://doi.org/10.1164/rccm.202004-1385ED.
6. Maslow A. Motivation and personality. New York: Harper and Row; 1970.
7. World Health Organisation (WHO). World Health Organization assesses the World's health systems. https://www.who.int/news/item/07-02-2000-world-health-organization-assesses-the-world's-health-systems. Accessed on 4 Sept 2021.

Chapter 7
Nursing

Robert Church, Raymundo M. Apellido, Angela Babaev, Alma Calandria, Mary B. Carmel, Brian J. Dolan, Donna L. Douglas, Ann C. Hennessy, Pauline A. Lattery, Clover Mclennon, and Courtney White

Introduction

This chapter explains the functioning and contributions of the nursing department at SBH Health System during the COVID-19 pandemic surge in the Spring of 2020, with important lessons learned about the indispensable role of nurses during a health crisis. This chapter highlights the various aspects of nursing including patient care, education, labor union matters, nursing administration, interdepartmental relations, and crisis planning, preparedness, and management.

R. Church (✉) · A. Calandria · M. B. Carmel · A. C. Hennessy · P. A. Lattery · C. Mclennon
C. White
Department of Nursing, SBH Health System, Bronx, NY, USA
e-mail: rchurch@sbhny.org

R. M. Apellido
Intensive Care Units, SBH Health System, Bronx, NY, USA

A. Babaev
Department of Nursing, SBH Health System, Bronx, NY, USA

CUNY School of Medicine, New York, NY, USA

Bloomfield College, Bloomfield, NJ, USA

B. J. Dolan
Department of Emergency Medicine and Department of Nursing, SBH Health System, Bronx, NY, USA

D. L. Douglas
Perioperative Services, SBH Health System, Bronx, NY, USA

© The Author(s), under exclusive license to Springer Nature Switzerland AG 2022
R. Shabsigh (ed.), *Health Crisis Management in Acute Care Hospitals*, https://doi.org/10.1007/978-3-030-95806-0_7

The Importance of Harmony and Coordination Between Hospital Nursing Leadership and Nursing Union Leadership During a Health Crisis

The majority of hospitals in New York City (NYC) are unionized, which means that labor unions have a voice and a say over the employees, salaries, benefits, and working conditions. Management maintains responsibility for operations, supplies, policies, and procedures. It is important to have a good working relationship with the unions and keep them aware of what is happening, soliciting nursing staff input whenever necessary. During the initial surge of the COVID-19 pandemic, the nursing department at SBH Health System experienced a sudden and mass increase in the number of patients; each nurse would usually care for 6–8 patients at a time, but during the pandemic, they had to manage 12–16. This quickly became difficult, and contact was made with the union to request help. Because the union works together with a variety of hospitals, it had quickly realized how expansive the pandemic situation was and how significantly overburdened departments had become. While the union worked on a plan to support hospitals, it was at the same time providing necessary emotional support to the hardworking nursing staff, reassuring them that they were working with the hospital to their maximal capacity in order to solve the issues, alongside providing honest communication about the fact that these problems were a reality across all hospitals. Instead of further compounding the situation with this information, the support given by the union was actually necessary encouragement for nursing staff to realize that, at that time, all they could do was take care of the "here and now." The importance of a hospital having a good relationship with its labor union never became more crucial than during the COVID-19 pandemic. Thankfully, the messages received by the nursing staff, from both the hospital and the union, were concise and constant. Nursing staff who were reassigned to other departments to help manage the crisis were overwhelmed by the changes but praised the union and the hospital nursing leadership for their consistent support and messaging during that time.

The Importance of Morale-Boosting Huddles

Within the nursing department, there were frequent safety calls which allowed nursing staff to get a pulse of what was going on in the rest of the hospital during the pandemic. The nursing department had its own daily (and sometimes hourly) communication strategies: "huddles" – an informal (often spontaneous) and formal gatherings of nursing staff with the aim of sharing information, providing updates, and allowing for an open dialogue among nursing staff and managers. Huddles before and after each shift lasted around 15 minutes and provided nursing staff with the opportunity to touch base and ask questions on any issues they may have had.

Huddles were also used to provide educational updates on new guidelines, equipment, or processes. SBH Health System used a formal education platform called "HealthStream" to deploy specific educational programs to train nursing staff; however, a huddle was also a great place to demonstrate a piece of equipment or a mask. The overall aim was to assure nursing staff that their voices were being heard in relation to leadership issues, any concerns, or other questions they might have. This was crucial since it ultimately affected the working environment. In response to the demands of the pandemic, not only was it necessary to expand the nursing staffing and ICU capacity, but it was vital to reassure and encourage existing nursing staff, reinforcing that their daily presence was significant and necessary (see Boxes 7.1 and 7.2).

Box 7.1 One of Several Frequent Communications Sent to the Nursing Staff from the Chief Nursing Officer (CNO)

On behalf of all of St. Barnabas leadership and the nursing department, I want you to know how thankful we are for you and your dedication to taking care of our patients and community during this COVID-19 event. As registered nurses, we care for sick patients every day, but it is not every day that we are faced with a new virus that we are learning more about every day. As registered nurses, we are the frontline nursing staff who provide care, who comfort, and who educate our patients. To do that, we must educate ourselves and communicate with our teams, and we must not panic.

Your safety and well-being is our highest priority. We are updating our guidelines each and every time the CDC and DOH make new recommendations. As you have heard, there is a national shortage of masks and other personal protective equipment. We monitor the amount we have daily to try to ensure you have what you need to keep you safe and care for our patients, but we need your help to prevent unnecessary waste of our supplies.

As a registered nurse you are invaluable and irreplaceable. No one else can do what you do. Please monitor your own health daily. If you develop a fever, cough, or breathing issues, notify your director immediately, and we will get you screened by employee health and tested if needed. If you are well, please come to work, please support your fellow nurses, ancillary nursing staff, and care team. We need you; your patients need you, and I personally want to thank you for your dedication. It is a privilege and honor to be a registered nurse, and it is because of times like this that the community hold us as the most trusted and respected profession in the country. I am available if you have any questions or concerns. Please feel free to email me at rchurch@sbhny.org and I will respond back to you as soon as possible.

Thank you again for all you do. Please be safe and stay healthy.
Rob Church, RN, CNO.

> **Box 7.2 A Message of Morale Support Coming from the CNO**
> *This message is for every single employee at SBH. **YOU MAKE A DIFFERENCE**. One of several frequent communications sent to the nursing staff from the Chief Nursing Officer (CNO).*
>
> *You are a Hero. Your dedication and sacrifice saves lives. Whether you're a nurse, a doctor, a respiratory therapist, a materials management handler, a housekeeper, a dietary worker, a facility person, a lab tech, a finance person....no matter where you work, **YOU MAKE A DIFFERENCE**. Whether you care for patients directly or you are supporting and providing resources for others to do so, **YOU MAKE A DIFFERENCE**!*
>
> *Here is feedback from someone who spoke to a COVID patient we all took care of and was discharged home:*
>
>> I spoke with a patient yesterday as a virtual visit at the adult medicine clinic, and the patient had recently been discharged from SBH after a hospitalization for COVID. He was doing great at home and expressed a tremendous amount of gratitude to the healthcare workers at SBH whom he credited with saving his life. He said that every person who entered his room, from nurses and doctors to phlebotomists, showed tremendous dedication and passion for helping patients and treated him as though he were their family member. He was so grateful and really overjoyed by his recovery. It was a real bright spot in an otherwise tough time and I wanted to share his gratitude with you and your nursing staff.
>
> *Thank you for all you do each and every day.*

The Qualities That Differentiate the Nursing Department and Stepping Up to Help Others

One of the factors that differentiates nursing from other departments is the affinity nurses develop with the patients. It is not just about the numbers of cases or figures of the deceased; the relationship between the patient and nurse and the journey they go through together become a story. And it is these stories that end up providing valuable lessons for others.

Flexibility and adaptability became of utmost importance during the pandemic. At SBH Health System, the Addiction Medicine Unit and one of two psychiatric units were closed with plans to convert them to medical units in preparation for the expectant rise in COVID-19 patients. Not only did this severely impact those significantly struggling with mental health who were being treated in these units, but it impacted the nursing staff as well. Nursing staff who had previously worked in behavioral health or addiction were now being reassigned to medicine. Instead of complaining or arguing about the truly significant changes to their careers, they went willingly, knowing the vast contributions everybody was making to help tackle this huge health crisis.

The Mandate to Expand Patient Capacity by 50%

Processes Undertaken to Review Nursing Units and Their Capacity/Services

As the need for increased capacity started to overwhelm, Governor Cuomo issued a mandate to increase patient capacity by 50%. Following this, a process was undertaken to review nursing units, their capacities, and services. This was a collaborative process between physicians, nurses, respiratory therapists, radiology, laboratory, pharmacy, facilities, IT, purchasing, the supply chain department, and others. There were three ways to expand the bed capacity of a hospital: the first was doubling single rooms or tripling the double rooms, the second was reopening closed units, and the third was repurposing already active areas. In some cases, a second bed could be added to a room, as long as there were sufficient utilities. This was often the case at magnet hospitals where there were many spacious, private rooms. However, since most of the rooms at SBH Health System were already double rooms with limited capacity for expansion, other solutions had to be explored. There were a number of services and units in the hospital that had been shut down due to the pandemic, such as the sleep lab. Some units had been converted to offices in the past. Other units were still in use such as the detox unit, but they were designated possible targets to create space and relieve pressure on the already overloaded critical care areas.

Collaboration During a Healthcare Crisis Is Vital

The nursing department was challenged to get the new units 'patient ready' within 5–7 days. This could often take weeks or months to be accomplished, as many of which had been shut down for a handful of years. Under this time pressure and in the absence of a specific manual or directive explaining how it could be done, it was vital to form a solid and collaborative team with expert representatives from several departments, including nursing, pharmacy, facilities, IT, purchasing, and housekeeping. Pharmacy was in charge of setting up a machine called Pyxis – an automated medication dispensing system – in every unit and ensuring that appropriate medications were in place. Facilities were responsible for electrical and structural repairs. IT identified where Pyxis machines, workstations, and computers would be needed and positioned and ensured that hookups and lines were in place. Since every unit had a supply room, supply chain and materials management worked feverishly to either find carts or match supplies from a similar unit, ensuring that each unit was equipped with sufficient equipment, stock, and PPE. Housekeeping ensured beds were obtained and that patient rooms and the nursing stations were cleaned and ready for occupancy. By being on location at the same time, the whole team developed an extremely well-organized and coordinated approach and was able to provide the necessary input which resulted in the rapid opening of these units.

In the beginning, almost every patient was a critical care patient. Initially, the hospital had just one ten-bed medical ICU unit and one six-bed surgical ICU unit. However, the hospital soon realized that the patient demand was increasing. Three new ICUs were created, which expanded ICU bed capacity by over 500%. Despite this significant increase in capacity, the nursing staff soon learned that having additional and separate ICUs in different areas made it difficult to staff, supply, and keep track of patients. Learning from the first surge of the pandemic and in anticipation of a second, the hospital leaders decided to create ICU-ready areas with central monitoring.

Increasing bed capacity was a significant achievement, but it also meant that equipment availability had to be expanded in parallel. Ventilator capacity increased substantially, and in parallel, so did the need for IV pumps, feeding pumps, sedation and paralytic medications, cardiac monitors and pulse oximeters, additional suction catheters, suction regulators, oxygen regulators, proning pillows, and additional oxygen tanks. In the beginning, a lot of time was spent on making sure there was enough PPE for all units. The need for IV pumps to regulate critical care medications, sedation, and analgesia became so dire at one point that the hospital ended up reaching out to nursing homes to borrow IV tubing with flow regulators, to help free up IV pumps that were needed for the more critical medications. The nursing leadership spent a lot of time collaborating with the supply chain department and clinical engineering.

The ethics committee, which the nursing leadership was a part of, created a "ventilator triage committee" to help with addressing issues related to ventilator shortages, if this should arise. All patients were scored using the SOFA (Sequential Organ Failure Assessment – see further details in the Chap. 5) calculator. SBH did successfully trial ventilator sharing and bi-level positive airway pressure (BIPAP) machine conversion to ventilators should such contingency arise.

How Nursing Staff Were Impacted and What SBH Health System Did About It

Changes in Nursing Staff Ratios and the Ethical Issues of "Price Gouging" When Obtaining Agency COVID-19 Crisis Workers

Despite the significant and rapid (within a day) change in nurse-to-patient ratio from roughly 1:6 up to 1:12, the daily huddles provided enormous support in enabling this transition to happen as smoothly as possible. Alongside huddles, the psychiatry and pastoral care departments stepped up to provide much needed moral support to the nursing staff who were starting to experience burnout, physical fatigue, and mental exhaustion. With the much sicker patients, ICU nurses, who normally care for one or two patients at a time, became part of a care team that cared for five or six patients. The teams – consisting of an ICU nurse, a med-surg nurse, ancillary nursing staff, and physicians – worked together in spite of the challenging circumstances, and even though some weren't trained in specific tasks, everybody stepped up to help and support each other. One of the key roles in helping these critically ill patients was respiratory therapy. Pre-COVID-19, the hospital utilized 18–20 ventilators a day. During the pandemic, up to approximately 100 ventilators were being used, resulting in a dramatic need for additional respiratory therapists.

The challenge of SBH Health System being a standalone hospital and not part of a large multihospital health system was that it wasn't possible to just pull nursing staff from other hospitals. SBH Health System was purely relying on agency nursing staffing. Under these desperate and overburdened situations, this ultimately led to price gouging. As hospitals started to compete on access to resources, the hourly rate for an ICU nurse soared to three times the pre-COVID-19 hourly rate. Not only was SBH Health System a one-hospital system, but it was also a safety net hospital that cared, with tight budgets, for a very large number of Medicaid patients. Lacking a strong financial backbone meant it wasn't possible to compete with other hospitals for nursing staff during the pandemic. The market was extremely fluid, and even after acquiring agency nurses for 8- or 12-week contracts, it was difficult to keep them since many would cancel their contracts and chase rapidly increasing rates offered by other hospitals. Eventually, the hospital had to offer the same rates and worry about the budget deficits at a later time.

After the worst part of the pandemic started to ease, the demand for agency nursing staffing settled, and nurses who had left their secure jobs ended up either returning to their jobs or searching for new ones. For the majority of dedicated nurses, many of whom had been working at SBH Health System for 20, 30, and some 40 years, the biggest resource the hospital had – the "extended family-like," caring and nurturing environment – prevented them from leaving.

Challenges Associated with Retraining Senior and Junior Nursing Staff Under a Pandemic

Not only was cost a factor associated with agency workers, but there was a significant amount of administrative onboarding work that had to be done in order to clear them for work (basic employee health, criminal background checks, orientation, training, among other things). What usually would have been a week-long orientation ended up being expedited and completed in 1 or 2 days, with basic instruction on computer systems and equipment so that the new nurses could start helping care for patients as quickly as possible. Included in the training was an introduction to all processes such as levels of observations and all the relevant procedures – a significant investment of time, coordination, and organization, with constant 24/7 support and facilitation; all of this was documented.

A previously existing plan was redeveloped and named "crisis orientations," and this, along with "fit testing," an important part of onboarding (and also for all existing nursing staff) – ensuring that N-95 masks fit correctly in order to prevent infection transmission – and cross-training, was all incorporated into the strategy. Over 40 people were trained to be part of the mobile proning teams (see more details in the chapter on proning and respiratory therapy).

The Critical Role of Nursing Leadership in Mentally Supporting Nursing Staff

The hallmark of being a nurse is being a patient advocate. The hallmark of being a nurse director is not just being a patient advocate but also an advocate for their nursing staff. Nurse directors often start their shifts early and/or stay after a shift, in order to support nursing staff, answer questions, provide feedback, or offer any other kind of mental support and strength they could to the clinical nursing staff. Nurse directors are department heads and as such have 24/7 responsibility but normally work the day shift, with nursing supervisors physically present on evenings and night shifts. Box 7.3 highlights some key talking points for nursing directors during the pandemic.

To help avoid physical and mental burnout of the nurse directors and the Chief Nursing Officer revised their work schedule, so shifts were staggered, enabling them not only to be visible and present for all shifts 7 days a week but also to provide the directors the opportunity to take 2–3 days off a week. Although they didn't always comply with this schedule, some still coming in on their days off; the initiative was securely in place. Despite some negative feedback about the new working schedule in the beginning, the overall effect it had on the nursing staff was significant, with the knowledge that hospital leadership saw their well-being as a top priority. Even the directors who were initially against the scheduling change felt this was the right decision. As a leader, you have to believe in yourself and trust your judgment. Often, making the right decision is not always the most popular decision.

Not only was the pandemic pressure a huge burden on nursing staff members while on site, but when nursing staff members became sick during the pandemic, this not only impacted available manpower but the anxiety levels of the nursing staff who were able to work. A few members of the nursing staff, many of whom had made invaluable contributions throughout their careers at SBH Health System, sadly perished during the pandemic. The loss of so many patients was demoralizing enough, but the loss of close colleagues impacted the nursing staff heavily. Alongside dealing with their working environment anguish, nursing staff members were also trying to protect family members at home, and many chose not to see their family for several months due to the risk and fear of transmission. The likelihood that PTSD now exists among the hospital community as a result of these considerable and compounded pressures is high.

Box 7.3 An Example of Talking Points Given to the Nursing Directors During the Pandemic
Informational Points

- At the start of COVID outbreak, the Governor of New York directed all hospitals to increase their bed capacity by >50%, which means we opened 5 additional units and added 95 new beds. So, nursing staff has had a much greater patient assignment than they normally would.
  - We received no additional nursing staff from the NYC, NY State, or the Federal Government or 1199.
  - SBH on our own had to execute 15 contracts with nursing staffing agencies at "crisis pay rates" to try and recruit ICU nurses, ED nurses, vent trained nurses, and respiratory therapists:

    This week, we have 13 nurses (3 ICU and 7 ED) and 15 per diem respiratory therapists onboarding.
    Next week, we have 12 more nurses (5 ED and 7 ICU) onboarding.

  - We have had a >15% sick call rate, not counting the employees who tested + and were out on quarantine.
  - To provide greater support and guidance to the nursing staff, the nurse directors have been working staggering shifts to cover 6 am–12 am, 7 days a week since April 5.
  - PPE: We have a good supply of PPE now. In the beginning, we never knew when our next delivery would come, so it was important to conserve PPE, but we were never without PPE:

    Masks are now being replaced as needed and at least every day.
    We are tight on gowns but expect a delivery this week.
    Nursing staff are seeing different gowns, masks, etc. weekly, because we are getting it from many different vendors, but it is all approved PPE.

- Early on, we asked 1199 to allow us to change the med-surg floors to 12-hour shifts; they could not come to an agreement to do so.
- We offered an increased pay incentive for nursing staff, double time for all overtime worked, but we are still waiting for 1199 to sign the agreement.
- The good news is 14 patients who were intubated on ventilators have been discharged, and we have discharged a total of 448 COVID-positive patients.

Education, Education, Education

The Role of Hospital-Wide Nursing Education, Refresher Training, Retraining, and Adhering to CDC Guidelines

After the pandemic hit, the nursing education department was responsible for creating basic isolation training for all hospital nursing staff – including nonclinical departments such as finance and registration – so that everybody understood how vital basic hygiene (handwashing) and wearing a mask was (mask use was tracked; see Table 7.1). Even though many of the nonclinical roles moved to working remotely, the education system was still crucial in managing response of all

Table 7.1 Mask count and record used to track all mask usage
Mask Count and Record Log

Date:_____ Unit:_____

Due to the national shortage of masks, and our need to protect our nursing staff now and in the weeks to come, we need to account for every mask.

Name	Role	Procedure mask count	Procedure mask with shield Count	N-95 Count	Reason	Prior mask returned
					1-assigned to unit (nursing and resident nursing staff)	
						1-yes
					2-assigned to airborne isolation patient (N-95)	2-no
						3-not provided, explain why
					3-mask contaminated	
					4-doing a procedure with risk of splash (shield)	
					5-doing a procedure with risk of aerosolization (N-95)	

nursing staff to the pandemic. As the pandemic developed, so too did the guidelines emerging from the Centers for Disease Control and Prevention (CDC) and New York State Department of Health (NYSDOH), as the understanding of how the virus spread changed from contact and droplet only to airborne and then both. The CDC and NYSDOH did a good job of keeping the department updated via daily calls, enabling a simple route of communicating new information to the nursing staff.

Alongside these aforementioned streams of education, refresher courses were also a significant part of responding to the pandemic; some psychiatric nurses who had previously worked in medicine and surgery more than 20 years ago had to now learn how to do this again.

Initially, most of the education happened via safety calls, huddles, or in-service sessions. Hands-on learning also played a huge role, allowing more experienced members from the nursing education department to train others in the use of new equipment. Coping with the volume of new nursing staff and new equipment in daily operation was only made possible because of the incredible coordination and communication displayed by the nursing staff in the education department. As the pandemic situation worsened and nursing staff became increasingly overwhelmed and short of time, the e-learning platform – "HealthStream" – became a vital tool in communicating new information and providing training in the most effective way.

As the crisis worsened, many noncritical care nurses and doctors were cross-trained in critical care. Dental residents, perioperative nurses, and residents, among others, were trained in skills they previously had no experience with: EMR documentation, phlebotomy, and the difficult task of transporting deceased patients to the morgue, the latter having substantial impact on the nursing staff. Acknowledging the willingness of all members of nursing staff to learn new skills and get stuck in during the pandemic is vital, since the capacity to cope would have been severely compounded without them.

Morale, Engagement, and Support

The Importance of Keeping Morale Up and Nursing Staff Engaged and Committed During Difficult Times

The devastation caused by a crisis such as the COVID-19 pandemic is widespread among the community and especially among the healthcare workers who have been directly involved in dealing with huge volumes of cases. Having mostly never experienced anything to this extent previously, nursing staff morale dipped quickly on dealing with the daily chaos and seeing the unexpected mass fatality the crisis brought with it. Understanding the immediate and crucial need for support was recognized by the senior nursing leadership and directors. They did their utmost to provide a solid foundation for their valued nursing staff members to lean on, 24/7. One of the hardest parts of the pandemic for many was having to make that phone call to the family member to say, "I am sorry." In the instance that a care provider felt overwhelmed, the directors would assist or ask another care provider to provide postmortem care to a deceased patient. If the member of nursing staff who had been caring for that person was simply unable to do so, another was found who could manage:

> I would work all day here with the team and go home and even on the way home or in the morning or during the night you would constantly hear the sirens from ambulances. I would not sleep because all I could hear was the sirens. Once COVID-19 subsided, those sounds lessened; but every time I heard a siren again, I would think 'oh my god, another person!'. Then you would count fingers and I remembered reflecting on how sad it was that the whole city completely succumbed to this.

Making sure individuals were fed on a regular and timely basis was important to keep energy and morale up, but also to show how appreciated the nursing staff were, not just by the hospital but also by the community. Donations were made by many community restaurants on Arthur Avenue in the Bronx, by the Girl Scouts, by the NY Mets and NY Yankees, and by Lizzo, the pop star who was from the Bronx. The cafeteria stayed open 24/7 in order to accommodate the hospital healthcare workers. The hospital also provided 3 months' worth of free parking for its healthcare workers; every little helps. One member of nursing staff brought in 24 roses one day, one for each member of the nursing staff. On April 10, 2020, the nursing staff started to play a song every time a COVID-19 patient was discharged to let everyone know they were making a difference, that patients were surviving and going home. The first song was written specifically for SBH Health System by a local musician.

Known as a hospital system with a "huge heart," SBH Health System revealed its true strength during the pandemic as people pulled together on so many levels to provide support and show how strong their teamwork was. Whether it was a smile, a joke, or just simply breathing together, the nursing leadership and the individual nursing staff members formed an immense and very special bond.

Reflection and Lessons Learned

It wouldn't be productive to emerge from such a devastating situation without engaging in some sort of reflective practice, contemplating how things could have been done better and how they might be done, should a health crisis occur again. Here are some perspectives from the nursing staff at SBH Health System:

- Your nursing staff are your greatest and most important resource; take extra good care of your nursing staff at the beginning of a crisis. Outside resources may not happen, but what you have is your surest resource. Take extra good care of it, protect it, nurture it, organize it, and utilize it efficiently.
- Engage psychiatric and pastoral care support early in a crisis to provide the most optimal level of mental support to anyone and everyone.

- Cross-training of general medical/surgical nurses in critical care can create a very valuable much needed contingency workforce during a crisis. Giving general medical/surgical nurses initial cross-training and subsequent periodic refresher training in critical care can help nursing staff expand ICUs during a crisis:

  > Always remain humble and humane, and never ask someone to do something you would not do yourself.

Case Study: Stepping up to Support the Whole Team

At one point during the pandemic, the Chief Nursing Officer (CNO) was pulled in to help move deceased patients. Here is his narrative:

> Once the morgue had reached full capacity, the New York City Office of Emergency Management (OEM) sent us a refrigerated tractor trailer to store bodies in. After about a week or so, we also reached capacity in that with 76 bodies. OEM delivered a second truck but told us we had to build two levels of shelving in the new truck, then move the bodies from truck 1 to truck 2, and build shelving in truck 1. Our facility management team built the shelves. I gathered a group of transporters and security guards and told them we needed to move the 76 bodies from truck 1 into the truck 2 with the shelves. I explained what had to be done and offered everyone the opportunity to be excused if they didn't feel able to help. Every single person volunteered to help. Remember, they were moving patients who had died of COVID-19. They had to wear full protection and lift the bodies, weighing anywhere from 100lbs to over 300lbs. As we began, I also helped moved the bodies. Some of the workers looked shocked and asked why I was doing this as a Senior VP, and I shared with them that my first job in my career was as a transporter and as a leader now; I would never ask them to do anything I wouldn't do myself. After 5 hours of moving the bodies, Dr. Perlstein, our CEO, came out and thanked everyone for helping and then purchased pizza and soda for the team.

Summary

In the face of a healthcare crisis, leadership and teamwork are at the core of survival. SBH Health System is a standalone hospital that lacked the financial strength needed to access highly priced agency nursing staff workers. Dealing with a very tired, understaffed, and stressed workforce and grappling with an insufficient supply of beds, ventilators, and other necessary equipment to take care of the huge influx of critically ill patients meant that the hospital had to find alternate methods to stay afloat, including reopening old wards and creating new ICUs and retraining non-critical nurses from other departments. All of this would have been implausible without the strong pillar of support that was provided by the nursing leadership, providing mental decompression outlets and multiple daily communications, among others. Despite the utter tragedy that has occurred, nursing staff emerged with a new set of tools, skills, and awareness, should they ever find themselves in such a dire situation again.

Chapter 8
Clinical Nutrition and Food Services

Cecilia Moy

Clinical Nutrition Services

> Let food be thy medicine and medicine be thy food. Hippocrates (400 BC).

Clinical nutrition services within acute care hospitals focuses on the prevention and treatment of disease with diet. Clinical nutrition is an essential aspect of healthcare, because it often involves bedside management of nutrition through individualized dietary recommendations and interventions to match patient needs right through to counseling services for outpatient recovery.

The components of clinical nutrition services in SBH Health System are twofold consisting of the diet office operation and clinical nutrition care. The functions of diet office operation are related to patient diet order transcriptions and meal ticket preparations as per physician's orders. These are coordinated via the interface between the two computer systems – Allscripts electronic medical record (EMR) and CBORD meal service systems. These systems integrate open-platform solutions with nutritional analysis and diet planning, connecting the healthcare workers and bringing all data sources together to improve efficiency of patient care.

Specific clinical nutritional care is performed by a registered dietitian and consists of a full comprehensive nutrition assessment for nutritional need evaluation, therapeutic diet education, and determining the patient's nutritional risk level, setting therapeutic goals and treatment plans for the patient. The care is ongoing and will continue during the patient's hospital stay. All clinical service lines are supported by the registered dietitians providing inpatient nutrition care to patients who are deemed at nutritional risk during admission or hospital stays in all medical, surgical, and critical care units. Likewise, they provide outpatient nutritional care

---

C. Moy (✉)
Department of Food and Nutrition, SBH Health System, Bronx, NY, USA
e-mail: cmoy@sbhny.org

including educational support to adults with chronic disease, pediatrics, and prenatal patients in the ambulatory settings.

In some cases, it may be sufficient for patients to receive broad recommendations such as the Dietary Guidelines for Americans (developed by the US Departments of Health and Human Services and Agriculture) [1] or those of the American Heart Association [2]. However, in complex multifactorial and chronic diseases with special concerns or risk factors, consultation with a registered dietitian is appropriate. Indeed, the role of clinical nutrition services is emphasized in the care of chronic diseases. This is highlighted by studies which demonstrate the effectiveness of clinical nutrition services improving the health outcome of the patient's disease through active intervention in the treatment of in-patients [3, 4].

Clinical Nutrition Delivery

The preferred route of nutrition provision is through oral consumption. However, critical illness is often associated with systemic inflammatory response coupled with catabolic stress and other disease-related complications. Some critically ill patients may experience problems with eating or digestion, such as loss of appetite or gastrointestinal (GI) intolerance, and unable to consume adequately to meet their anticipated nutritional needs. In these cases, it is sometimes necessary to provide nutrition with artificial formulated food which ensures the provision of the right balance of key nutritional fats, proteins, carbohydrates, vitamins, and minerals. The delivery of these artificial preparations can be achieved in two main ways (Fig. 8.1).

Enteral nutrition therapy is preferred for patients with functional GI tract, but their volitional intake is insufficient to meet their anticipated nutritional needs. Nutrition is delivered directly into the gut through a feeding tube and to be absorbed via the normal absorption mechanism. This is the preferred way of delivering nutritional support due to factors such as comparative ease of application, less risk of complications, and cost. In some patients who can tolerate oral diets, rather than feeding through a feeding tube, oral medial nutrition products can be provided to boost nutritional intake in addition to the regular meals if the patient is able to manage. The formulated enteral nutritional products are designed to provide adequate calories, protein, fats, carbohydrates, vitamins, and minerals based on the recommended daily intake (RDI). Certain enteral nutrition products also contain specialized nutrients, such as the peptide-based amino acids, arginine and omega-3 fatty acids in the form of DHA/EPA to promote anabolism and immune support. In the event when patient illness prevents consumption of food or drink, enteral nutrition may have to be delivered into the gut through a tube via a feeding pump which is to regulate the feeding rate [5].

When a patient is at high nutritional risk, severely malnourished and enteral feeding route is not feasible due to hemodynamic instability, escalating vasopressor support or significant GI intolerance; alternatively, the use of *parenteral nutrition* is

Parenteral and enteral nutrition

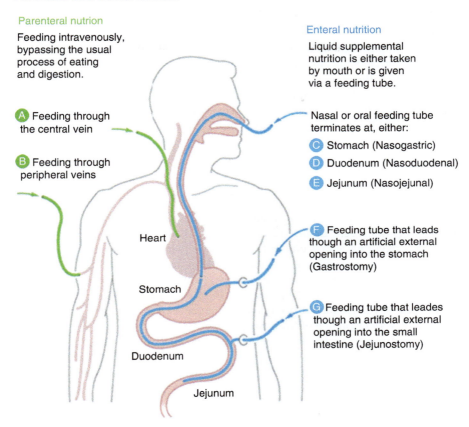

Fig. 8.1 Clinical nutrition can be delivered in several different ways, that can be divided into two main types; enteral and parenteral nutrition. (Image with permission from the Crohn's & Colitis Foundation, www.crohnscolitisfoundation.org)

indicated. With parenteral nutrition, nutrition in the form of amino acids, dextrose, and fat emulsion along with vitamins, minerals, and electrolytes is being delivered directly into the blood stream bypassing the gastrointestinal tract digestion and absorption. These specially formulated products containing specific nutritional requirements are slowly infused into the blood stream via a drip through a central venous line. Large veins near the heart (upper arm, chest, or neck) are usually selected to reduce venous irritation. Parenteral nutrition can also be delivered through the peripheral lines using formulary products with lower osmolarity under 900mOsmol/L if the central line is unavailable to be used. Parenteral nutrition patients need intensive monitoring and sterile technique as sometimes blood infections or biochemical abnormalities can occur [5].

Expanding Nutrition Services: Strategic Planning Aligning with the Challenges During the Evolving COVID-19 Crisis

During the rapid surge of incoming COVID-19 patients, many were critically ill requiring ventilation therapy and enteral tube feedings. These patients were at high acuity level of illness needing intensive nutrition therapy. Their needs for critical service were well above the normal routine care causing a high demand of clinical nutrition professionals for COVID-19 management needs.

Staffing

The biggest challenge that the department faced was how to maintain adequate staffing to provide the same high-quality care and to meet the nutrition service demands of critical care, despite the rapid rise of patient census, increasing numbers of patients requiring high acuity of care, and meanwhile dealing with staff outage due to virus exposure and/or quarantine. Another issue was how to protect the staff from the virus while performing their work duties, particularly during the PPE shortage in the beginning of the pandemic. To resolve these staffing situations and to minimize any potential adverse impact on patient care, several key actions were taken at the very beginning of the crisis.

The department obtained an additional dietitian from a local agency to provide clinical coverage secondary to the increased patient load and clinical staff outage. It was possible to recruit additional clinical dietitians from noncritical areas, such as the bariatric program, and cross-trained noncritical care dietitians, such as those situated in the outpatient clinic and renal dialysis center. This greatly assisted the critical care coverage that was needed.

Telecommuting was set up to allow work from home rotations for all dietitians. This meant half of the dietitians would work from home, while the other half would work on site to reduce the number of dietitians in the office for proper physical distancing and to minimize the risk of virus exposure. Daily tasks were reassigned for on-site and off-site dietitians to ensure all required tasks were addressed and shared among the dietitians. All face-to-face interactions would be handled by on-site dietitians. Of these tasks, outpatient virtual consultations were transferred to a telehealth nutrition service mode of delivery allowing continuity of service while reducing patient contact.

Complementing this, a telecommuting communication system between dietitians, diet office staff, and the unit healthcare team was put in place via telephone and secure privacy-compliant work emails to ensure collaboration and clear lines of communication. During the early stage of pandemic when the PPE supplies were limited, the dietitians mostly relied on EMR and other healthcare team members, including doctors and nurses, for the needed information in addition to phone "visits" to patient room for phone interview and education purposes.

Despite these important actions being implemented, the biggest challenge in staffing was related to the schedule of the inpatient dietitians telecommuting from home. A few dietitians often called out or requested time off during their on-site assignments causing an imbalanced work force to handle the on-site clinical duties. This resulted in adding extra workload and stress to the on-site dietitians. In response to this, the telecommuting ratio between dietitians was adjusted to ensure adequate on-site staffing to handle the required in-person clinical duties. This decision came from management and was respected as one of fairness to team members. At the same time, for staff protection, Flexi-Glass dividers were installed in the office between dietitian's desks.

Critical Care Expansion and Room Revisions

To accommodate the rapid increase of census during the health crisis surge and to ensure a smooth flow of patient information, namely, diet order transcriptions, food allergies, and preferences to the currently used meal system, the hospital quickly set up new units, expanded the existing units and bed capacity, and interfaced the patient information from the facility's electronic medical record system into the CBORD meal service system. Some general medical/surgical and behavioral units were converted to house the influx of COVID-19 patients as well as to add new units by converting other areas, such as ambulatory surgery, cardiac lab, and endoscopy, into temporary intensive care units. With close collaborations between the two departments – nutrition services and information technology – the entire process of adding more beds, rooms, and units to the CBORD meal service system and the interface between the two EMR and CBORD systems were smooth and successful.

Supply Chain and Procurement

The supply chain and procurement were a huge concern very early in the pandemic as the critically ill COVID-19 patient admissions were increasing at an alarming rate. Many of these patients often developed acute respiratory distress syndrome (ARDS), required ventilator support, and were placed on artificial nutrition, mostly enteral nutrition or parenteral nutrition. The need for tube feedings skyrocketed to at least five times of the usual usage, causing high consumption and shortages in both feeding pumps and enteral feeding products.

As the feeding pumps were at high demand at that time, during the period of late March to April 2020, the hospital soon experienced feeding pump shortage due to the sheer number of tube-fed patients accelerating far beyond the number of feeding pumps available in house. As the department and supply chain reached out to the suppliers and vendors for additional pumps, it was realized the issue of feeding pumps had grown beyond the local area. Numerous inquiries from other in- and out-of-state facilities were observed, asking for pumps. It became a nationwide issue secondary to the rapid surge of COVID-19 patients requiring intubations and tube feedings around the country.

While the supply chain was out to compete with multiple other healthcare systems for additional feeding pumps and tubes, with joint effort, the clinical nutrition team along with the critical care team developed a strategic plan to review the feeding pump utilization, should the number of tube-fed patients exceed the number of feeding pumps available in-house. This inevitably could have led to very difficult decisions to be made by healthcare workers on the frontline. The goal, however, was to prioritize and reserve the feeding pumps for the most needed and most vulnerable patients. The guidance within SBH was that during the feeding pump shortage, the feeding pumps were to be reserved for critically ill patients who had not yet stabilized and/or for those patients who had not yet developed tolerance to their feeding regimens. For those patients who had been stabilized and feeding tolerance had been established, gravity feeding or intermittent feeding was then used to alleviate the need for feeding pumps when not available. Advance ordering and increased inventory par level for enteral formulary products was put in place along with daily monitoring on product usages. This allowed projections for need to be made in a timely fashion, and plans were established for minimizing the impact of shortages. Gravity feeding instructions and chart information were provided to nursing staff which included the product name and number of drips per minute per product. Through early planning and forecasting, supply chain was successfully able to recruit additional pumps, quickly bringing the total number of available feeding pumps to 90 pumps in-house.

In addition to the necessity for an increased number of feeding pumps, the need for enteral feeding products also increased drastically as a secondary effect of the rapid surge of patients requiring alternate route of enteral nutrition. There were months long back orders and shortages on certain high-demand products, such as the peptide-based high-protein formulas utilized for critical care patients. To ensure product availability, we strategically changed the enteral product procurement practices from weekly ordering to advance ordering with daily monitoring on product usage, inventory, and usage projections based on actual orders.

Par level on the most commonly used products was increased with the aim of keeping at least 1 month worth of supplies on hand at all times. Despite this effort, in late March and early April 2020, demands for certain enteral products were far exceeding the manufacturing pace causing frequent back orders on common widely used products during the pandemic surge. To manage the back-order situation and to ensure product availability, products in different package sizes or other nutrient comparable products were utilized to minimize any impact on a patient's nutritional care. This "product replacement" was carefully undertaken by the clinical nutrition department and greatly extended the ability to provide continuity in nutritional care to the growing number of critically ill patients. Table 8.1 summarized the various measures taken during the health crisis to address potential shortages of nutritional needs of critically ill patients.

Table 8.1 Challenges and solutions of critical care nutrition demands during a health crisis

Item	Challenge	Solution
Feeding pumps and feeding tubes	Shortage due to high demand by critically ill patients	Feeding pumps to be prioritized for those who were unstable and/or those whose feeding tolerance had not yet been established Gravity feeding for those who were stable and their feeding tolerance had been established
Nutrition products	Shortages	Advanced ordering Daily monitoring of usage and inventory Frequent adjustment of need projections Product replacement strategies Inventory par level increase to at least 1 month based on actual usage data analysis

Specific Nutrition Challenges in Managing COVID-19 Disease

Nutritional Guidelines

For clinical nutrition services, educational and practice guidance resources on COVID-19 and their impact on patient nutrition were scarce and rarely available particularly in the very beginning of the crisis. The most common concerns were related to muscle atrophy, weakness, difficulty of weaning the patients from the ventilators, and out-of-range laboratory values related to the hyper-inflammatory disease state and the metabolic responses. Many of the COVID-19 patients presented signs of malnutrition, such as muscle weakness, and did not respond well to the routine enteral feeding regimens. The prolonged illness prior to hospital admission might have played a role in this. Some of the main COVID-19 symptoms such as fever, difficulty in breathing, vomiting, diarrhea, etc. often lead to poor oral intake of nutrition and dehydration, which in turn might have led to catabolism and malnutrition before hospital admission. Since most patients admitted to the hospital had some degree of sepsis and also required mechanical ventilation, the clinical nutrition team chose to follow the ASPEN 2016 Critical Care Guidelines for Sepsis and ARDS [6]. These guidelines advise using high-protein, hypocaloric regimens with a peptide-based formula as a safe start for newly admitted patients with such a condition as COVID-19 who required enteral nutrition feedings.

As knowledge of the disease was rapidly evolving, professional groups, such as the Academy of Nutrition and Dietetics, American Society for Parenteral and Enteral Nutrition (ASPEN), Baxter, Abbott Nutrition, and Nestle, became resources for continued guidance and any available clinical resources. Between the months of late March to May 2020, the dietitians at the SBH Health System nutrition department had participated in many COVID-19-related workshops and support groups held by Baxter and Abbott Nutrition. The "Helping Empower Recovery – the Online Series (Heroes)" sponsored by Baxter Healthcare [7] and the online COVID-19 support group discussion sponsored by Abbott Nutrition [8] proved very helpful and informative in providing much insight into the pathology of this disease and nutrition management of it.

In early April 2020, the Society of Critical Care Medicine and ASPEN issued new practice guidelines for managing and delivering the nutritional support for COVID-19 patients. Furthermore, the "Nutrition Therapy in the Patient with COVID-19 Disease Requiring ICU Care" issued by ASPEN in April 2020 provided clear guidelines on nutrition management for COVID-19 patients. Its guiding principles were related to the care of critically ill COVID-19 patients and delivery of nutrition in intensive care units. It focused on cluster care, adherence to the Centers for Disease Control and Prevention (CDC) recommendations to minimize exposure and transmission, and the correct use of PPE. It outlined the recommendations for key aspects of nutritional support including:

- Nutrition assessment.
- Timing of nutrition delivery
- Route, tube placement, and method of nutrition delivery
- Nutrition dose, advancing to goal and adjustments
- Formula selection
- Monitoring nutrition tolerance
- Nutrition for the patient undergoing prone positioning
- Nutrition therapy during ECMO

The ASPEN guidelines were detailed and specific in each of its recommendations. The clinical nutrition team employed these ASPEN recommendations for in-house nutrition practices in managing the special needs and challenges faced by the COVID-19 patients. Box 8.1 highlights the nutritional observations of COVID-19 patients.

Box 8.1. The Most Common Nutritional Concerns Observed Among the COVID-19 Patients
- Poor oral intake due to the prolonged illness prior to hospital admission which could potentially lead to protein-calorie malnutrition and micronutrient deficiencies.
- Catabolic state – due to severe inflammation and increased protein needs to fight the infections, the body turned to muscle mass for energy leading to increasing lean muscle loss.
- Decrease in muscle strength and functional level related to inadequate oral intake to support the increased protein needs and the prolonged inactivity during illness.
- Possible dehydration if patients exhibited symptoms of fever, vomiting, and/or diarrhea.
- Abnormal laboratory values related to the illness – such as hyperglycemia, hypernatremia, hyperphosphatemia/hypophosphatemia, elevated lactate dehydrogenase, hyperkalemic/hypokalemic.

In May 2020, the Academy of Nutrition and Dietetics Evidence Analysis Center issued further nutrition guidelines on managing COVID-19 patients. It focused on the importance of nutrition screening and assessment of malnutrition in COVID-19 patients. Other recommendations were aligned with the previous ASPEN guidelines and recommendations. Taken together, these comprehensive guidelines allowed a high level of patient care.

The Need for PPE

With the limited supply in the beginning of pandemic, to preserve the PPE, the dietitians were often not entering the COVID-19 patient rooms. Rather, the dietitians relied on other providers, such as the physicians and nurses to collect the nutritional data, the patient's EMR to collect the assessment data, and calling the patient or family to perform data collection and/or education. The dietitians then documented the findings, collaborated and coordinated with the patient's healthcare team to develop a safe, feasible nutrition intervention strategy plan. This was an adopted practice wherever possible; however, in some cases where in-room support was necessary, the full recommended PPE measures were undertaken.

The SBH Health System Nutritional Response

During a critical care contingency meeting in May 2020, the critical care physicians raised questions pertaining to the chronicity of the disease and clarified that muscle atrophy was identified as an issue causing difficulties in weaning COVID-19 patients off mechanical ventilation. The clinical nutrition team was involved in addressing this issue by emphasizing early nutritional intervention and education to the healthcare providers on nutrition management for COVID-19 patients. Key strategy is highlighted in Box 8.2.

Box 8.2. Key Actions to Address Nutritional Needs of COVID-19 Patients
- Collaboration with the hospital IT department to set up daily printout reports providing a list of patients admitted to the hospital with a COVID-19-positive diagnosis. This report was set up in tableau available to the dietitians and other healthcare providers. The dietitians would review the COVID-19 printout report to identify the newly admitted COVID-19-positive patients for timely assessment and intervention. This included patients on oral, enteral, and parenteral nutrition regimens.
- Creation of a revised nutrition risk screen which added COVID-19-positive diagnosis to the nutrition high-risk list and therefore necessitated the

patient to be visited by a dietitian within 48 hours of admission. Oral nutrition supplement would be recommended for COVID-19 patients as part of the medical interventions provided.
- Development of an education module in the hospital education portal – HealthStream – on "Nutrition Therapy for COVID-19 Patients" to address the ASPEN guideline recommendations for all healthcare providers including physicians and dietitians to access.
- Creation of a poster on nutrition therapy for managing COVID-19 placed in each COVID-19 unit to serve as a reference for the healthcare providers. Likewise, a pocket size mini post card was created for the physicians to be easily carried in the pocket to allow easy access to critical nutritional information.

Enteral Nutrition Provision

For the enteral nutrition product selection, SBH chose to use a peptide-based, high-protein (more than 20%) product along with Omega-3 Fatty Acids in the form of DHA/EPA to reduce oxidation injury and attenuate inflammatory response while the peptide-based formula aided in GI tolerance. In addition, arginine supplementation was frequently used on the COVID-19 patients for its anti-inflammatory functions in T&B cell production and reduction in cytokine production, while the use of arginine in sepsis is still controversial. Vital and Pivot were commonly used products for the COVID patients while on enteral nutrition feedings. The commonly used oral supplement was Ensure Enlive for containing HMB (calcium β-hydroxy-β-methylbutyrate) to promote muscle health or Ensure High Protein for its high-protein hypocaloric content.

One particular challenge was the use of enteral nutrition feeding during prone positioning that feeding patients during pronging was inconsistent. Feeding often stopped while the patient undergoing prone positioning causing underfeeding. The requirement for pronging may last for a day or up to weeks, and duration of each pronging would last for hours. Not feeding patient while in prone positioning could translate to underfeeding leading to increased risk of malnutrition. The clinical nutrition team would continue the effort of coordinating with physicians to consider the use of other means, such as prokinetic agents, post-pyloric feeding if necessary to maintain the patient's nutritional status during this time.

Parenteral Nutrition Provision

For the parenteral nutrition provision, higher-protein and lower dextrose formulas were available for patients meeting the high-protein hypocaloric ASPEN nutrition recommendations. To do this, SBH used a central line formula consisting of 8%

amino acid and 10% dextrose (80 grams protein/100 grams Dextrose per 1000 ml). Peripheral formula contained 4.25% amino acid and 5% dextrose (42.5 grams protein/50 grams Dextrose per 1000 ml). Additionally, the fat emulsion formula was changed from Intralipid, which is constituted of 100% Soy based Omega-6 fatty acids and considered potentially pro-inflammatory and immunosuppressive, to Clinolipid, which is composed of comparatively 80% of Olive based Omega-9 fatty acid which is known to be inflammatory-neutral and cause less interference with normal inflammatory response. These changes were ultimately made to further reduce inflammation.

Additional Nutrient Requirements

There were many discussions about the use of certain micronutrients and antioxidants, such as vitamins A, D, and C and zinc, and their functions in immune response. Vitamin D was of particular interest related to its impact on COVID-19 patients and the findings that worse outcomes in-patients with COVID-19 were seen in those with lower circulating levels of vitamin D metabolites [9]. Indeed, Vitamin D has known potent antimicrobial and anti-inflammatory effects in vitro [10], and specifically, vitamin D metabolites also have direct action on angiotensin-converting enzyme 2 (ACE2) upregulating expression in pulmonary microvascular endothelial cells in animal models of acute lung injury [11]. As ACE2 is the cell surface entry receptor for SARS-CoV-2, enhanced expression could theoretically increase viral entry into cells. However, it is considered that it may paradoxically have beneficial effects in COVID-19 patients already infected because SARS-CoV-2-mediated downregulation of ACE2 may actually worsen lung injury [12].

Many of these theoretical considerations for the use of micronutrient supplementation were still inconclusive. Of note, the largest published randomized, double-blind, placebo-controlled trial of vitamin D3 administration among hospitalized patients with COVID-19 was unable to show any significant differences between the treated group and the placebo group for factors including hospital length of stay, in-hospital mortality, admission to the intensive care unit, or need for mechanical ventilation [13]. Despite this, at SBH Health System, some COVID-19 patients received the micronutrient cocktails, such as the combination of vitamins C and D and zinc as part of their treatment plan. In these cases, the clinical nutrition team suggested to reassess the benefits and needs of the patients after 2 weeks if micronutrient supplements were given.

Lessons Learned

Many lessons were learned from the SBH response to the initial surge in the health crisis as knowledge of the disease developed. These are summarized in Box 8.3.

Box 8.3. The Key Points for Nutrition Support for Managing COVID-19 Patients
- Start nutrition support and intervention as early as possible with the goal meeting the patient's nutritional needs to prevent further muscle wasting and deterioration.
- If oral intake is inadequate, consider oral nutrition supplementation early.
- As suggested by ASPEN guidelines, most COVID-19 patients will tolerate intragastric enteral nutrition feeding. Sepsis or circulatory shock alone are not a contraindication of trophic feeds, and therefore this should be used in suitable patients.
- Maintain a lower threshold for switching enteral feeding to parenteral feeding. Accordingly, consider early parenteral feeding when enteral feeding is contraindicated, and reverse back to enteral feeding when conditions improve and enteral feeding is once again suitable.
- Supplement enteral feeding with parenteral nutrition if unable to progress enteral feeding to goal in 5–7 days.
- Consider prebiotic fiber or probiotic supplement for the patient once stable.
- There is no firm recommendation for the use of micronutrient supplementation.
- Know the daily intake for protein energy adequacy with the goal to achieve nitrogen balance.

References

1. Dietary Guidelines for Americans: https://www.dietaryguidelines.gov/. Accessed 10 Aug 2021.
2. Eckel RH, Jakicic JM, Ard JD, de Jesus JM, Houston Miller N, Hubbard VS, et al. 2013 AHA/ACC guideline on lifestyle management to reduce cardiovascular risk: a report of the American College of Cardiology/American Heart Association task force on practice guidelines. Circulation. 2014;129(25 Suppl 2):S76–99. https://doi.org/10.1161/01.cir.0000437740.48606.d1.
3. Chima CS, Pollack HA. Position of the American Dietetic Association: nutrition services in managed care. J Am Diet Assoc. 2002;102(10):1471–8. https://doi.org/10.1016/s0002-8223(02)90326-3.
4. Collins J, Porter J. The effect of interventions to prevent and treat malnutrition in patients admitted for rehabilitation: a systematic review with meta-analysis. J Hum Nutr Diet. 2015;28(1):1–15. https://doi.org/10.1111/jhn.12230.
5. Institute of Medicine (US) Committee on Nutrition Services for Medicare Beneficiaries. The role of nutrition in maintaining health in the nation's elderly: evaluating coverage of nutrition services for the medicare population. Washington (DC). 2000.
6. McClave SA, Taylor BE, Martindale RG, Warren MM, Johnson DR, Braunschweig C, et al. Guidelines for the provision and assessment of Nutrition support therapy in the adult critically ill patient: Society of Critical Care Medicine (SCCM) and American Society for Parenteral and Enteral Nutrition (A.S.P.E.N.). JPEN J Parenter Enteral Nutr. 2016;40(2):159–211. https://doi.org/10.1177/0148607115621863.
7. Baxter: https://www.baxterglobal.com/nutrition_hero_series. Accessed 10 Aug 2021.

8. Abbot Nutrition: https://static.abbottnutrition.com/cms-prod/abbottnutrition-2016.com/img/Nutrition%20and%20COVID-19_Abbott%20products%20v2.pdf. Accessed 10 Aug 2021.
9. Ali N. Role of vitamin D in preventing of COVID-19 infection, progression and severity. J Infect Public Health. 2020;13(10):1373–80. https://doi.org/10.1016/j.jiph.2020.06.021.
10. Liu PT, Stenger S, Li H, Wenzel L, Tan BH, Krutzik SR, et al. Toll-like receptor triggering of a vitamin D-mediated human antimicrobial response. Science. 2006;311(5768):1770–3. https://doi.org/10.1126/science.1123933.
11. Xu J, Yang J, Chen J, Luo Q, Zhang Q, Zhang H. Vitamin D alleviates lipopolysaccharide-induced acute lung injury via regulation of the renin-angiotensin system. Mol Med Rep. 2017;16(5):7432–8. https://doi.org/10.3892/mmr.2017.7546.
12. Imai Y, Kuba K, Rao S, Huan Y, Guo F, Guan B, et al. Angiotensin-converting enzyme 2 protects from severe acute lung failure. Nature. 2005;436(7047):112–6. https://doi.org/10.1038/nature03712.
13. Murai IH, Fernandes AL, Sales LP, Pinto AJ, Goessler KF, Duran CSC, et al. Effect of a single high dose of vitamin D3 on hospital length of stay in patients with moderate to severe COVID-19: a randomized clinical trial. JAMA. 2021;325(11):1053–60. https://doi.org/10.1001/jama.2020.26848.

Chapter 9
Rehabilitation

Jovito S. Sabino, Josephine S. Dolera, and Glenn H. Constante

The Initial Response

The initial response within the department of rehabilitation was to identify space or offices that could be converted into hospital rooms. The rehabilitation staff were educated on the proper use of personal protective equipment (PPE) according to the established guidelines by the hospital. Infection control procedures were reviewed most specifically getting in and out of patient rooms, handwashing, use of hand sanitizers, and cleaning of equipment. The rehabilitation stock rooms were arranged to make ample space for additional PPE and cleaning products for staff use. When the first COVID-19 patient was admitted to the hospital in March 2020, things escalated to borderline panic among the rehabilitation staff. The "unknown" nature of the disease made the rehabilitation staff apprehensive in providing the necessary care knowing the risk of potential exposure. The staff were coached according to the standards of infection control making sure they had sufficient supply of PPE to ease their anxiety. The goal was to continue providing rehabilitation services to the patients regardless of their diagnosis even with COVID-19 infection.

Inpatient Bed Management

All hospitals within New York State were mandated by the state governor to increase bed capacity by 50%. As a result, several inpatient offices were converted to additional patient rooms to accommodate two hospital beds. The rehabilitation

---

J. S. Sabino (✉) · J. S. Dolera
Rehabilitation Services, SBH Health System, Bronx, NY, USA
e-mail: jsabino@sbhny.org

G. H. Constante
Physical Therapy, SBH Health System, Bronx, NY, USA

© The Author(s), under exclusive license to Springer Nature
Switzerland AG 2022
R. Shabsigh (ed.), *Health Crisis Management in Acute Care Hospitals*,
https://doi.org/10.1007/978-3-030-95806-0_9

department at SBH Health System was one such space that was considered for this expansion. Several years ago, the space that the rehabilitation department was using had been a patient unit. The hospital administrators once again designated the rehabilitation unit to be accessible for patient use. Prior to the pandemic, the rehabilitation department had a total of six rooms and an entire nurses' station for its use. As a result of the pandemic, the rehabilitation department was downsized to a total of four rooms, and the rehabilitation staff were placed in a single room. This was done to create a new patient unit to accommodate the expansion of the inpatient bed capacity during the COVID-19 surge.

Inpatient Rehabilitation

The rehabilitation full-time staff consisted of one director of rehabilitation, three physical therapists (PT), one physical therapist assistant (PTA), one speech-language pathologist (SLP), two occupational therapists (OT), and one rehab technician. On a routine day, prior to the pandemic, each rehabilitation therapist would see an average of 10–12 patients a day which consisted of evaluation of new patients and the revisits for patient treatment sessions. There were also a number of per diem therapists that would cover the late afternoons. They would cover if the total number of patients needed to be seen by the rehabilitation staff surpassed what was capable of the full-time staff. The rehabilitation department was seeing patients with a broad variety of diagnosis.

At the beginning of the pandemic, rehabilitation consult requests declined across disciplines with the cancellation of elective surgeries. Over the course of a few days, the number of COVID-19 cases exponentially increased. To avoid direct contact and control the transmission of the disease, all departmental and interdisciplinary meetings were held over conference calls, and all in-person interactions were minimized. A decision was made to suspend the student clinical rotations, including those for physical therapy, occupational therapy, and speech-language pathology. Most nonclinical staff were directed to work from home, in order to reduce travel time and minimize risk of potential exposure. Visitors were prohibited within hospital premises. Ambulatory rehabilitation services closed for a few weeks, and staff were reassigned to assist in what was considered essential departments. Any patients who required continued rehabilitation services were transferred in a timely manner. Figure 9.1 shows the weekly rehabilitation census during the peak of the pandemic.

Outpatient Rehabilitation

The outpatient rehabilitation department under Union Community Health Center (Union) consisted of two locations within the Bronx. They averaged about 140 in-person visits per day managed by a total of 11 physical therapists, 6 occupational therapists, and 3 rehab technicians. During the initial surge of COVID-19, the number of patients going to therapy decreased due to their fear of contracting the

9   Rehabilitation

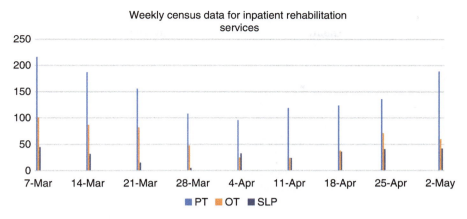

Fig. 9.1 Inpatient rehabilitation census at SBH Health System

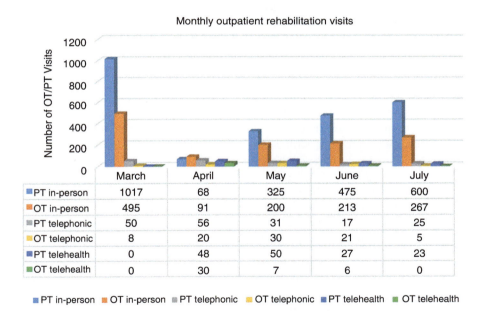

Fig. 9.2 Outpatient rehabilitation census at Union Community Health Center, Bronx, New York, from March 2020 to July 2020. (With permission from Union Community Health Center)

disease. The number of patients in the waiting area and within the workout area/gym had to decrease. The exercise equipment was to be sanitized before and after every use. These guidelines when adhered to offered the staff and the patients a sense of security. Physical and occupational therapists became the principal providers of physical care and had to adjust their workflows to ensure quality care and maintain patient safety. Figure 9.2 shows the outpatient census data for UCHC from March 2020 to July 2020.

Due to the pandemic, telehealth outpatient services became preferable to face-to-face interactions [1]. The transition was not as easy as it sounds. Many challenges were encountered before telehealth was successfully established. Firstly, it was unclear whether any given facility was ready to provide telehealth services. The hospital administration was tirelessly prepping for the telehealth platform and began acquiring electronic orders due to an extensive worldwide demand for telehealth equipment. Secondly, it wasn't sure which platform would be best suited for the practice. It needed to be a single platform that allowed the patients to conveniently connect from personal devices. It was recommended that rehabilitation services carefully review the patient types that would be seen via telehealth and undertake an analysis of the various interactions they will have with these patients in order to make informed decisions on which platform they will choose. In addition, the rehabilitation staff was provided with a checklist to identify the type of patient suitable for telehealth visits. Table 9.1 is an example of patient checklist that is used in outpatient rehabilitation.

Physical rehabilitation had always been a form of healthcare service that required hands-on assessment, and the therapists were perplexed about how to provide the best care via phone. Several passive rehabilitation techniques required direct physical contact and close proximity, but the pandemic challenged rehabilitation professionals to adopt to different modes of delivering care, without endangering the safety of patients or clinicians [2]. Therapists had to be trained on how to effectively manage telehealth intake. A telehealth visit consisted of contacting the patients and asking them for their current level of pain. Any corresponding physical symptoms were to be reported, and they were asked if they had any emotional concerns. Patients who were provided with a home exercise program during their previous in-person visits were encouraged to continue with it to achieve or maintain the pain-free level of function.

One major hindrance to having a telehealth visit was that patients were often unable to remember their home exercise program or to perform the exercises without any verbal cueing or physical assistance. Often, they had misplaced a paper copy or email of the exercise program that had been provided. Therapists would

Table 9.1 Telehealth patient checklist in outpatient rehabilitation

Questionnaire	Yes	No
1. Does the patient have a minimum baseline hearing, vision, and cognitive capacity to interact effectively with the screen?		
2. Does the patient have the ability to connect with a device with video access such as computer, iPad, or smart phone?		
3. Does the patient have sufficient understanding on how to connect or access the program through video call?		
4. Does the patient have the ability to safely perform a series of physical activities alone or with the assistance of a family member or caregiver?		
5. Does the patient have good internet connectivity or network access?		
*The patient should be able to answer *yes* to all questions to be eligible for telehealth visits		

9 Rehabilitation

Table 9.2 Advantages and disadvantages of telehealth for rehabilitation services

Advantages	Disadvantages
(1) maintain continuity of musculoskeletal care, directly educating patients through remote consultation in their own home environment	(1) limited ability to use an electronic device and limited access to a computer, laptop, iPad, or smart phone
(2) perform a physical assessment, and plan a targeted therapeutic exercise program	(2) limited ability to receive a proper physical assessment, which compromises validity and reliability
(3) monitor patients' progress, providing them with continuous feedback and supervision	(3) lack of proprioceptive input and absence of manual therapy management
(4) adapt the intensity, frequency, and duration of rehabilitation programs in accordance with patients' needs	(4) difficulties for children in maintaining engagement and attention during telehealth appointments
(5) increase care efficiency while containing costs	(5) financial impact due to decreased rate of reimbursement
(6) guarantee adequate and continued services for both acute (e.g., postsurgical) and chronic (e.g., degenerative) conditions	(6) absence of exercise equipment and other exercise tools, such as weights, weighted balls, TheraBands, etc.

patiently explain the step-by-step movements over the phone or refer them to YouTube videos for those who had Internet access. Therapists demonstrated innovation by using household items as exercise tools, such as a can of soup as a substitute for a weighted dumbbell, using a stair banister for support while doing balance exercises, and engaged a family member to help provide assistance or physical queuing. Furthermore, the therapists ensured that they prescribed exercises that were easy and safe to perform in the confines of the patients' homes. Table 9.2 outlines the advantages and disadvantages of telehealth for rehabilitation.

Conversations with the patients had their share of challenges, and often language was a hindrance as 80% of the patient population spoke Spanish. There were a few bilingual therapists and the use of language interpretation services were often utilized. Despite the barriers, telehealth consults still provided a temporary substitute to help improve or maintain patient's ability to perform their daily activities.

Telehealth was another tool in the box that was considered a great resource for clinicians to use, especially during this COVID-19 pandemic. Telehealth helped limit the spread of contagions, promotes safety for patients and clinicians, decreased the use of scarce PPE, and improves patient satisfaction due to one-on-one interactions.

Telehealth was the principal resource for rehabilitation at the peak of the pandemic. It maintained continuity of musculoskeletal care, educating patients through remote consultation, directly in their own home environment, performing a physical assessment, planning a targeted therapeutic exercise program, monitoring patients' progress, providing them continuous feedback and supervision, and guaranteeing adequate and continued services to both acute (e.g., postsurgical) and chronic (e.g., degenerative) conditions.

Since the transition from face-to-face visits to telehealth encounters, outpatient services experienced both positive and negative financial impacts from the

COVID-19 pandemic throughout 2020 and 2021. The telehealth reimbursement was initially significantly lower for both Medicaid and Medicare. This significantly lowered the average payment per visit. Telehealth reimbursement eventually improved among all payers, making it more financially sustainable for the department and allowing outpatient services to sustain a threshold level of revenue that would have otherwise been completely erased due to reduction of in-person patient visits during the pandemic.

Protecting the Frontline Staff

The rehabilitation department, along with the rest of the hospital, experienced the tight supply of PPE and other supplies during the first surge of the COVID-19 pandemic. PPE was distributed in calculated quantities on a weekly basis to each department. Regular surgical masks were asked to be worn over N95 and also to be kept for as long as possible.

Rehabilitation of COVID-19 Survivors in Acute Care

Prone Positioning of Patients

One of the clinical manifestations of severe COVID-19 infection was the presence of acute respiratory distress syndrome (ARDS) that often required intubation, ventilator support, and admission to the ICU. ARDS was first described in the 1960s during the Vietnam War [3]. It could begin either by direct (pulmonary) injury to the lung parenchyma or by indirect (extrapulmonary) blood-borne sources into the lungs. The subsequent insults could lead to diffuse alveolar damage leading to non-cardiogenic pulmonary edema and atelectasis [3]. Evidence shows that most patients with ARDS managed with prone positioning had improved oxygenation regardless of the etiology of the disease [4]. Prone positioning results in a more even alveolar size throughout the lung while reducing the compressive forces of the heart and the abdomen [5].

As the number of ventilated patients and ICU beds increased exponentially, the need for supportive care for these patients followed suit. The department of rehabilitation was asked to be part of a team that turned patients form supine to prone position, or vice versa. Prone positioning was a nursing-driven program introduced early in the pandemic to help ventilated, sedated patients improve oxygenation to their lungs. The rehabilitation department participated with other departments in the proning team. More details on proning are in the chapter on physical therapy and proning.

Clinical Management

The primary goals of rehabilitation are to optimize cardiopulmonary and neuromuscular function in order to minimize loss of functional abilities, maximize independence, and facilitate ventilator weaning. Sometimes, it can be as simple as performing passive range of motion, turning from side to side, providing splints for prevention of contracture, and adjusting bed height to a more upright position. But it is important to remember that mobility does not only pertain to getting the patient out of bed and performing ambulation. The interdisciplinary involvement is crucial as everyone has a role in ensuring the safety of the patient and feasibility of mobilization activity. Rehabilitation in the ICU is best delivered by multidisciplinary specialists using the expertise of PTs, OTs, and SLPs to build a compassionate therapeutic alliance with the patients and their family.

As with any patient in the ICU, successful clinical management of COVID-19 included treating both the medical condition that initially resulted in admission and other comorbidities and nosocomial complications. As the pandemic continued over weeks, there were a few extubated COVID-19 patients who were in such a deconditioned state that rehabilitation services were all the more important. In the weeks that followed, the rehabilitation department started to receive increasing referrals for PT, OT, and SLP services. At this point, rehabilitation staff were more comfortable treating COVID-19 patients, focusing mainly on getting the patients back on their feet due to significant deconditioning and lack of endurance. Most patients required oxygen supplementation to complete a simple task. The department also took on a major role in determining discharge recommendations and to what extent the patient would require further rehabilitation services.

Mobilization

A study states that "prolonged immobility and bed rest are associated with physical weakness, functional decline and higher mortality rates" [6]. It is well-documented that bed rest is associated with many complications that may affect patient survival from critical illnesses [7]. The consequences of immobility and bed rest include muscle atrophy, delirium, pressure ulcers, atelectasis, bone demineralization, and deconditioning. Despite of all the valuable research, it is still a common practice in ICUs worldwide to put critically ill patients on bed rest, especially if they are mechanically ventilated. Studies have shown that young healthy adults can lose 5–9% of quadriceps muscle mass and 20–27% of quadriceps muscle strength in just 2 weeks of immobilization [7]. In older adults, the effect is about three to six times greater. The effect is accelerated for mechanically ventilated patients where about 12.5% decrease of muscle mass occurs in just the first week of immobility [7]. Compounded with comorbidities, single or multiple organ failure, bed rest can lead to rapid deconditioning and muscle atrophy and is considered to be the single most important risk factor in developing muscle weakness of critically ill patients [7].

The responsibility of mobilization of severely deconditioned patients in the acute care setting due to COVID-19 did not fall solely on the shoulders of the rehabilitation team (PT, OT, SLP) and should also include intensivists, critical care nurses, respiratory therapists, nursing assistants, and rehab assistants. Social workers and case managers also play an integral role in planning the patient post-acute care. The role of rehabilitation was to rebuild endurance throughout mobility and every day activity for outpatients. Progress was slow and required patience from both the therapist and the patients themselves due to their level of fatigue and shortness of breath they experienced. What would normally be a 30–45-minute session of exercises and activity turned out to be minimal accomplishments of mobility such as attempting to get out of the bed, attempting to stand, and a possible attempt to ambulate if the oxygen saturation levels maintained a stable percentage. Rehabilitation proved to be an essential service for most COVID-19 patients and was instrumental in their recovery (Box 9.1).

Box 9.1 Essential Mobilization Considerations for COVID-19
1. Complete bed rest for prolonged periods should be avoided
2. Turn patients every 2 hours while on bed rest as tolerated
3. Maintain head of bed (HOB) of mechanically ventilated patients at least 30 degrees unless contraindicated
4. Perform range of motion (ROM) to patients who cannot actively participate in their care.
5. Order PT/OT/SLP consult as indicated.
6. Evaluate tolerance to activity for safe mobilization process

---

Comorbidities and Challenges

Cognitive impairment including delirium is common in ARDS and affects many COVID-19 survivors with persistent long-term impairments after hospital discharge [8]. Delirium, described as a brain-organ dysfunction characterized by disturbance in consciousness, has a rapid in onset, and is marked by fluctuating course of inattention, and impaired ability to receive, process, store, and recall information [9]. Delirium can affect approximately 80% of ICU stay and is more commonly associated with sepsis, multiple comorbidities, and older population [9]. It is associated with worse functional outcomes and a higher mortality rate [9]. Prevention is the primary treatment for ICU-acquired delirium.

The ability to swallow and communicate is always a concern for patients who require mechanical ventilation for airway protection. The primary reason for SLP referral for COVID-19 patients was due to oropharyngeal dysphagia (OD) resulting in increased risk of aspiration pneumonia and subsequent mortality. Cough reflex is a strong airway protective mechanism; however, this is absent or diminished for patients who are intubated or recently extubated [10]. Communication is also a great concern for many patients in critical care, especially when they are awake and intubated. The ability of the patient to communicate their needs to the staff is important for obtaining consent for essential medical procedures. For patients who are cognitively aware, the SLP may devise/recommend augmentative and alternative communication (AAC). AAC encompasses any communication method used to supplement or replace speech and writing and covers a wide range of nonverbal communication methods from picture and alphabet boards to speech-generating devices, including those accessed via eye gaze. It is the role of the SLP to identify the communication needs for each patients and advise the right tools to restore communication [11].

Rehabilitation of COVID-19 Survivors Post-acute Care

For COVID-19 survivors, the residual deficits would affect their ability to perform activities of daily living, delayed executive functioning, delayed return to employment, and impaired quality of life. In COVID-19 survivors who required mechanical ventilation, the added residual physical symptoms might include neuropathy, myopathy, dysphagia, joint stiffness, and pain [12]. Another factors to consider are mental health issues which are reported by between 8% and 57% of survivors [13]. These include anxiety, depression, and post-traumatic disorder (PTSD) which can still be present in about 20% of patients on a follow-up visit 1 year later [14]. As mentioned previously, between 30% and 80% of survivors will have cognitive impairments including memory loss, impaired executive function, difficulty in concentration, comprehension, and critical thinking [15]. Cognitive deficits are attributed to the effects of hypoxemia and direct involvement of the central nervous system [12]. The patients who became severely ill to COVID-19, typically with ARDS, will have more disabling effects requiring prolonged rehabilitation and multidisciplinary inpatient and outpatient follow-up after hospital discharge.

A comprehensive discharge plan is typically coordinated and prepared by an integrated team of case managers, social workers, rehabilitation specialists, and physicians prior to hospital discharge (Fig. 9.3). The emphasis has been creating a discharge plan on the day of admission, which anticipates the possible post-acute care needs of the patient, whether the patient is going to a facility for continued care or home. The physician initiates the process by recommending early rehabilitation, where the patient receives a comprehensive assessment and appropriate discharge disposition from the therapists. The case managers and social workers will then prepare the necessary paperwork and identify possible barriers to discharge.

Most insurance companies do not require authorizations as the federal government provided temporary relief on the required paperwork for placement in subacute care facilities. Rehabilitation services can also be provided at home with PT,

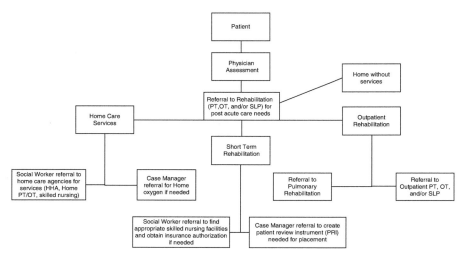

Fig. 9.3 Coordinated discharge planning post-acute care

OT, and/or SLP services together with nursing care and a social worker. Outpatient rehabilitation services with specialized pulmonary rehabilitation are another option for continuing care.

Adjusting to the "New Normal" and the Lessons Learned

The COVID-19 pandemic shifted the way rehabilitation services were delivered at SBH Health System. Having to wear an N95 mask and a face shield for every patient encounter became the new normal. Although telehealth services were an unpopular form of providing services, it continued to be in place. It was unpopular due to the absence of face-to-face interaction, as well as manual therapy manipulations and a hands-on approach that is necessary for providing outpatient rehabilitation services. Social distancing remained a challenge as space within the hospital and at Union sites continues to be limited. Despite these obvious challenges, the rehabilitation department became better equipped with knowledge and expertise as one looked ahead beyond the pandemic.

One example of how the rehabilitation department continued to strive in assisting with patient care was the creation of a special task force that created comprehensive policies and procedures for proning. There was a heightened awareness among physicians regarding mobilization. The rehabilitation needs of each individual patient were identified early throughout their hospital stay. The rehabilitation department became more involved, and consultations increased on a regular basis. The positive aspect to this change was that a greater number of patients were getting mobilized earlier within their hospital stay. However, the negative aspect was that the inpatient rehabilitation department was not appropriately staffed to meet the increased demand.

Having physicians, administrators, and staff champion, the use of telehealth services was imperative for the successful implementation and transition to telehealth. Additionally, a strong IT department that was able to pivot toward new technologies in a quick but efficient manner would continue to be key as new methods of delivering healthcare become available. Patient interaction remained a challenge as most of them preferred in-person interaction compared to virtual rehabilitation. Despite the unpopularity, the rehabilitation staff adapted to telehealth as part of their clinical tools and continues to be used as needed or if it is requested by the patient. Referral to outpatient services of COVID-19 patients remained limited as most of the patients discharged required a higher level of care whether in a rehabilitation facility or home care.

The creation of an integrated discharge planning process with interdisciplinary involvement remained to be successful in transitioning patients from the hospital to an appropriate discharge disposition. The early identification and referral to rehabilitation, with the appropriate discharge recommendation, were the key to a safe discharge planning process. The social workers and case managers initiated the referral process to facilities, agencies, and medical device suppliers. This process continued although insurance companies continued to require prior authorization for rehabilitation or medical equipment orders. These challenges often led to a delay of patient discharge.

There are several lessons to be learned from this experience. First, the resilience of the rehabilitation staff was important in helping patients who needed rehabilitation services. The staff were dealing with all the possible risks to their own health while helping others. The hospital provided support for the staff on a daily basis by providing appropriate PPE, mental health services, and support groups. The hospital administration also provided other benefits to help the staff manage their stress better. Second, there was a need to proactively anticipate new clinical needs of patients. Early mobilization in the ICU was part of the management of critically ill patients. Third, the interdisciplinary involvement with clearly defined roles and early identification of the patient's personal, social, economic needs contributed to a smoother transition from the hospital to their home. Lastly, the use of technology-mediated, or virtual rehabilitation, became a new norm during this pandemic. The use of technology during PT, OT, and SLP visits along with relaxing the rules and reimbursement for this kind of service was very helpful and should remain available in the foreseeable future.

Conclusion

Rehabilitation is an essential part of management of major health conditions. The goals of rehabilitation are to assist individuals in preventing loss of function, restore function, and maintain current function in order to actively participate in their environment as independently as possible. The COVID-19 pandemic highlighted this important role. Early mobilization of patients can avoid the deleterious effect of bed rest and has been found to be safe and feasible for patients who are on mechanical ventilation. These patients have been found to have better outcomes and quality-of-life post-discharge from acute inpatient episode. Prone positioning of patients with ARDS is effective in increasing oxygenation to the lungs while reducing the compressive forces of the heart and abdomen. The role of rehabilitation during post-acute care varies from short-term rehabilitation in skilled nursing facilities to virtual rehabilitation using telehealth. The focus of health crisis management is to stabilize the patients and save lives, but without rehabilitation professionals, health service delivery will be less efficient leaving more people impaired and disabled.

References

1. Eastman P, Dowd A, White J, Carter J, Ely M. Telehealth: rapid adoption in community palliative care due to COVID-19: patient and professional evaluation. BMJ Support Palliat Care. 2021; https://doi.org/10.1136/bmjspcare-2021-002987.
2. Tenforde AS, Hefner JE, Kodish-Wachs JE, Iaccarino MA, Paganoni S. Telehealth in physical medicine and rehabilitation: a narrative review. PM R. 2017;9(5S):S51–S8. https://doi.org/10.1016/j.pmrj.2017.02.013.
3. Koulouras V, Papathanakos G, Papathanasiou A, Nakos G. Efficacy of prone position in acute respiratory distress syndrome patients: a pathophysiology-based review. World J Crit Care Med. 2016;5(2):121–36. https://doi.org/10.5492/wjccm.v5.i2.121.
4. Henderson WR, Griesdale DE, Dominelli P, Ronco JJ. Does prone positioning improve oxygenation and reduce mortality in patients with acute respiratory distress syndrome? Can Respir J. 2014;21(4):213–5. https://doi.org/10.1155/2014/472136.
5. Kallet RH. A comprehensive review of prone position in ARDS. Respir Care. 2015;60(11):1660–87. https://doi.org/10.4187/respcare.04271.
6. Fraser D, Spiva L, Forman W, Hallen C. Original research: implementation of an early mobility program in an ICU. Am J Nurs. 2015;115(12):49–58. https://doi.org/10.1097/01.NAJ.0000475292.27985.fc.
7. Hashem MD, Nelliot A, Needham DM. Early mobilization and rehabilitation in the ICU: moving back to the future. Respir Care. 2016;61(7):971–9. https://doi.org/10.4187/respcare.04741.
8. Sasannejad C, Ely EW, Lahiri S. Long-term cognitive impairment after acute respiratory distress syndrome: a review of clinical impact and pathophysiological mechanisms. Crit Care. 2019;23(1):352. https://doi.org/10.1186/s13054-019-2626-z.
9. Girard TD, Pandharipande PP, Ely EW. Delirium in the intensive care unit. Crit Care. 2008;12(Suppl 3):S3. https://doi.org/10.1186/cc6149.
10. Tanaka A, Isono S, Ishikawa T, Nishino T. Laryngeal reflex before and after placement of airway interventions: endotracheal tube and laryngeal mask airway. Anesthesiology. 2005;102(1):20–5. https://doi.org/10.1097/00000542-200501000-00007.
11. Mohapatra B, Ccc SLP, Mohan R, Ccc SLP. Speech-language pathologists' role in the multidisciplinary management and rehabilitation of patients with Covid-19. J Rehabil Med Clin Commun. 2020;3:1000037. https://doi.org/10.2340/20030711-1000037.
12. Carda S, Invernizzi M, Bavikatte G, Bensmail D, Bianchi F, Deltombe T, et al. The role of physical and rehabilitation medicine in the COVID-19 pandemic: the clinician's view. Ann Phys Rehabil Med. 2020;63(6):554–6. https://doi.org/10.1016/j.rehab.2020.04.001.
13. Biehl M, Sese D. Post-intensive care syndrome and COVID-19 – implications post pandemic. Cleve Clin J Med. 2020; https://doi.org/10.3949/ccjm.87a.ccc055.

14. Rabiee A, Nikayin S, Hashem MD, Huang M, Dinglas VD, Bienvenu OJ, et al. Depressive symptoms after critical illness: a systematic review and meta-analysis. Crit Care Med. 2016;44(9):1744–53. https://doi.org/10.1097/CCM.0000000000001811.
15. Filatov A, Sharma P, Hindi F, Espinosa PS. Neurological complications of coronavirus disease (COVID-19): encephalopathy. Cureus. 2020;12(3):e7352. https://doi.org/10.7759/cureus.7352.

Chapter 10
Respiratory Therapy and Proning

Angela Babaev, Tracey Martin-Johnson, and Mark Klion

Respiratory Therapy

The respiratory therapist profession has been recognized for many years and is still an emerging allied health profession. Respiratory therapists have an extensive knowledge of the pathophysiology of the cardiopulmonary system. This understanding enables the therapist to assist physicians in treating patients, especially during a pandemic of an infectious respiratory virus [1, 2]. Along with understanding the cardiopulmonary system, the respiratory therapist must also be proficient in the devices used to deliver respiratory care. Respiratory therapists work alongside physicians in areas including intensive care units (ICUs), emergency departments, outpatient departments, and home care settings to provide essential respiratory care services tailored for a wide range of patients with varying levels of disease. Within this provision of care, the role of the respiratory therapist can be quite varied (Box 10.1).

A. Babaev (✉)
Department of Nursing, SBH Health System, Bronx, NY, USA

CUNY School of Medicine, New York, NY, USA

Bloomfield College, Bloomfield, NJ, USA
e-mail: ababaev@sbhny.org

T. Martin-Johnson
Respiratory Therapy, SBH Health System, Bronx, NY, USA

M. Klion
Division of Orthopedics, Department of Surgery, SBH Health System, Bronx, NY, USA

© The Author(s), under exclusive license to Springer Nature
Switzerland AG 2022
R. Shabsigh (ed.), *Health Crisis Management in Acute Care Hospitals*,
https://doi.org/10.1007/978-3-030-95806-0_10

> **Box 10.1. The Role of a Respiratory Therapist**
> - Managing life support mechanical ventilation devices
> - Managing noninvasive respiratory devices
> - Analyzing blood samples to determine levels of oxygen
> - Maintaining artificial airways
> - Delivering aerosol therapy
> - Assessing vital signs
> - Reviewing chest X-rays
> - Collecting and reviewing sputum specimens
> - Educating patients and families on purpose and procedures of respiratory equipment
> - Engaging in diagnostic evaluation and treatment of patients with physicians
> - Educating patients on cardiopulmonary health such as smoking cessation and asthma education
> - Performing test and studies related to cardiopulmonary such as rehabilitation and pulmonary function testing

Respiratory Therapy in the COVID-19 Crisis

The high importance of respiratory therapy becomes clear in the face of an infectious crisis, especially with a virus that attacks the respiratory system. The spectrum of the disease caused by SARS-CoV-2 can range from symptoms of a common cold to severe pneumonia, as defined according to the American Thoracic Society criteria [3]. Early reports from China estimated this incidence of severe pneumonia to be not insignificant in 15% of patients [4]. Indeed, ARDS [5], the life-threatening form of respiratory failure, is a frequent complication in COVID-19 [6]. Depending on the degree of hypoxemia in a patient as an indication of infection severity, ARDS can be categorized into mild, moderate, and severe [5]. Patients with moderate-to-severe ARDS frequently require invasive mechanical ventilation (IMV) and have a poor prognosis. A survey of clinical studies reporting COVID-19-associated ARDS in hospitalized patients since the beginning of the COVID-19 pandemic in January until the end of July 2020 showed a mortality rate in COVID-19-associated ARDS at 45% and the incidence of ARDS among non-survivors of COVID-19 at 90% [7]. Therefore, infections and infectious pandemics like COVID-19 that cause ARDS requiring intubation and mechanical ventilation or noninvasive ventilation place a high demand on respiratory therapy services.

Tom Kallstrom, the Executive Director of the American Association for Respiratory Care (AARC), said in March 2020: "Now, more than ever before, the role of the respiratory therapist is vital to the health of our nation" [8]. As the demand on respiratory therapists skyrocketed in the initial surge, it was evident that "respiratory therapists sacrifice and dedicate themselves to helping their patients and their communities during this time of COVID-19" said Kallstrom [8].

In response to the initial crisis in March of 2020 which saw the rapid increase in the incidence of COVID-19 patients and consequent saturation of the capacity of the intensive care units (ICUs), the SBH Health System had to increase more than fivefold the bed capacity for adult intensive care with mechanical ventilation. This was due to the dramatic increase in-patients with ARDS. The initial and most important aim was to prevent mortality in the severely affected patients. Standard supportive care along with lung-protective mechanical ventilation became the cornerstone of treatment for COVID-19 patients. To enable this, many challenges were faced along the way.

Challenges with Equipment

As the need for respiratory care services increased, the respiratory care supplies began to diminish due to escalating consumption. There was a dire need to have enough mechanical ventilators on hand to support the patient census. There were back orders on essential respiratory supplies which required research to find alternative and compatible substitutes. The respiratory therapy department role expanded at that time as it had to learn the dynamics of working with the Department of Health Emergency Management Division. Ventilators and supplies had to be tallied and tracked multiple times every day, spreadsheets completed, meetings held, and requests submitted for additional ventilators. The supply of new ventilators kept up closely with the rapidly increasing demand for mechanical ventilation at the time of the COVID-19 crisis (Fig. 10.1). A delay of 1–2 days in the delivery of ventilators

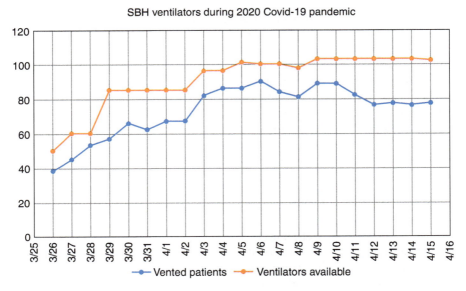

Fig. 10.1 The number of available ventilators (orange) and patients on ventilators (blue) at SBH Health System in March and April 2020

could have resulted in a shortage requiring drastic measures such as ventilator sharing or rationing of ventilators.

With a possible shortage of equipment, alternative methods of ventilation were increasingly discussed. The possibility of using noninvasive equipment in an invasive setting was considered, if additional ventilators did not arrive at any given crucial moment. Research, time, effort, and performing a test run prior to a real emergency helped to understand the risks and benefits of the alternative methods. Although SBH Health System had planned such contingencies, it was fortunate that it never had to use these alternative methods.

Staffing Concerns

Health crisis planners should not only include in their planning equipment and supplies, such as ventilators and high-flow nasal cannulas, but also expand staffing with respiratory therapists, supplemental staffing, and cross-trained health workers. At SBH Health System, the respiratory department's staff was small in number. Prior to the COVID-19 crisis, there were approximately two dozen therapists with a definitive need to increase the departmental staff. Part of the respiratory therapy scope is to be knowledgeable in all aspects of neonatal, pediatrics, adults, and geriatrics respiratory care and equipment. When the COVID-19 pandemic surge hit in the Spring of 2020, the demands for respiratory therapy services presented challenges due to the limited number of staff.

Due to the lean staff numbers, the workload became overwhelming as the pandemic unfolded. There were not enough therapists to take care of the rapidly increasing number of patients requiring respiratory services. Therapists were multitasking as best as possible while also concerned about both personal and patient safety. As the New York area, the Bronx and SBH Health System, became inundated with patients with ARDS and hospitals were starting to go overcapacity, there was a great need to bring in outside staff to assist. However, due to the competitive market and limited number of respiratory therapists available in New York City, significant challenges in hiring new staff were encountered.

The department was able to rise to the occasion by rallying together, alternating days, and working extended hours. As elective procedures were halted, the therapists were able to join forces with other departments to carry out the workload. It was fortunate to have the opportunity to work with residents and physicians from the dental department, a registered nurse from the anesthesia department, as well as an out-of-state dental anesthesiologist. Every individual who joined forces with the respiratory department truly assisted the department without hesitation. The respiratory therapy service used a checklist to help guide the residents, physicians, nurses, and volunteers. The list consisted of showing where all the respiratory equipment was stored, how the ventilators were set up, an overview of the different models of ventilators, and reminders to always remain paired up with a respiratory therapist for guidance. Due to the rapid increase in-patient census, training was hands-on, which made it more imperative for the dual team. It's not often to find different disciplines with different backgrounds coming together without resistance. SBH Health System staff was able to pull together successfully in a time of need.

Emotional and Psychological Impact

Emotional and psychological support for the frontline respiratory therapists, nurses, and physicians is of paramount importance during and after a health crisis. Under normal circumstances, respiratory therapists see and experienced an array of emergency situations on any given day. However, the pandemic presented them with an uncertainty about their healthcare decisions and about their own safety. The emotional impact emanated from a number of factors such as possibility of transmitting the virus to their own families, stress related to their own health, and the health of the patients. Questions such as "Why weren't we able to save the patients with ARDS even though we were putting them on mechanical ventilators? Why were the patients with ARDS appearing to get better and then decompensate so quickly?" reverberated in the minds of many respiratory therapists. A larger proportion of the staff was still struggling with the number of lives lost. The physical impact of working long continuous hours and not having downtime to de-stress also played a part in the psychological well-being of therapists throughout the pandemic [9]. To help the staff overcome these overwhelming challenges, the respiratory therapy service incorporated the following: open discussions for any questions or concerns, staff huddles at the beginning and end of shifts to provide support, counseling sessions provided by the psychiatry department, one-on-one sessions if staff were more comfortable speaking on an individual basis, making sure the staff was able to step away from the bedside, and taking a break for self-care and checking in on staff on their days off.

Personal Protective Equipment (PPE) Challenges

During the pandemic, the Centers for Disease Control and Prevention (CDC) guidelines on PPEs changed several times and continued to be modified: from requiring only surgical/droplet masks to using N95 respirators and then needing eye protection for every patient encounter. Guidelines on quarantine changed as well, for healthcare workers and the general population. Although updates were provided regularly, these frequent adjustments caused confusion on how to protect the staff properly. This brought about fear and anxiety, because no one wanted to contract the virus or become a silent spreader, keeping in mind that at the time there were no vaccines or specific therapeutics for COVID-19. Through ardent supply chain acquisition efforts, SBH Health System never ran out of PPE. As a frontline discipline, respiratory therapy was in constant contact with supply chain to determine what type, quality, and quantity of PPE was required. The respiratory therapy department was able to receive the allotments in a timely fashion every week. The SBH supply chain team was also able to have the PPE hand-delivered to departments so workflow would not be interrupted. As part of the frontline staff, the respiratory therapy department was always able to receive appropriate PPE.

Proning

With the increase in COVID-19 patient volume that required critical care and respiratory support, the hospital started to expand its ICU capacity from 16 beds to almost 100. All elective surgeries were halted, and new "satellite ICUs" were created to accommodate those critical care patients. As the number of patients with COVID-19 started to rise, so did the acuity of care increase in the ICUs. It was like a tidal wave that just hit the hospital.

The majority, if not all, patients requiring ICU level of care had acute hypoxemic respiratory failure requiring mechanical ventilation for ARDS. Standard principles were initially implemented to treat the ARDS, which included mechanical ventilation with positive end expiratory ventilation (PEEP). Proning patients, which is to place a patient lying flat with the chest down (prone position), has been reported to improve oxygenation, as early as 1976 [10].

In a supine position, the heart, diaphragm, and liver cause pressure on the lungs and can cause the alveoli to collapse in-patients with respiratory complications. In the prone position, the lung tissue is free from compression, and more alveoli are employed for gas exchange eventually improving oxygenation (Fig. 10.2). Indeed, prone positioning considerably reduces mortality by increasing functional lung volume and decreasing atelectasis by recruiting alveoli, improving dependent aeration, and mobilizing secretions [11–13]. In a prospective, randomized controlled trial with 237 severe ARDS patients assigned to the prone positioning group and 229 patients to the supine-positioned group, Guerin et al. [14, 15] showed that prone positioning in conjunction with ventilation is associated with reduced mortality. At 28 days, mortality was higher in the supine-positioned group (32%), compared to the prone-positioned group (16%). The clinical outcome for the prone-positioned group was also better at 90 days, with observed mortality of 23.6% compared to 41% for the supine-positioned group [14, 15].

While prone positioning was not a common practice at SBH Health System, early reports on the treatment of ARDS in symptomatic COVID-19 patients led to its introduction into the treatment plan. With additional hospital units transformed to "ICU" and the increased number of patients indicated for proning, staffing and education needed to be implemented at an accelerated pace. Strategies to increase prone positioning under crisis were needed. Even though prone positioning is not an invasive procedure, it is a complex process requiring careful synchronized coordination and collaborative approach to avoid many potential complications. The Nursing Department and the Hospital Leadership initiated a "homegrown" educational program including prone positioning protocol based on "best practice," educational classes, and creation of a "mobile prone team" to address the increased demand.

Supine position　　　　　　**Prone position**

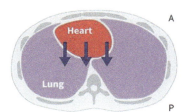　　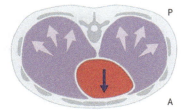

Gravitational pressure of heart and mediastinum on the lungs.　　Decreased gravitational pressure of heart and mediastinum on the lungs.

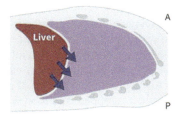　　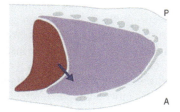

Compressive effects of the abdominal organs on the lungs.　　Decreased compressive effects of the abdominal organs on the lungs.

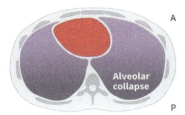　　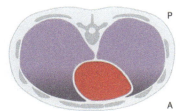

Expansion of the chest wall and overall less homogeneous chest wall compliance.　　More homogeneous chest wall compliance due to restriction of anterior chest wall movement.

Fig. 10.2 In supine position, at functional residual capacity (FRC) and FRC plus tidal volume (V_T), the alveoli are small due to pleural pressure, compression from the heart, and abdominal contents (arrows), compared to prone position [16]. (Reprinted from Canadian Medical Association Journal, vol. 192 (47) (2020) E1532-E1537, Kevin Venus, Laveena Munshi and Michael Fralick, Prone positioning for patients with hypoxic respiratory failure related to COVID-19, with permission from AMC Joule)

The Proning Procedure

Patient preparation was essential prior to proning, and a safety checklist was created to standardize the preparation and the proning procedure. This checklist included steps for the pre-proning, during proning, and post-proning procedures, with dedicated roles for each team member involved [17].

Pre-proning Procedure

Based on the defined criteria, patients who required proning were identified during the morning rounds and communicated to the senior charge nurse. This list was then communicated to the proning team every morning. Daily communications and reports maximized efficiency and minimized wait times for the mobile prone team. The pre-procedure steps included ensuring the MD order was in place; explaining the procedure to the patient; cleaning the eyes; instilling drops/lubricating gel if needed; securing the feeding tube if present; removing electrocardiography (ECG) pads; securing the endotracheal tube or, if there was a tracheotomy in place, ensuring that it was secured and sutured; inserting bite block; and ensuring that all central lines are secured, nasogastric tube feeding was stopped, and the patient would be kept nothing-by-mouth for 45–60 minutes prior to the proning procedure. If proning was to be done emergently, then tube feeding would be stopped, and food would be aspirated via nasogastric suction before turning.

The availability and preparation of the equipment needed for placing a patient in the prone position was an essential task that was done prior to entering the room. Supplies included proning pillows for positioning under patients' chest, face supports, appropriate mattresses (kinetic therapy bed or equivalent), airway box, and code cart. A proning cart was created (Fig. 10.3) that contained bedsheets used for turning the patients, closed circuit suctioning and endotracheal tube tapes, ECG electrodes, absorbent pad to place on and under the patient, skin cream, and skin protective pads [18]. A proning safety checklist was also attached to the cart which served as a "time-out" list similar to what is used in the operating room. This moment of pause, prior to initiation of proning, was vital to improve team coordination and ensure safety to patient and staff.

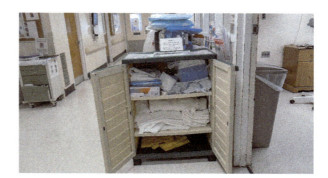

Fig. 10.3 Proning cart: a cart is assembled outside of the patient room with all necessary proning supplies. Affixed to the cart is the proning checklist

Procedure While Proning Patient

Initially when critical patients were placed in the prone position, the staffing included a respiratory therapist, a primary nurse, a proning team led by a physician, and at least two more staff personnel to assist. There was also an anesthesiologist present in case there was a need to re-intubate if the endotracheal tube was dislodged, a known possible complication of proning. Sedation was an essential element to placing a patient in the prone position – to prevent agitation and resistance to staff attempting proning. During turning to the prone position, all lines were capped and placed in the midline position to prevent tangling and disconnecting. A respiratory therapist pre-oxygenated the patient to 100% prior to proning. Furthermore, it was the respiratory therapist's responsibility to position the endotracheal tube and manage the airways prior to and during the turning of the patient. A "time-out" safety checklist was performed. Once the "all ready" was called, the patient was lifted in unison and moved over to the edge of the mattress away from the ventilator and tilted 90 degrees onto the sides. Chest rolls or pillows were then placed in position to allow for an unrestricted abdomen. The patient was subsequently turned to the prone position toward the ventilator. See Figs. 10.4, 10.5, 10.6, 10.7, 10.8, 10.9, 10.10 through 10.11 for the sequence of the proning procedure.

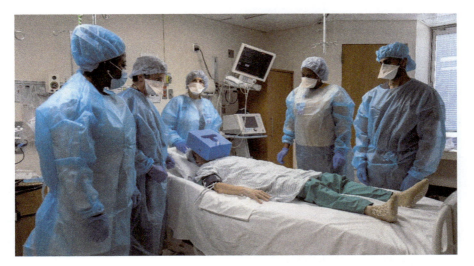

Fig. 10.4 The proning team is assembled at bedside, with a minimum of five people including a respiratory therapist at the head of the bed. Ample room is needed around the bed. A head and face protector pad is placed over secured endotracheal tube. All intravenous and arterial lines are capped (except lines for sedation). EKG leads and pulse oximeter are removed. Rectal tubes, urinary catheters, and chest tubes are managed by placing the lines between the legs if possible

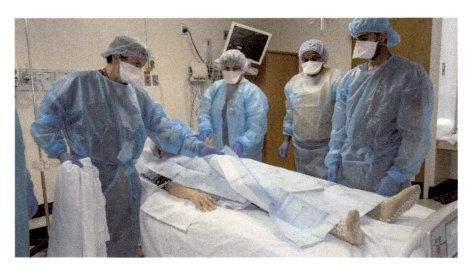

Fig. 10.5 After skin care, clean absorbent pads are placed on the undressed body against the skin

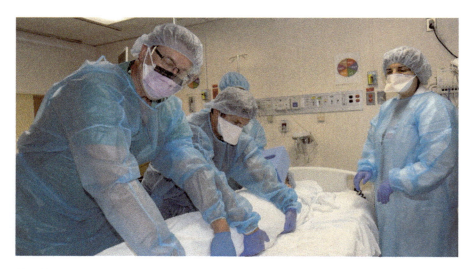

Fig. 10.6 A full sheet is then placed on the patient and tucked on the side toward the ventilator, and the side that the patient will be turned onto. This will allow the removal of the soiled linen from the bed and facilitate turning the patient

Post-proning Procedure and Maintenance

Following prone positioning, the lungs are auscultated bilaterally to ensure that the endotracheal tube (ETT) or the tracheostomy was not displaced. Proning pillows were adjusted to keep the head in a neutral position and to ensure proper padding and skin protection at extremities. Checks were made to ensure the eyes were not

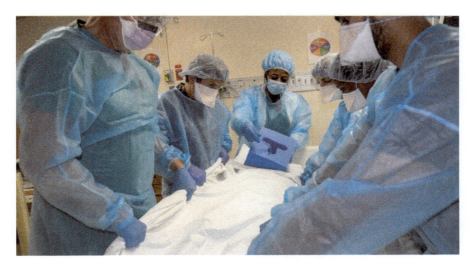

Fig. 10.7 The team leader at the head of the bed initiates and controls the first maneuvers in turning the patient. The head and face protector is secured. The endotracheal tube is disconnected from the ventilator. Team members take the bottom sheet and in unison move the patient 50% away from the ventilator to place the patient ready to turn onto his/her side toward the ventilator

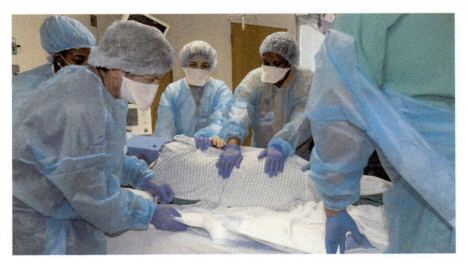

Fig. 10.8 All soiled linen and pads are removed at this time, and the sheet that was tucked on the side of the patient is grabbed. The latter will be used to complete the proning turn toward the ventilator

obstructed, the neck was in a neutral position, ears were not compressed, and the nose was free of pressure. The bed was put in a slight reverse Trendelenburg (the head slightly higher) position to keep the eyes slightly above the right atrium to

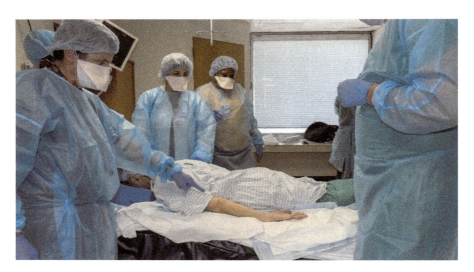

Fig. 10.9 The patient is now in the prone position. The endotracheal tube is reconnected to the ventilator. The head position is adjusted to ensure no excess pressure is placed on the eyes and the tube is securely in place

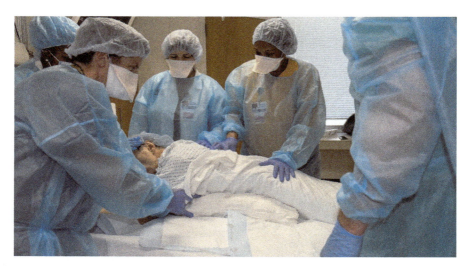

Fig. 10.10 Two chest rolls, one on each side, are then placed by rolling the patient from side to side to suspend patient and allowing for decreased pressure from the abdomen and improved ventilation. The patient is also placed in mild reverse Trendelenburg position

provide for venous drainage and decrease edema. Every 2 hours, the arms position of the patients was changed, and an assessment was conducted to check for wrinkles under the patient. The respiratory therapist continually monitored ventilation settings and pressures throughout the maneuver, and chest therapy was initiated to help mobilize secretions.

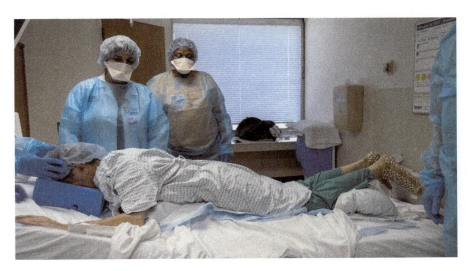

Fig. 10.11 Final padding is placed under the knees and the feet to prevent skin breakdown. The arms can be placed at the side or alternated in the swimmer's position to avoid skin breakdown. Chest physical therapy is done at this time to help mobilize secretions. All leads and lines are reconnected. The patient is observed over the next 10 minutes or until stability is confirmed

Finally, a post-proning safety checklist was completed. This includes checking the patient to ensure optimal positioning of pillows tailored to the patient's body habitus to assure comfort, to check pressure areas meticulously, and to make sure there was no pressure on the eyes or ears and that the endotracheal and nasogastric tubes were not compressed. It was also ensured that the urinary catheter is secured and any lines and tubing not pressed against the skin to prevent any skin injury. Skin care was meticulously performed at the end of the procedure. Over the next 5–15 minutes, the patient was monitored by the team to ensure patient stability of respiration, with preparations for emergency deproning (supining) always in place prior to proning. A successful proning procedure takes time, approximately 30–60 minutes per patient, as long as the setup was correct and no post-proning complications or respiratory instability occurred. It required a well-coordinated team approach. The SBH Health System proning checklist is shown in Box 10.2.

Box 10.2. Proning Checklist at SBH

1. Assemble adequate team:
   - Four proning staff.
   - One respiratory therapist.
   - Critical care nurse assigned to patient.
2. Identify patient/confirm they are "stable for proning."
3. Confirm feeding was stopped 45 min to 1 hr prior to procedure.

4. Check adequate bedside supplies:
   - Three to four chucks.
   - Clean gown/sheet for proning.
   - Skin care materials.
   - Face pads.
   - Eye guards.
   - Line caps.
   - Two pre-rolled bumps.
   - One pillow for the head.
   - Sheets or pillows for padding legs.
   - New ECG pads/pulse oximeter probe.

- *At bedside*
  1. Flatten bed.
  2. Pull away from the wall to allow respiratory therapist to gain access to the head.
  3. Adjust respirator to appropriate settings.
  4. Document vitals for post-proning assessment.
  5. Cap lines: Leave sedation/pressors and other essential lines.
  6. Do skin care.

- *Pre-proning*
  1. Place chucks on patient.
  2. Release bottom sheet.
  3. Place top sheet to cover chucks and patient.
  4. Tuck sheet under the arm on the side of the respirator over the chucks but not over the sheet on that side.
  5. Protect eyes.
  6. Place head cover: Allow respiratory therapist to ensure tube is secure and controlled.
  7. Patient suction.
  8. Foley and rectal tube between legs/all other lines placed toward the head.

- *Proning*
  1. Respiratory therapist calls the prone on the count of three.
  2. Pull bottom sheet with patient on the side of the bed away from the respirator to the edge.
  3. Rotate patient in one motion onto their side.
  4. Protect all lines.
  5. As the patient is turning to prone position, look for the top sheet that was tucked. Use that to continue to prone the patient.
  6. Always have head and tube secured.

7. Discard dirty sheets.
8. Place body rolls under the chest one side and then the other rolling patient each time.
9. Pad knees and ankles.
10. New pillow with chuck under the face.
11. Respiratory PT to the back.
12. Skin care.
13. Apply ECG leads/reattach lines.
14. Assess vitals for stabilization and document.

- *Maintenance*

    1. Arm position swimmer: Change every 2 hr

Challenges Faced at SBH

The greatest number of patients placed in the prone position was between March and June 2020 which coincided with the initial surge in cases seen in the Bronx, NY. On a daily basis, the ICU physicians identified ventilated patients that were indicated for proning. The procedure involved placing the patients in the prone position around 1 pm and then turning them back in the supine position 16–18 hours later around 8–9 am the next day. This schedule allowed for adequate patient preparation and equipment procurement. If a patient needed to be emergently repositioned outside in the absence of the proning team, the primary nurses and the staff, who were responsible for the patient, would reposition the patient. The checklist (Box 10.2) became an important guidance for successful proning and deproning. Nevertheless, there were some challenges faced and lessons learned in the implementation of proning.

Training and Education of Staff

The challenges of implementation of proning were generally the lack of standardized proning techniques, resource utilization (i.e., staff, supplies, etc.), communication, and team mobilization. Nursing education trained all the people that were identified as potential mobile proning team members. This was accomplished with a classroom training session and subsequent production of a training video now available to all team members on the internal web portal e-learning system called HealthStream. The video provided step-by-step guide and techniques in placing a patient in prone position. Initial techniques and resources were revised several times until a standard protocol was developed.

The rapid expansion of educational efforts allowed the staff to increase confidence and approach the issue with established processes and protocols. The training and use of other clinical services during the crisis avoided additional strain on nursing personnel and other clinicians on the units who were already understaffed. Additionally, the ability to focus the training on a group of individuals dedicated to proning worked well by improving care, competence, expertise, and safety. The success of prone team led to the development of the policies and protocols for both ventilated patients and non-intubated patients in order to sustain and expand proning capabilities across the hospital in case of future crises.

Staffing Concerns

The lack of personnel needed to reposition the patient safely was often an issue. The first few patients were proned with an anesthesiologist present to monitor and ensure patient safety and to prevent loss of airway. As protocol and processes were better defined, a minimum of four to six competent proning team members were essential, which included a respiratory therapist for managing the head and airways during the maneuver. The nursing shortage was particularly an issue due to staff exposure, illnesses, and burnout during the crisis. As elective orthopedics cases were cancelled, the orthopedic team was able to support the nursing division by supplementing the proning team. Orthopedic surgeons had extensive experience in understanding patient positioning, as this was a commonplace procedure that is performed in the operating room [19]. The orthopedic service inclusive of all surgeons and physician assistants and the podiatry residents along with the physical therapists became an integral part of the mobile proning team that rotated on a day-to-day basis to help minimize exposure to COVID-19 patients. This group of redeployed healthcare workers created a large resource of personnel that could be called upon in case of staff shortages.

Conclusions

The respiratory therapy services were at the forefront of the SHB Health System response and were critical to COVID-19 patient care. During this response, respiratory therapy services learned valuable lessons in management of resources, staff logistics, as well as their emotional and psychological well-being of team members. This experience equipped the department with a confidence to overcome any such future crises. In particular, the success of the multidisciplinary proning team rested on the collaborative cohesive approach that was taken by a dedicated leadership team with focus on continuous process assessment and improvement. Effective and rapid implementation of an education and training program proved vital in building staff skills and confidence to meet the challenge. Furthermore, the immediate development and implementation of a mobile proning team and standardized protocols allowed for increased capacity to prone all critically ill patients with ARDS. The great teamwork and astonishing efforts of the nurses, clinicians, respiratory therapists, occupational therapists, and the orthopedic team were critical to overcome the tidal wave of severely ill COVID-19 patients (Box 10.3).

> **Box 10.3. Key Lessons Learned in Respiratory Therapy**
> - For health crisis planning and preparation, it is highly important for any hospital to have contingency planning for expanded staffing with respiratory therapists. This is especially important in preparation for an infectious viral pandemic which can cause respiratory failure.
> - Dedicated leadership teams need to prioritize the multidisciplinary team approach to ensure a collaborative cohesive approach with focus on continuous process assessment and improvement of patient care.
> - Planning and preparation must include the provision of adequate and even redundant equipment and supplies, not only for the initial response to a health crisis but also to sustain the care of large numbers of severely ill patients with long hospitalizations. Equipment should include mechanical ventilators and ventilator alternatives such as high-flow nasal cannulas.
> - Effective and rapid implementation of an education and training program is vital in building staff skills and confidence in new and developing techniques such as proning. Standardized protocols resulting from this are hugely beneficial.
> - Emotional and psychological support of the frontline respiratory therapy staff is of utmost importance.

References

1. Sawadkar MM, Nayak VR. Respiratory therapists: the unnoticed warriors during COVID-19 pandemic in India. Can J Respir Ther. 2020;56:57.
2. Tu GW, Liu K, Su Y, Yu SJ, Ju MJ, Lou Z. The role of respiratory therapists in fighting the COVID-19 crisis: unsung heroes in Wuhan. Ann Palliat Med. 2020;9(6):4423–6.
3. Metlay JP, Waterer GW, Long AC, Anzueto A, Brozek J, Crothers K, et al. Diagnosis and treatment of adults with community-acquired pneumonia. An official clinical practice guideline of the American Thoracic Society and Infectious Diseases Society of America. Am J Respir Crit Care Med. 2019;200(7):e45–67.
4. Guan WJ, Ni ZY, Hu Y, Liang WH, Ou CQ, He JX, et al. Clinical characteristics of coronavirus disease 2019 in China. N Engl J Med. 2020;382(18):1708–20.
5. ARDS Definition Task Force, Ranieri VM, Rubenfeld GD, Thompson BT, Ferguson ND, Caldwell E, Fan E, Camporota L, Slutsky AS. Acute respiratory distress syndrome: the Berlin Definition. JAMA. 2012;307(23):2526–33. https://doi.org/10.1001/jama.2012.5669.
6. Wu C, Chen X, Cai Y, Xia J, Zhou X, Xu S, et al. Risk factors associated with acute respiratory distress syndrome and death in patients with coronavirus disease 2019 pneumonia in Wuhan, China. JAMA Intern Med. 2020;180(7):934–43. https://doi.org/10.1001/jamainternmed.2020.0994. Erratum in: JAMA Intern Med. 2020 Jul 1;180(7):1031.

7. Tzotzos SJ, Fischer B, Fischer H, Zeitlinger M. Incidence of ARDS and outcomes in hospitalized patients with COVID-19: a global literature survey. Crit Care. 2020;24(1):516. https://doi.org/10.1186/s13054-020-03240-7.
8. American Association for Respiratory Care. 2020. https://www.aarc.org/nn20-respiratory-therapists-warriors-in-the-fight-against-covid-19/. Accessed 16 Aug 2021.
9. Miller AG, Roberts KJ, Smith BJ, Burr KL, Hinkson CR, Hoerr CA, et al. Prevalence of burnout among respiratory therapists amidst the COVID-19. Respir Care. 2021:respcare.09283. https://doi.org/10.4187/respcare.09283.
10. Piehl MA, Brown RS. Use of extreme position changes in acute respiratory failure. Crit Care Med. 1976;4(1):13–4.
11. Albert RK. Prone ventilation for patients with mild or moderate acute respiratory distress syndrome. Ann Am Thorac Soc. 2020;17(1):24–9.
12. Bellani G, Laffey JG, Pham T, Fan E, Brochard L, Esteban A, et al. Epidemiology, patterns of care, and mortality for patients with acute respiratory distress syndrome in intensive care units in 50 countries. JAMA. 2016;315(8):788–800. https://doi.org/10.1001/jama.2016.0291.
13. Scholten EL, Beitler JR, Prisk GK, Malhotra A. Treatment of ARDS with prone positioning. Chest. 2017;151(1):215–24. https://doi.org/10.1016/j.chest.2016.06.032.
14. Guerin C, Beuret P, Constantin JM, Bellani G, Garcia-Oliveras P, Roca O, et al. A prospective international observational prevalence study on prone positioning of ARDS patients: the APRONET (ARDS Prone Position Network) study. Intensive Care Med. 2018;44(1):22–37. https://doi.org/10.1007/s00134-017-4996-5.
15. Guerin C, Reignier J, Richard JC, Beuret P, Gacoin A, Boulain T, et al. Prone positioning in severe acute respiratory distress syndrome. N Engl J Med. 2013;368(23):2159–68. https://doi.org/10.1056/NEJMoa1214103.
16. Venus K, Munshi L, Fralik M. Prone positioning for patients with hypoxic respiratory failure related to COVID-19. CMAJ. 2020;192(47):E1532–7. https://doi.org/10.1503/cmaj.201201.
17. Oliveira VM, et al. Safe prone checklist: construction and implementation of a tool for performing the prone maneuver. Rev Bras Ter Intensiva. 2017;29(2):131–41.
18. Jackson ME, Piekala DM, Deponti GN, DCR B, Minossi SD, Chiste M, et al. Skin preparation process for the prevention of skin breakdown in patients who are intubated and treated with RotoProne. Respir Care. 2012;57(2):311–4.
19. Rahman OF, Murray DP, Zbeda RM, Volpi AD, Mo AZ, Wessling NA, et al. Repurposing orthopaedic residents amid COVID-19: critical care prone positioning team. JB JS Open Access. 2020;5(2):e0058.

Chapter 11
Pharmacy

Ruth E. Cassidy

Alone we can do so little; together we can do so much. – Helen Keller

Pharmacy as an Integral Component of a Healthcare System

The World Health Organization (WHO) describes six building blocks that contribute to the strengthening of a healthcare system: service delivery, health workforce, health information systems, access to essential medical products/technologies, financing, and leadership/governance [1]. Leadership/governance provides the foundation for policies and protocols that the other blocks stand upon for stability and guidance, and it also forms a framework for patient-centered excellence (Fig. 11.1).

Regardless of the size of a crisis, it represents a very dynamic situation, and effective crisis management – which must be called upon in response – should be perceived as a living system *within* an organization [2]. A healthcare system is accustomed to coping with small-scale crises. However, in times of a large-scale crisis, the building block framework is shaken to its fundamental core, and this calls for swift and accurate decision-making in order to restabilize it.

The Department of Pharmacy is a clinical support service that plays a dynamic role in each of the six critical building blocks of a healthcare system. This chapter will outline the elements of pharmacy practice that are impacted by a crisis and can disrupt the foundational building blocks of a healthcare system. It will further delineate, in a prescriptive manner, the methods used to implement a plan of action for

R. E. Cassidy (✉)
Clinical Support Services and Pharmacy, SBH Health System, Bronx, NY, USA
e-mail: rcassidy@sbhny.org

© The Author(s), under exclusive license to Springer Nature Switzerland AG 2022
R. Shabsigh (ed.), *Health Crisis Management in Acute Care Hospitals*,
https://doi.org/10.1007/978-3-030-95806-0_11

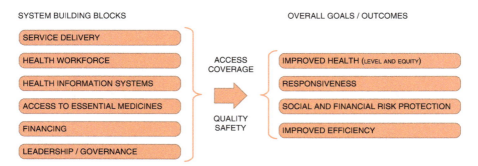

Fig. 11.1 The WHO health system framework. (Reproduced from: World Health Organization (WHO) [3] with permission from the WHO)

the four phases of crisis management: mitigation, preparedness, response, and recovery [4]. Finally, the chapter will describe an effective crisis management response, both established and implemented, by a health system pharmacy department during the 2020 COVID-19 pandemic.

As the epicenter of medication expertise, the pharmacy department is responsible for the delivery of safe, effective, and quality medications as well as pharmacotherapeutic services that achieve optimal health outcomes for all patients. Led by the chief pharmacy officer (CPO) or director of pharmacy, pharmacy provides an essential service to the healthcare system and reports to an executive leader of the healthcare system.

Comprehensively, the practice of pharmacy can be categorized into five key elements of performance: (1) supply chain/procurement, (2) distribution/security of medications, (3) ordering and prescribing, (4) preparation/administration, and (5) monitoring. Each of these elements has the capacity to impact the stability of one or more of the building blocks in the health system framework.

The department consists of two main branches: operational services and clinical services (Fig. 11.2). The operational services branch focuses on three of the key elements of performance mentioned above: (1), (2), and (4). The clinical services branch focuses on two of the other elements: (3) and (5).

Pharmacy: The Support Pillar of Health Crisis Management

In order to establish an effective crisis management response, it is critical to fully understand how each of the key elements comprising the medication process impact the stability of the health system framework when a crisis ensues.

As previously described, the building block of leadership/governance is the overarching segment that serves as the main foundation, the essential driver and central stabilizer of all other building blocks. In essence, they provide the compass to steer

11 Pharmacy

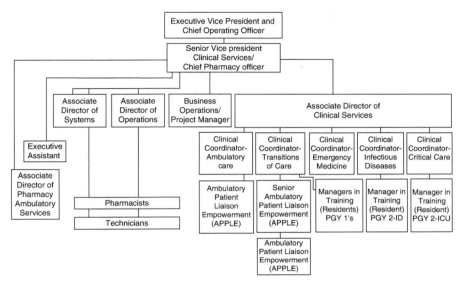

Fig. 11.2 The organizational structure of the Department of Pharmacy

the health system and stipulate direction via detailed policies and guidelines. Although there can be some traverse, the remaining five building blocks can be correlated to the elements of pharmacy practice. Examples of how the elements of pharmacy practice can disrupt a specific building block and impede the overall goal of improved health and optimal clinical outcomes are provided in Table 11.1.

A healthcare crisis is typically an unforeseen event that presents itself in a dramatic fashion, customarily accompanied by disorganization and chaos. During these tumultuous times, it is essential to thwart extreme variabilities in processes. Having a comprehensive list of specific disruptors to the elements of pharmacy practice will assist the pharmacy leaders in several ways: in outlining the four phases of a crisis management plan, in helping to reorient the support service, and, lastly, in realigning the building blocks of the health system.

Outline of the Crisis Management Plan at SBH Health System

To ensure excellence inpatient care in the midst of a crisis, each department within the health system must design a crisis management plan and be ever ready to call upon that plan when a tumultuous situation arises. An effective crisis management process plan consists of four main phases (Fig. 11.3). Two of the phases must be implemented prior to the crisis situation, and two are to be implemented after the crisis situation. The crisis management process plan for the pharmacy department of a health system is similarly engineered.

Table 11.1 Consequences and impact of disruptions to key elements of pharmacy performance

Element of Pharmacy Practice/ Building block	Disruptive Force
Supply chain/ procurement/ *Access to Medicines and Financing*	1. Break down in supply chain ≫ limited or no availability of essential medications 2. Restricted access to novel research medications 3. Constrained financial resources 4. Manufacturers/wholesalers diminished ability to meet supply and demand 5. Competition on both a local and a national level for products
Distribution/ security of medications/ *Service Delivery*	1. Units expanded rapidly – e.g., critical care 2. Units closed – e.g., med-surg units/pediatrics/geriatric 3. Major expansion of the Emergency Room Department: (a) Above three items complicate the distribution of medications and raise an issue for continuity of security/storage of meds across the health system 4. Ensuring safety of staff during delivery and exchange of medications (on units (Pyxis) and within pharmacy (returns/crash carts)) – e.g., biological or infectious disease crisis

Ordering and prescribing/ *Health Information Systems*	1. Novel medications brought to formulary
	2. Developing new medication guidelines and protocols
	3. Obtaining access to research medications:
	  (a) Issues with order sets assigned to specific service lines may need immediate expansion
	  (b) Increase in volume of IV orders skyrocket
	  (c) CPOE build issues that were minor are exacerbated due to increased volume of orders entered
	  (d) Availability of IT hardware

Administering/ preparation/ *Health Workforce*	1. Operations within pharmacy related to distribution dramatically challenged:
	  (a) IV room capacity
	  (b) Staffing challenges

Monitoring/ *Health Workforce*	1. Clinical staff centralized – challenge to optimal communication with physicians 2. Uncertain or novel treatment modalities 3. Real-time clinical decision support 4. Real-time drug utilization and projections for need

Mitigation Phase

During the mitigation phase, the pharmacy department constructs strategies that aim to minimize the impact of the crisis by reducing vulnerability [5]. To do this, the department must ensure that the CPO is included in the emergency planning committee and is privy to all internal as well as external public communications. Moreover, strategies to maintain constant lines of communication with all pharmacy stakeholders, and to minimize any financial impact of the crisis, should be created. Designated lead coordinators should be in place for all areas of pharmacy practice including supplies, staffing, operations, and clinical and IT systems. Finally, processes should be developed so that a command center can be deployed rapidly, if and when necessary.

Fig. 11.3 The crisis management process at SBH. (Image provide by Presenter Media www.preserntermedia.com with permission)

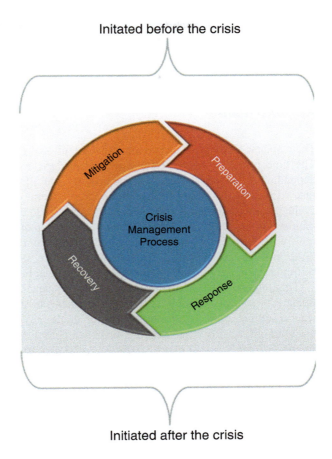

Preparedness

During the preparation phase, the pharmacy department will attempt to anticipate the financial and operational resources it may need during the crisis situation. Some disasters occur rapidly and offer little to no time for preparation. Other crisis situations can be so immense and unpredictable that the elements of preparation are difficult to forecast, such as in the case of a pandemic. To ensure preparedness to overcome any crisis, the department must create a plan for rapid expansion and scale-down of pharmacy services. To do this, it is essential that there are regular assessments of current equipment, potential additional equipment which may be needed, and the ease at which equipment can be redeployed. This should be done in conjunction with an assessment of the current staffing complement and the ability to flex up or down. The department should also create strategies for onboarding alternative staffing and establish systems for virtual communications and remote functioning of CPOE and pharmacy IT applications/systems. Systems should be created to efficiently track financial resources and expenses to prevent the department becoming overstretched during a crisis. A multidisciplinary committee could also prove useful in ensuring that the department is prepared for a crisis.

Response Phase

The response phase is the period immediately following the onset of the crisis event. The time frame of the response phase can endure over days, weeks, or months, depending on the crisis situation. The primary goal of the health system and pharmacy department is to address the immediate concerns of patients and staff, as well as the resources needed for business continuity. To do this effectively, regular communication between the leadership and the management is vital. This may include reviewing checklists regularly, daily huddles with frontline staff, and open communication channels with all stakeholders. Furthermore, systems and processes should be in place for communication with peers at external health systems.

Triaging can help identify the most critical issues during crisis and allocate the limited resources efficiently [6]. Daily assessments of staffing needs, budgets, medication supplies, and changes to medication guidelines need to be conducted, since these are all crucial in an effective response phase. Additionally, the department should also put together plans to educate and train current and alternative staff and maintain a strong awareness of their well-being.

Recovery Phase

The recovery phase occurs after the crisis situation has abated. During this phase, the health system and pharmacy department focuses on rebuilding, with a primary goal of a "return to normal" or a "new normal." A reevaluation of staffing, supply, and operational requirements must occur following the crisis. Transition plans must be drawn up to de-escalate to normal or a new normal functioning of the department, and this may require redeployment of staff, understanding the financial impact and organizing access to recovery funding and offering continued support to staff to maintain their well-being. It is also essential that the department highlights lessons learned during the crisis, along with analyzing its overall performance, adjusting future training needs accordingly. Finally, celebrating the achievements of the pharmacy staff and stakeholders is essential to keep morale high.

When a crisis situation ensues, the health system pharmacy department runs the risk of being thrown into utter chaos due to the dramatic shifts in resource requirements associated with the volatility of the circumstances. Significant demands on medication supply, an immediate increase in staffing requirements, and an increased need for equipment hardware to store and manage patient's medications effectively are all forced upon the department in rapid succession. To be best prepared for the mercurial events that identify a crisis, the health system pharmacy department should have a policy clearly stating that a crisis management process plan should be in place at all times. Furthermore, the pharmacy leadership should ensure all staff are thoroughly educated on that crisis management plan.

Expansion of Pharmacy Services and Operations During the Crisis

In crisis situations, concurrent information comes to the healthcare organization from multiple sources, both public and private. Additionally, the multiple sources often provide conflicting information that is frequently modified. Therefore, incoming data needs to be assessed for relevance and reliability and then integrated into the healthcare crisis management response or discarded [7]. Incorporating all leaders of each healthcare discipline and obtaining their input are crucial to establish a comprehensive crisis response plan. Moreover, the flow of information must be continuous and bidirectional from each discipline. Most often, this is done through establishing a command center within the organization specific to the crisis at hand.

The CPO takes the lead for the Department of Pharmacy within the command center. Within the command center, the CPO can ensure the pharmacy crisis response is directly aligned with the health system's overall crisis response. This information is then communicated from the officer to the designated coordinators who lead all pharmacy areas and who in turn communicate to the frontline staff.

As previously discussed, the elements of performance for pharmacy operations focus on procurement of medication, its preparation, its administration, and its security and distribution. In the wake of a catastrophic event such as a disaster or pandemic, the pharmacy department's routine operational processes are significantly disrupted. The department must respond methodically and rapidly to the immediate increase in demand for operational resources.

Distressed Supply Chains

Under normal circumstances, the pharmacy medication budget is one of the largest budgets for a health system. During a disaster or crisis situation, the supply chains become stressed at both a national and a local level. Instability in procurement of medication becomes a paramount concern as all health systems are competing for similar essential medications. National manufacturers and wholesalers are most often unable to keep up with the significant increase in demand. Figure 11.4 is an illustrative example how spending in the pharmacy in the immediate aftermath of the COVID-19 pandemic begins to impact two of the six building blocks of the health system, by placing a burden on financial resources and access to essential

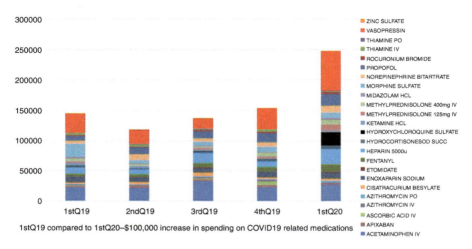

Fig. 11.4 Increase in pharmacy expense during the pandemic in Q1 of 2020 at SBH Health System

medications. This stress can cause the health system framework to buckle. If these unstable building blocks are not addressed in a timely fashion, there will be a negative effect on the overall goals of the health system, i.e., to improve health and optimal clinical outcome.

Secured Access to Medication and Automated Dispensing Cabinets

It is essential that the pharmacy department remains synchronized with the expansion of the larger health system. As a crisis develops, critical care units are opened in rapid succession. All federal and state regulatory bodies (Joint Commission, CMS, Boards of Pharmacy, DEA) require medications to be stored safely and securely. The CPO and the designated area coordinators must adhere to the regulatory requirements while meeting the new increased demand for secure medication access in these critical care units. As each new critical care unit comes online, pharmacy meets this demand with a very meticulous and systematic process to allow the provision of medication. A key element to this continuity in provision is the use of automated dispensing cabinets (ADC) for medication. ADCs enable improved medication safety and quality of care, mainly by decreasing medication errors. Additionally they save time and costs by removing large amounts of physician and nurse time during the medication process. This saving of health worker time in a pandemic is vital, as is the potential reduction of errors from overworked, tired, and emotionally drained hospital staff.

Each step of the systematic process allowing pharmacy to meet the growing demands of critical care unit expansion is outlined below:

- The command center provides an updated list of all hospital units that are converted to critical care units.

- The pharmacy coordinator for IT systems assesses how many additional ADCs are needed to meet the new demand for essential medication.
- Calls are made to vendors to acquire additional ADCs.
- ADCs are procured and deployed to hospital units.
- ADCs are configured and connected with network interfaces.
- Pharmacy buyer procures the essential medications to stock the ADCs.
- The pharmacy coordinator of operations works with frontline staff to stock the ADCs with essential medications.

Increase in Orders Received and Processed

In a crisis situation, the number of critical patients increases. The medical care required for improved outcome is extensive and complex. Moreover, requirements for medications for these critical patients are often urgent, and consequently the number of orders the pharmacist needs to verify increases significantly. Figure 11.5 illustrates how the number of STAT IV orders increased threefold within a 60-day period during the peak of the COVID-19 health crisis first surge in 2020.

Staffing Concerns During the Crisis

Depending on the type of healthcare crisis and its duration, the impact it has on personnel may affect adequate staffing complements. Staff shortages can result due to staff illness, stress, burnout, or care responsibilities. Therefore, it is important for the operations coordinator to assess staffing needs and staffing complements daily for the duration of the crisis period.

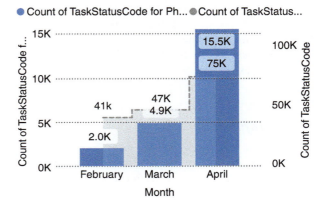

Fig. 11.5 STAT IV orders received by pharmacy operations from the COVID-19 floors in the spring of 2020 at SBH Health System

In a widespread healthcare crisis, state governments will invoke executive orders to permit licensed professionals, as well as retired professionals, to cross state lines in order to work in areas that are most impacted. Rapid onboarding and training of alternative staffing can bolster bench strength within the department to protect business continuity.

Integrated tiered team staffing is a very effective and essential strategy to ensure adequate staffing in a crisis situation [8]. The integrated tiered team maximizes utilization of limited resources and broadens staff coverage, especially when rapid expansion of critical patient care units is warranted. The tiered staffing model allows a department to capitalize on all potential alternative staffing and involves utilizing one well-trained pharmacist or pharmacy technician to work alongside newly hired pharmacists and pharmacy technicians, as well as other licensed professionals assigned to assist in pharmacy operations. To allow for quick implementation of the tiered staffing model, all the pharmacists and pharmacy technicians should be cross-trained to work in any area of the pharmacy department (Box 11.1).

Box 11.1 Everyone Can Contribute During the Crisis
For the creation of additional pharmacy staff force from non-pharmacy staff, help was enlisted at SBH Health System from:

- *Dentists and dental residents for pharmacy delivery and granting access to ADCs*
- *Medical students, residents, and fellows*
- *Pharmacy residents, interns, and students*

Pharmacy Clinical Services

As pharmacy increases procurement of medication and commences to methodically augment its medication distribution to the new patient care units, the clinical services arm simultaneously enhances its services to these new patient care units too. The focus of the clinical pharmacy services is on the remaining two performance metrics of the medication process: ordering/prescribing and medication monitoring. Health information systems and the health workforce are the two building blocks of the patient care framework which most impacted the performance of clinical pharmacy services.

Health Information Systems

In the event of a widespread healthcare crisis, the health information coming from the public health sector changes frequently. Pharmacy clinical services must respond to these updates expeditiously and judiciously. The medication protocols and guidelines must be reworked in accordance with the new information and redistributed and reeducated across all disciplines. Subsequent to the newly revised protocols and guidelines, downstream pharmacy information systems must also be modified: computerized physician order entry must be configured with new treatment modalities; knowledge-based medication barcoding system databases must be reconfigured; medication order sets must be restructured; drug libraries for medication infusion pumps must be amended and uploaded to all medication pumps on the network. Essentially, all pharmacy IT applications must be updated with new information as and when it becomes available.

A key factor to ensuring that all new health information is accurately and concurrently configured in all pharmacy information systems and then precisely communicated to all disciplines is the formation of a *multidisciplinary pharmacy committee*. The primary goal of this committee is to ensure all pharmacy applications and medication libraries are rapidly updated with new medication protocols or guidelines as rapidly as the information is disseminated from the public health sectors. With a focus on critical care, every discipline and service line should be represented on this committee, and everyone should be kept abreast of new information on a weekly basis.

Without such a timely and prompt response of pharmacy clinical services, the health information system building block of the patient care framework would be severely and negatively impacted, imposing significant detrimental consequences upon health outcomes. It is prudent for the health system pharmacy and clinical services to outline a clear crisis management process plan to protect against any destabilization of the patient care framework involving pharmacy informatics.

Health Workforce

Over the last decade, clinical pharmacy services have become highly specialized with many clinical pharmacists earning board certifications in specific areas. During any health crisis scenario, there are three specialty areas of clinical pharmacy services that are most likely to be impacted: pharmacy critical care services, pharmacy emergency services, and pharmacy transitions of care services.

Pharmacy Critical Care Services The Society of Critical Care Medicine (SCCM) guidelines for critical care services and personnel deem that pharmacists are essential for the delivery of quality care to critically ill patients [9]. Today, pharmacists are viewed as a vital element to the multidisciplinary team in the intensive care unit by providing monitoring of therapeutic medication, nutritional support, and actively participating in the patient care rounds [9].

During a crisis situation, pharmacy critical care service is one of the first specialty pharmacy services to be called upon. The resource requirement for pharmacy critical care service can expand quite rapidly in the wake of a crisis. It is important that the health system pharmacy department has the ability to flex up on critical care pharmacist resources when a crisis ensues. The burden placed on the pharmacy critical care team can range from minimal to significant, depending on the extent of the crisis at hand. For example, during the COVID-19 pandemic, critical care beds within the SBH Health System increased sixfold. Implementing an integrated team approach to critical care pharmacist staffing will assist in meeting the substantial increase on human resource demand.

Pharmacy Emergency Services The American College of Emergency Physicians together with the American Society of Health-System Pharmacists have long recognized the importance of clinical pharmacists in the emergency medicine setting [10]. In this fast-paced, highly complex environment, clinical pharmacists work alongside emergency medicine practitioners, optimizing medication protocols, ensuring medication safety, verifying all aspects of medication orders specific to each patient, participating in medical and trauma emergencies, and educating physicians, nurses, residents, and students on drug information.

Pharmacy emergency service is front line when a crisis initially enters the doors of the health system. The medication process often involves high-risk medications administered in time critical procedures. The emergency clinical pharmacist has proven to be a highly valued member of the emergency department multidisciplinary team with reduced patient mortality and improved patient outcomes well documented in scholarly literature [11, 12]. From the onset of a health crisis, whether acute or widespread, the pharmacy emergency clinical service must remain in place and be readily available to assist with the typically overburdened environment of high-risk patients.

Pharmacy Transition of Care Services Medication management is crucial to optimal patient care outcomes, not only throughout the inpatient experience but also during transitions of care to the ambulatory setting or assisted living environments. The pharmacy transition of care service therefore plays a critical role in the health system framework for patient-centered excellence. Throughout a healthcare crisis, patients can be triaged to be discharged or stepped down to an intermediate level of care unit or facility. The pharmacy transition of care services include medication reconciliation, discharge medication dispensing and counseling, as well as medication management post-discharge, in person or via telehealth visits.

In the aftermath of a healthcare crisis, pharmacy clinical care services are immediately overburdened. An overburdened health workforce can jeopardize the stability of the health system framework yielding negative effects on patient quality and patient clinical outcomes. The health system pharmacy department must delineate a clear crisis management process plan to guarantee continuity of care for these services lines.

Case Study: The SBH Pharmacy Response to COVID-19 and Expansion of Pharmacy Services

Almost immediately following the announcement by the WHO at the end of January 2020 that COVID-19 was a public health emergency [13], SBH Health System senior leadership held a meeting to discuss the potential impact on the hospital. The pharmacy department within SBH Health System is led by the chief pharmacy officer and consists of a total of 50 employees evenly split between pharmacists and pharmacy technicians. The pharmacy department had to confront many challenges as the SBH Health System adapted to the ensuing health crisis.

Expansion of Critical Care Patient Care Units

Over the course of the next few weeks, the SBH Health System was required to increase the critical care bed capacity significantly. For pharmacy operations, this resulted in an increased need for equipment, to secure medications; an increase in processing, preparation, and distribution of medication orders; and an increase in human resources to perform the increase in work tasks. Specifically, three key adaptations were made: (1) Five medical/surgical units were converted to critical care units, and three additional units were to be configured for immediate transition to a critical care unit – automated dispensing cabinets were procured and/or configured for these new critical care units. (2) Total medication orders processed by pharmacists increased by 2000 orders in a 1 month period (Fig. 11.6), and the total IV products compounded by pharmacists increased by 27,000 during the same month.

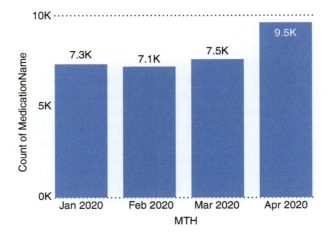

Fig. 11.6 Medication orders processed by pharmacists per month in 2020 at SBH Health System

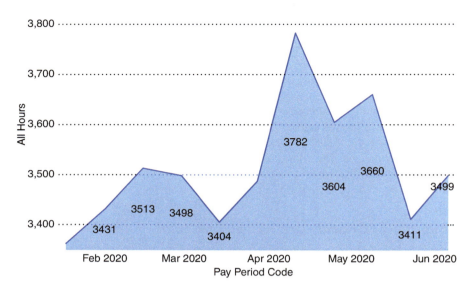

Fig. 11.7 Staff pharmacist biweekly hours per month at SBH Health System. These hours did not include hours worked by pharmacy technicians, any alternate/ancillary staff, clinical pharmacists, or managers

(3) The number of hours worked by staff pharmacists increased by almost 400 hours in a 1 month period (Fig. 11.7). Moreover, the pharmacy clinical services simultaneously had new work responsibilities added on to their daily routines (Table 11.2).

Gaining Access to Essential Medications

Treating COVID-19 was a challenge. Many of the medications required to treat patients were not FDA-approved. Others were difficult to procure due to the fact that all healthcare systems across the country required them.

The medications that were not FDA-approved required access to research study protocols with the manufacturers. The clinical infectious disease service pharmacist was assigned to coordinate access to all necessary study protocols with the various manufacturers. A further challenge was that SBH Health System was not currently participating in any of the research studies; it took a lot of fast maneuvering and coordination to gain access to essential medications.

Later that year (November 2020), the COVID-19 vaccine was made available to health systems. This presented with a new challenge in its administration and distribution since deep-freezer storage was needed to maintain the stocks, IT reports and interfaces needed to be built for the required DOH data collection, and appointments for first and second doses needed to be coordinated.

Table 11.2 Added responsibilities for each pharmacy clinical service area

Pharmacy emergency clinical services	Pharmacy critical care and infectious disease services	Pharmacy transition of care services
Created a cath lab diversion thrombolytic protocol Created critical care infusion dosing charts due to pump shortage (propofol, midazolam, ketamine, dexmedetomidine, norepinephrine, epinephrine, dobutamine, dopamine) to convert standard rates to ml/hr and drops/minute Bedside care for up to 25 intubated patients/shift (~5–7 new intubations/shift) Optimized ED automated dispensing cabinets to ensure adequate stock of critical medications Provided daily updates to ED leadership regarding medication shortages and recommended alterative RSI/sedation recommendations Off-hour prospective order review Bedside ACLS CPR participation Nursing and provider education for paralytic infusions	Remdesivir compassionate use and expanded access programs Data entry and clinical trial paperwork for remdesivir studies COVID-19 treatment guideline creation EMPACTA trial participation Tocilizumab criteria and utilization Anticoagulation protocol development Concentrated drip protocols List of preferred drugs for decreased nurse requirement, e.g., once/twice daily drugs Steroid alternatives Ketamine utilization in addition to fentanyl Order set creations Monoclonal antibody protocol – ED, Room 601, outpatient hemodialysis Provide clinical medication decision support on rounds daily in the ICU Attended infectious disease consults daily for COVID-19 patients	Ensure safe transitions of patients being relocated to Javits/naval ship Verified and dispensed a 5-day supply of medications for all patients being transferred to other sites on a daily basis during the surge Order verification in EMR on shift and remote order verification during off hours Assisted with additional staffing requirements on evenings and weekends Drug inventory/shortage management Provide clinical medication decision support on rounds in med/surg units

Maintaining Adequate Staffing Levels

State and federal regulatory agencies recognize that maintaining appropriate staffing levels is a key component to providing a safe environment for workers and patients, but also essential to achieving optimal outcomes in-patient-centered care [14]. During the peak of the surge, pharmacy personnel were working hours far beyond a normal work week (see Fig. 11.7). In addition to physical exhaustion from long hours of extreme workloads, workers or their families, who had been exposed to COVID-19, had to be quarantined. Some employees were also physically ill. With remote learning in place and daycare closures, some workers had to be home to care for young children, and others were suffering from the mental strain for fear of exposing themselves and/or family members to the virus, due to their hospital-based work and therefore exposure.

Regardless of the focused efforts by the department's leadership on staffing complements, maintaining adequate staffing levels was a daily challenge during the COVID-19 surge months. One of the primary strategies utilized to assist with staffing was to cancel nonessential procedures. This allowed the freed staff to be floated to the pharmacy department. One great resource of ancillary staff was the dental residents. Dental residents were able, with quick training, to assist with many pharmacy technician work responsibilities such as restocking of airway trays and medication deliveries to the pharmacy automated dispensing systems.

Furthermore, a policy to halt personal time off, vacation and work-related travel, was put into effect by executive leadership. Pharmacy residents and interns were pulled off their normal rotations to assist with pharmacist work responsibilities. Emergency waivers were granted by the state to allow both out-of-state licensed pharmacists and retired pharmacists to work during the COVID-19 surge. All supplementary staff needed to be onboarded through human resources as quickly as possible. Additionally, the new staff had to be quickly educated and trained on the various work and workflow processes. As previously described, an integrated tiered approach to staffing was utilized to maximize resource effectiveness. Finally, VPN access was granted to clinical pharmacists to allow virtual working from home off hours.

The challenges the pharmacy department was confronted with during the months of the surge had to be assessed and immediately addressed by leadership. Effective strategies and solutions had to be rapidly implemented to sustain business continuity and to restabilize the health system's framework for patient-centered excellence. The greatest factor in meeting all the pharmacy department challenges was having the mitigation and preparedness components of an effective crisis management process plan already established.

Successes Realized by the SBH Pharmacy Department

The most remarkable success of the pharmacy department, related to the pandemic, was that the leaders were able to directly align expansion of and de-escalation of services with that of other departments of the health system, in a highly effective manner. This alignment is attributed to the department having all the elements of the mitigation and preparedness phase of a crisis management plan in place prior to the pandemic.

Additionally, the level of success is attributed to a wonderful group of individual pharmacists and pharmacy technicians that were fully committed to ensuring safe and optimal care for every patient with a collaborative culture and superb work ethics. Each member of staff who supported the pharmacy workload made a heroic effort.

Key Lessons Learned

The principal lesson learned by the SBH Health System Department of Pharmacy is that preparation in itself is never enough; however, it is critically important to remain "ever ready" for that unforeseen event which may occur. The CPO and all the pharmacy department leaders are certified in FEMA disaster response and regularly participate in FEMA disaster response training drills which are immensely useful. It is clear that the facility's regular training drills contributed to the preparedness and success to overcome the pandemic.

The primary takeaway related to pharmacy operational services is twofold. First, the pharmacy manages a very tight medication budget with a medication surplus to sustain the health system's normal population of patients for approximately a 7-day supply, very close to just-in-time inventory (a form of inventory management where raw materials arrive just as production is scheduled to begin). With the pandemic surge, the health system patient population increased by at least 50%. Procuring and maintaining an adequate supply of critical care medications essential for the treatment of COVID-19 patients was one of the most significant challenges pharmacy operations was confronted with. Keeping slightly larger stocks of essential medications is one of the main lessons learned. The second lesson is to have a larger number of per diem pharmacists and technicians who are trained in the policy and procedures of a health system pharmacy department. Although there is a financial impact related to on-boarding and training, this will be largely offset by a higher level of emergency preparedness.

The lesson learned related to clinical pharmacy services is the continued need for full-time board-certified clinical pharmacists in the specialty areas of critical care and infectious diseases. This becomes more evident to the service line lead physicians, and as a result of the clinical pharmacist contributions, two additional full-time clinical pharmacists were added to the pharmacy staffing budget.

Conclusion

Health crises will often arrive unexpectedly and can cause significant disruption to health system service lines. This chapter illustrates that the magnitude of disruption is dependent on how well department leaders have prepared their department and staff in crisis management. Having a crisis management plan is critical to successfully abate the disruptive forces and thwart variability in processes. The ultimate goal of the pharmacy crisis management plan is to maintain the stability of the building block framework of the health system that guarantees improved clinical outcomes for the patients. Preparedness for an emergency is a journey for the pharmacy department, not a destination. The pharmacy department will continue to be "ever ready" for the next eventual healthcare crisis, continually learning and educating the necessary stakeholders.

References

1. World Health Organization (WHO). Monitoring the building blocks of health systems: a handbook of indicators and their measurement strategies. Geneva: WHO; 2010.
2. Paraskevas A. Crisis management or crisis response system? A complexity science approach to organizational crises. Manag Decis. 2006;44:892–907.
3. World Health Organization (WHO). Everybody's business - strengthening health systems to improve health outcomes: WHO's framework for action. Geneva: WHO; 2007. http://www.who.int/healthsystems/strategy/everybodys_business.pdf.
4. Chadha P. The four phases of crisis management. https://agb.org/. 2020. [cited 2020]. https://agb.org/blog-post/the-four-phases-of-crisis-management/. Accessed 21 July 2021.
5. Rose DA, Murthy S, Brooks J, Bryant J. The evolution of public health emergency management as a field of practice. Am J Public Health. 2017;107(S2):S126–S33.
6. Moore B, Bone EA. Decision-making in crisis: applying a healthcare triage methodology to business continuity management. J Bus Contin Emer Plan. 2017;11(1):21–6.
7. St. Pierre M, Hofinger G, Simon R. Crisis management in acute care settings. 3rd ed. Springer International Publishing; 2016. XXII. p. 433.
8. Halpern N, Tan K. Critical connections blog [Internet]: Society of Critical Care Medicine. 2020. [cited 2021]. https://sccm.org/Blog/March-2020/United-States-Resource-Availability-for-COVID-19. Accessed 21 July 2021.
9. Position paper on critical care pharmacy services. Pharmacotherapy. 2000;20(11):1400–6.
10. Morgan SR, Acquisto NM, Coralic Z, Basalyga V, Campbell M, Kelly JJ, et al. Clinical pharmacy services in the emergency department. Am J Emerg Med. 2018;36(10):1727–32.
11. Zhai XB, Gu ZC, Liu XY. Effectiveness of the clinical pharmacist in reducing mortality in hospitalized cardiac patients: a propensity score-matched analysis. Ther Clin Risk Manag. 2016;12:241–50.
12. Newsome AS, Jones TW, Smith SE. Pharmacists are associated with reduced mortality in critically ill patients: now what? Crit Care Med. 2019;47(12):e1036–e7.
13. Archived: WHO Timeline - COVID19 20 Avenue Appia, Geneva, 2020 [updated April 27].
14. CDC. Strategies to mitigate healthcare personnel staffing shortages 2021. https://www.cdc.gov/coronavirus/2019-ncov/hcp/mitigating-staff-shortages.html. Accessed 21 July 2021.

Chapter 12
Laboratory

Richard R. Hwang and Muhammad F. Durrani

Laboratory's Role, Response, and Continuity Plan During a Healthcare Crisis

Laboratory plays an integral role in providing quality, accurate and reliable services and valuable information in a timely fashion to satisfy clinicians' needs, help improve patient outcomes, and maximize benefits of healthcare delivery, patient safety, and safeguard public health. About 70% of today's medical decisions are based on results produced by clinical laboratory tests [1]. This is a substantial contribution and signifies the importance of laboratory services being able to endure despite overwhelm caused by any health crisis. During a crisis, laboratory becomes the first line of defense, after hospital emergency units, to perform screening and diagnostic testing, and if, under these high-pressure situations, laboratory is struggling with human and financial resources, to perform training, testing, logistics, and biosafety and to test equipment enabling the support of patient management, the system may collapse. This theory became a reality during COVID-19 pandemic when there was a shortage of labor force, necessary tools, personal protective and testing equipment, and supplies to ensure safety and provide laboratory services in a timely fashion.

R. R. Hwang (✉)
Laboratory Services, SBH Health System, Bronx, NY, USA

CUNY School of Medicine, New York, NY, USA

M. F. Durrani
Laboratory Services, SBH Health System, Bronx, NY, USA
e-mail: mdurrani1@Northwell.edu

© The Author(s), under exclusive license to Springer Nature Switzerland AG 2022
R. Shabsigh (ed.), *Health Crisis Management in Acute Care Hospitals*,
https://doi.org/10.1007/978-3-030-95806-0_12

Conducting a Comprehensive Risk Assessment and Identification of Disruption in Services

Every crisis behaves differently and may not end as expected; therefore, a comprehensive risk assessment, including identification of all possible elements/events that may cause disruption in services, is key in managing or overcoming a crisis. Incorporating a routine risk assessment into the schedule prior to a crisis occurring may aid in the development of a laboratory healthcare crisis management plan. Strategic planning, flexible remedial actions, and immediate implementation of the developed plans may then help mitigate risks and overcome problems, allowing for a successful outcome. Risk assessment in anticipation of, and during a crisis, is different than a routine assessment since it requires a more robust and immediate approach, with careful actions to allow for continuation of services. It should include, though not be limited to, a critical and realistic analysis of the current processes, procedures and status (situation analysis), identification of gaps, continuation/improvement of quality practices, and how to mitigate disruptions and minimize errors, and it should include the development of plans for continued and effective laboratory services (accuracy, reliability, and quality).

To increase efficacy of a risk assessment, it can be beneficial to develop a checklist of the problems (what has happened and expectations of what can happen on a scale from best to worst), perform a SWOT (strength, weaknesses, opportunities, and threats) analysis, and do a needs assessment. All such tools were effectively used during COVID-19 crisis management at the SBH Health System Laboratory. The laboratory was fortunately able to continue providing effective services without any disruption in services or a struggling supply chain. The risk assessment anticipated a labor force shortage due to excessive sickness, supply chain issues, and reagent availability due to manufacturing shortages, transport and communication, storage problems, and intradepartmental/section communications. Being able to foresee these issues and successfully execute the laboratory healthcare crisis plan was extremely valuable for the SBH Health System Laboratory. These guidelines can now confidently be used in the future for any laboratory setup, to help ensure effective continuity of services during a healthcare crisis.

Developing a Laboratory Crisis and Continuity Management Plan

Having a crisis and continuity management plan is crucial in order to manage circumstances arising during a crisis that may otherwise impair laboratory operations and functionality. By conducting a comprehensive risk assessment, a realistic plan can be created which allows a degree of flexibility for forecasted unforeseen events that could occur at any stage during a crisis. The following are some guidelines for developing a laboratory crisis and continuity management plan.

Expanding and Prioritizing Laboratory Services During a Healthcare Crisis

It is important to review the current test menu and subsequently create a prioritized test menu, which should be followed during crisis management. Furthermore, emphasis should be put on adopting a value-based approach for new testing services and technologies and a more robust system of testing in order to streamline existing processes. Expanding the current capacity of testing for optimal and rapid care in the immediate care areas can be achieved through rapid diagnostics and point-of-care testing (POCT) ambulatory laboratory services, or patient nearside testing services. Finally, having a list of the support activities/services that need to be continued during a crisis is of great value.

Setting Up Dedicated Laboratory Team and Capacity Building

Setting up a dedicated laboratory team and capacity building is vital to cope with the increased demand for testing, training, competency, proficiency of staff, and allowing for continuation of services during a crisis. Setup of this dedicated team involves delegation of tasks and responsibilities to individual members or the team as a whole, providing a clear description of the tasks to be completed and resources required, and there should be a continued review and documentation of these assigned tasks. Where relevant, training, retraining, or in-service of staff to assess competency (formal or nonformal) and proficiency should be conducted, alongside coaching and mentoring personnel on the continuity plan, to prepare staff well and encourage resolution of issues in a timely fashion. A list of all contact numbers for key resources, entities, and staff, plus their roles in crisis management and unexpected events, should be readily available. In order to increase efficiency and effectiveness of the services, a review of the existing testing capacity should be carried out.

Setting Up and/or Coordination with an Incident Command Center

Setting up an incident command or coordination with a command center is a vital important part of the continuity plan. The command center provides a line of actions, updated information, guidelines, receiving information, and reports. It also assesses all incidents and operations and monitors core activities to help maintain efficiency. Where appropriate, the center will ensure contact with external agencies and coordination of services, including notification for implementation of recovery processes when the crisis is over.

Mobilization of Staff During Healthcare Crisis

Staff resource management during a healthcare crisis is crucial to staying afloat. Individuals may be identified for appropriate (and often new) tasks/roles based on their capacity and capabilities. In order to help support activities and critical value reporting, it may be necessary to reschedule, cross-train, and reassign duties. Of utmost importance in any crisis is assessing and protecting the emotional, physical, and psychological health of staff members. Ensuring easy and equitable access to resources, and that staff needs are fairly and effectively included in the plan, is a necessity.

Resource Management

Resource management is vital for the smooth operation, quality, and reliability of laboratory services. Laboratory must have resources including facilities, materials, equipment, and instruments available at all times in order to provide appropriate services as required for the continuity of operations plan. It should also be possible to describe laboratory testing services or conduct alternative arrangements during a crisis. The following describes requirements and suggestions to support resource management:

- Inventory management (procurement, supplies, specimen collection kits, instruments, reagents, test kits, and personal protective equipment (PPE))
- Utilities and backup arrangements (backup power supplies, fire suppression systems, safety, building and/or strengthening security systems, internal and external safety measures e.g., if services need to be temporarily shifted to another area). In addition, arrangements such as dedicated space/accommodation, storage and environmental requirements, or the shifting of core activities
- Maintenance of required processes/procedures and acquiring necessary resources for the continuity of essential core functions
- Validations and verification, interface and computer system maintenance, security, and functionality
- Storage capacity (short term and long term) for supplies, specimens, and dead bodies
- Workload assessment in various sections of laboratory and redistribution of workload and staff in various sections
- Admissible and appropriate remote access and resources
- Exploring the possibilities of new vendors for provision of supplies and testing materials
- Budgeting for the continuity of services and flexibility for acquiring resources

Developing a Communication and Reporting Plan

The communication and reporting plan are vital to ensure effective and accurate transmission of information. It should include the following information:

- Arrangements for communication with clients regarding status of laboratory services and reporting results
- Contact information and communication of information among laboratory staff
- Internal communication structure (using existing multidisciplinary committees and dedicated laboratory teams, holding meetings, communication with physicians, and other providers with specification of method for communication, memo, e-mail, or phone call)
- External communication strategy with outside laboratories, vendor, community organizations, and regulatory agencies
- Collection and dissemination of critical information
- Instructions for reporting and providing status updates to government and regulatory agencies and national and local authorities
- Communication to stakeholders when the crisis is over, normal routine processes will be resumed, and work will be started on recovery processes

Networking, Linkage Development, and Identifying Sources of Information and Help

Collaboration during a crisis can be critical in determining the success of the response by the healthcare sector, in particular the laboratory. One way of doing this is to develop linkages with other laboratories, organizations/government agencies (local, public health and state/federal laboratories, reference laboratories), facilities, new stakeholders, and vendors. By doing so, it may be possible to share experiences and seek help from other laboratories or organizations. Alongside establishing a laboratory outreach communication system, it is important to identify sources from where laboratory will get information. For example, SBH Health System Laboratory worked closely with the mayor's office in New York City, the New York City Department of Health and Mental Hygiene, and the New York City Health and Hospitals Corporation laboratory pandemic response committee to do value analyses and select vendors for supplies, collection resources, reagents, and test systems for quality, reliable and effective services for the laboratory continuity plan. Committee conference calls were conducted at least twice a week and were deemed helpful and effective in sharing experiences, doing value-based analyses, and managing supply resources.

Emergency Succession Plan

Development of an emergency succession plan is a vital component of the laboratory crisis and continuity management plan, in case of temporary disruption, or a partial or even full shutdown of laboratory services, the goal being to ensure essential and continued provision of services, either through internal or external sources. The emergency succession plan should contain instructions for finding alternate arrangements for both short- and long-term storage of specimens or for diverting testing services to either reference and contract laboratories or established government facilities. In addition, the laboratory may practice plan deviation (deviating from approved policies and procedures) if required and only when approved by the laboratory director, medical community, or ordinances.

Emergency Succession Plan in Case of Temporary Disruption of Laboratory Services

During a temporary disruption (e.g., fire alarm or some other short-term emergencies), employees must be trained to react in an appropriate way and evacuate when required. Procedures should be established and staff trained/instructed to follow these established policies and procedures. During unexpected interruption of services, each section of the laboratory should follow specific departmental procedures including downtime procedures, staff safety, temporary storage and preservation of samples and test materials, and communication with staff, providers, and emergency responders in order to determine the best way to work closely with each other under these circumstances. Supervisors and laboratory management/directors must also be notified. In the situation that a temporary termination of routine services is put in place, it is important to create a list of laboratory tests or STAT tests that meet patient needs. Maintenance of an effective communication plan, laboratory section-wise supplies, and documentation showing approval of planned deviation from services/policies, if required, is essential. In addition, alternative arrangements for reference testing should be made using the current reference testing laboratory or exploring the possibilities of other reference laboratories in case either internal testing is not possible or there are challenges with the current reference laboratory.

Emergency Succession Plan in Case of Partial Shutdown of Laboratory Services

The following are some general guidelines for an emergency succession plan in case of partial shutdown of laboratory services, many of which overlap with procedures during a temporary disruption. Below are laboratory section-specific guidelines.

General guidelines:
- Prepare a list of responsible personnel who are designated and trained to be liaison personnel.
- Conduct training and drills on emergency plans.
- Create a list of laboratory tests or STAT tests that meet patient needs.
- Determine the best way to work closely with the emergency/critical areas or responsible medical staff.
- In addition, arrangements for alternative reference testing should be determined (using current reference testing laboratory or exploring the possibilities of other reference laboratories to have a backup plan in case of incapacity to do internal testing or because there are challenges with current reference laboratory).
- Ensure the location and availability of emergency equipment in the laboratory (fire extinguishers, emergency lights, emergency shower, eyewash, and spill kit and fire blanket if available).
- Ensure procedures are in place to continue partial services and protect employees.
- Prepare and share primary and secondary evacuation routes/plans.

Phlebotomy and Specimen Receiving Areas

- Ensure appropriate supplies are available for ordering, labeling, and blood collection, and inform supervisor(s)/laboratory management or director. Secure/store more supplies, other than required to overcome shortages, when there is disruption in supply chain.
- Communicate service disruption to staff, and relocate services if needed.
- Follow instructions from the command center or laboratory.
- Help coworkers and patients then properly secure and immediately send samples to a designated location primed for receipt.
- Ensure tracking/records of ongoing events, specimens, patients, times, dates, records, and problems or contacts made.

Anatomic Pathology

- Ensure sufficient emergency supplies, secure all hazardous and flammable supplies, and only complete STAT specimens. If possible, process all specimens before shutdown.
- Evaluate specimens in process; if completion is not required, they can be secured in recommended preservatives (e.g., 95% alcohol or formalin as appropriate) for later processing or alternatively sent to a reference laboratory.
- Follow downtime procedures, and inform relevant departments so that the specimen collection process can be delayed.
- During the recovery processes, fix all unfixed cytology specimens immediately with 95% alcohol in order to maintain specimen integrity.
- Plan with the medical examiner to transfer any deceased bodies or other materials from the morgue refrigerator.

Blood Bank

- Evaluate blood supplies, and ensure that at least 2 weeks of appropriate blood products are in stock or easily accessible, especially O-negative blood supplies.
- Assure issuing of blood in a timely fashion on an emergency basis, and monitor stability and storage conditions of the issued blood.
- Communicate information about current supplies to the supply chain and laboratory staff and future needs, and request cancellation/postponement of nonemergent procedures.
- Activate emergency use protocols and downtime procedures only if required.
- Alternate arrangements of blood supplies from vendors and other resources.

Core Laboratory: Chemistry, Hematology, and Immunology or Others

- Make sure there are sufficient supplies of reagent grade water and other required materials for testing.
- Evaluate whether completion of in-process specimens is needed, and only process STAT samples moving forward. Efforts shall be made to complete in-process specimens.
- If possible, initiate and prepare for downtime procedure.
- Secure supplies, and preserve specimens according to the requirements if they cannot be processed immediately.

Microbiology

- Evaluate whether completion of in-process specimens is necessary. If possible, only process STAT specimens, and initiate or be prepared for downtime procedure.
- Properly secure QC organisms and cultures in process to avoid hazardous conditions.
- Secure supplies, and preserve specimens according to the requirements if they cannot be processed immediately or send specimens to the reference laboratory.

Point-of-Care Testing

- Routinely continue and emphasize POC testing. POC testing shall be continued if the laboratory is not functional in any capacity.
- POC testing may be extended to whole patient care areas, and POC testing instruments capable of performing other necessary laboratory tests can be utilized under planned deviation, in case of emergency, to avoid life-threatening situations.

- Reagents, consumables, and supplies should be moved and stored according to the manufacturer's instructions, in an easily accessible place for use.
- Acquire more POC testing supplies, enabling laboratory to provide services at the patient near side as well as in the laboratory.

Emergency Succession Plan in Case of Full Shutdown of Laboratory Services

In case of complete shutdown of laboratory services, specific actions should be taken to avoid unnecessary damage to laboratory structure and equipment and prevent safety issues. All equipment must be shut down and unplugged; clients and regulatory agencies should be notified, as appropriate; and the feasibility of establishing a satellite location to preserve products along with moving to another location should be researched.

Recovery Processes

Strategies for the initiation of recovery processes should be established following crisis management to assess what tasks need to be accomplished on a priority basis. A comprehensive activity report should be compiled once the emergency is over, consisting of documents that can be used for future reference, e.g., lessons learned, strategies and plans that worked successfully, bottlenecks, and obstacles and challenges during crisis.

Mass Fatality Management

The COVID-19 pandemic thus far has resulted in significant fatality. The majority of this fatality happened during the first wave of the pandemic (March–June 2020). During the peak of the pandemic, funeral homes, crematoriums, and cemeteries were unable to handle the mass fatality. Bodies in the hospital morgues weren't removed fast enough, and eventually, the overflow became a considerable burden to hospitals and communities.

Managing mass fatalities is challenging since the number of bodies usually exceeds what can usually be managed with existing resources. All jurisdictions should have a mass fatality management plan, and this should include governments in local and state and at the federal/national level. Every healthcare facility should also have a mass fatality plan which is in line with the plan of local health authorities. Frequent revision of the plan should be performed to ensure the plan is executable, effective, and practical and is sensitive to the cultural or religious practices for the deceased. The plan should also address issues about how to provide care with respect and dignity for the deceased and their families

Initiation of the SBH Health System mass fatality plan granted contact with the Office of Chief Medical Examiner (OCME) and New York City Emergency Management Department (NYCEM), which subsequently initiated help from the local authorities. However, although these government agencies could provide significant assistance with BCP operations at healthcare facilities, a large portion of responsibility was on the hospital staff. Therefore, this should be part of hospital's mass fatality planning.

Since the pathology department usually oversees the hospital morgue, it is imperative that the morgue count be closely monitored. This can be accomplished by working closely and collaboratively with the admitting (patient access), security, facility, nursing, and housekeeping departments. If mass fatality is identified, this should be reported to the hospital command center. The decision to activate the fatality surge plan via the command center will be made by the senior leadership in the hospital. At this point, the hospital should request the refrigerated trailer (body collection point (BCP)) from the emergency management department of the local government. This refrigerated trailer is a temporary refrigeration unit used to store decedents until transport can be arranged and is considered an extension of the hospital morgue. A BCP can support a healthcare facility by providing additional space to augment their fixed facility morgue capacity. This resource will allow the healthcare facility to store a larger number of bodies until they can be released to families/funeral homes or until government authorities such as OCME take custody.

Request and Preparation of Body Collection Points

When a mass fatality occurs, the governments of national/federal, state, or local levels take the lead and work collaboratively with healthcare facilities, hospitals, private sectors (funeral homes, crematoriums), and faith-based communities. In New York City, OCME and NYCEM took initiatives and started running weekly virtual meetings with hospital management teams. In these meetings, the hospitals presented their needs and limitations, and in return, OCME and NYCEM aided and guided. BCP were one of the most crucial forms of assistance provided by OCME and NYCEM [2].

Hospitals were instructed to submit the BCP requests through the appropriate healthcare association, for example, NYC Health + Hospitals (H + H) or Greater New York Hospital Association (GNYHA), who then contacted NYCEM.

The following information must be submitted when requesting a BCP:

1. Facility name
2. Facility address
3. Date and time of requested delivery

4. Point of contact for mortuary operations or fatality management operations (including name, position, phone number, and email)
5. Designated location for the BCP

Once a refrigerated trailer is requested, an area (usually in the loading dock area) should be predesignated for parking of the trailer. Upon arrival, a ramp may have to be built by the hospital engineering department for easy access and transportation of the bodies.

Managing the Body Collection Points

As an extension of the hospital's morgue space, the hospital is responsible for properly managing the BCP in the facility. As mentioned, this will be a collaborative effort between various departments in the hospital. In most hospitals, additional staff should be added for this task, either from internal mobilization or new hire.

Handling and Transport of the Human Remains

Decedents should always be handled with a manner of respect and care. To prevent leakage, it is advised to use a clearly labeled heavy-duty body bag. At least two patient identifiers (decedent's name, medical record number, date of birth, or date of death) must be used. A body bag tag and patient label will also be affixed to the bag. Claim-only cases, claimed remains, and unclaimed remains can all be stored in the BCP, both COVID-19- and non-COVID-19-related cases. Cases which fall under the jurisdiction of OCME (medical examiner (ME) cases) must be stored in the hospital morgue and cannot be stored in the BCP. ME cases must be reported to OCME, according to normal protocols.

Staffing in Morgue/BCP Management

Due to the massive increase in workload in managing a mass fatality, the hospital should preemptively increase the number of staff available, either by mobilizing internally or by hiring temporary staff. These staff will be distributed to security, admitting office, and transportation and will aid in cleaning/disinfection, helping to ensure efficient ongoing management of the situation.

Infection Control Procedures

According to the World Health Organization (WHO), personnel who have contact with human remains, including those performing autopsy and collecting or handling specimens, are at risk for exposure to infectious agents, such as SARS-CoV-2, since it may be present in tissues, blood, and other bodily fluids of the deceased person. Measures should therefore be taken to reduce the risk of transmission of disease associated with handling human remains. Standard precautions are essential for those handling human remains with the assumption that every decedent is potentially infected or colonized with an organism that could be transmitted. When handling human remains, these precautions include:

- Appropriate PPE such as gloves, masks, eye protection devices (goggles or chin-length face shields), and protective clothing (gowns, aprons) must be used.
- PPE should be disposed of appropriately.
- Hand hygiene with soap or hand sanitizer immediately after removing PPE.
- Vehicles used for transportation should be cleaned and decontaminated as indicated.

Storage of Bodies in the Body Collection Point

Decedents should be treated with dignity and should never be stacked. Bodies should always be placed face up and arranged on each side of the BCP, leaving a center aisle for walking. For effective use of the BCP in a mass casualty, decedents should be properly positioned to allow for maximum storage. A 53-foot trailer can store approximately 40–50 decedents. During the peak of a pandemic, emergency management or OCME may require a doubling of storage capacity, or approximately 100 bodies, before the BCP can be picked up. In this case, shelving can be pre-built by the hospital engineering department, if not already done so, to accommodate more bodies. Factors determining the need for shelving include the local situation, the number of bodies, and the speed of handling/retrieving the bodies. Body handlers should use sliding boards and other lifting devices, when applicable, to make it easier to move bodies and also to prevent back injury. Gurneys should be lowered, if possible, before moving decedents and placing them on the BCP floor.

Temperature Monitoring

Human remains should be stored within the temperature range of 37–44 °F, and this must be monitored and ensured by the hospital.

Fuel Management

The trailer is fueled by diesel and usually refueled every 2–3 days. Hospitals are responsible for monitoring fuel levels and refueling units.

Security

The healthcare facility must ensure that the unit is secure 24 hours a day. The refrigerated trailer must remain locked at all times and guarded by security. Other security measures may include deploying lighting elements or security cameras, restricting access to the BCP, and preventing photography of the interior of the BCP (by the public or others). Funeral directors should never be given direct access to a BCP. The retrieval of decedents from the BCP should be completed by hospital staff.

Personal Effects

The hospital is responsible for the management of personal effects and will ensure that personal effects are properly collected, documented, packaged, vouchered, and secured in a safe, respectful, and dignified manner.

Morgue Census

In the daily morgue census survey, OCME requests that all hospitals provide their daily morgue census which includes hospital morgue and BCP (if one is deployed). This assists OCME in monitoring case storage capabilities and managing transport resources citywide. The hospital should provide all three of the following to OCME for each case as it is stored in the BCP [3]:

- Healthcare facility face sheet (required) which is produced by the admitting department. This contains basic patient information (name, gender, date of birth, medical record number, contact information, next of kin, etc.)
- A signed and registered work copy of the death certificate (required)
- Completed OCME clinical summary worksheet 3.0 (preferred)

Case Management/Tracking

Hospitals must maintain a morgue census for all cases stored in the BCP, as mentioned above. A tracking form should be used for this purpose.

Family Management

The hospital should communicate notification of death to the family of the deceased and enable arrangements for final disposition. The hospital admitting department must verify the current contact information for the next of kin and document the family's intention for final disposition, either a private service or city burial.

A general overview regarding the process for case storage and release to the funeral home/city burial should be provided to the family of the deceased. It should be indicated that if timely case release to a funeral home is not possible, OCME will take custody of the case to maintain case tracking and storage until arrangements can be made. If city burial is requested, it should be communicated that this will occur once the case is transferred to OCME. If family is unknown, the hospital must follow protocol to report the case to the public administrator. In addition, the hospital should coordinate with the family to provide them with all decedent's personal effects in hospital custody. Upon taking custody of decedents from a hospital, OCME will communicate with the known family and the chosen funeral home to enable case release for final disposition.

Release Cases to Funeral Homes

Hospitals should release cases to funeral homes on demand and in accordance with normal procedures.

Retrieval of the Body Collection Point

When the BCP is nearing capacity, the healthcare facility must reach out to OCME to coordinate pickup of the refrigerated trailer and replacement with an empty unit. All required decedent paperwork must be submitted to OCME as decedents are placed into the BCP and must be complete before case pickup can occur. Once all the required information is confirmed, the hospital will be authorized to fax the final BCP manifest to OCME.

Once a date has been scheduled for retrieval of the BCP, the hospital may continue to remove (and document) any listed cases as they are released to funeral homes. However, no more cases may be added into the BCP once the manifest is submitted. In order to prepare a trailer for removal, the hospital must:

- Maximize BCP storage capacity within the unit.
- Confirm BCP manifest is current and correct.
- Verify that all cases in the BCP are properly labeled (including a body tag, tag on the bag, and documentation on the exterior of the body bag).
- Ensure all case paperwork has been submitted to OCME and corrections requested have been made.

Upon case paperwork approval, OCME will dispatch a team to perform an audit of the BCP and its contents. Once the state of the BCP has been approved and case reconciliation of the manifest has been made on site, OCME will take custody of the remains by locking and sealing the BCP and then approve for transport. Following relocation of the BCP, funeral directors will be able to utilize the funeral director portal to locate and submit documentation to facilitate case release at the family's request. In case the decedent's family is unable to locate a body, OCME and NYCEM will work with the police department and 311 phone system to support them in their search.

Summary

The laboratory plays an integral part in providing quality, accurate, and reliable services to help improve patient outcomes and safeguard public health. However, the COVID-19 pandemic put a staggering and unforeseeable pressure on the entire laboratory profession, resource, and staffing requirements beyond any scale that clinical laboratories had previously had to face [4]. New York City experienced a shortage of labor force, necessary tools, personal protective equipment and testing equipment, supplies, and an inability to store bodies in response to mass fatality caused by the COVID-19 pandemic. In the absence of some form of a continuity plan, the risk is that the whole system will sink. Having a laboratory response plan in place is not only to support continuation of laboratory services but also to support those at the crux of it: the staff. The clinical laboratory workforce is a highly trained resource that cannot be easily or quickly replaced, and the importance of maintaining and supporting the clinical laboratory workforce is therefore paramount [4]. Having a defined laboratory response during a crisis involves not only a comprehensive risk assessment, expansion of services, and resource management, among others, but also developing linkages and networking with public health entities is crucial to gaining an external support system.

References

1. Silverstein MD. An approach to medical errors and patient safety in laboratory services. In: A White Paper. Atlanta: The Quality Institute Meeting; 2003.
2. NYC Office of Chief Medical Examiner: Hospital Body Collection Point Guide for COVID-19, Version 3.0 April 24, 2020. 20200423_HCF_BCP_Guide_FINAL.pdf (nysfda.org) https://www.nysfda.org/images/COVID-19/20200423_HCF_BCP_Guide_FINAL.pdf.
3. Durrani M, Hwang R. Resource management. Laboratory General policies and procedures, Department of Pathology and Laboratories, SBH Health System, Bronx, New York. 2020; SOP # LABG 4.
4. Jackson BR, Genzen JR. The lab must go on. Am J Clin Pathol. 2021;155(1):4–11. https://doi.org/10.1093/ajcp/aqaa187.

Chapter 13
Radiology

Brian Bobby Chiong, Steven B. Epstein, and Razia Rehmani

A Radiologist's Reflection on the Start of the Pandemic

Brian Bobby Chiong recalls: "As the year 2019 turned into 2020, I was on a beach in Phuket, Thailand. I flew home a few days later with a layover in Hong Kong. I didn't know it at the time, but a worldwide pandemic was starting in China that would change all our lives forever. I still had plans to attend a radiology conference in Seattle, Washington, which was scheduled for March 2020. It feels silly thinking about it now, but during the months of January and February, there was still a sense of 'it could never happen to us here in NYC.'

I remember being at a meeting that first week of March 2020 with the department chairs of SBH Health System. The chief medical officer was laying out the four possible levels of impact that COVID-19 could have on us. To paraphrase what he said: 'Level 1, nothing changes; it's just like a bad flu season. Level 2, the surge comes; we get tested to the max; we survive. Level 3, we can't keep up and we have to ration care. Level 4, zombie apocalypse, tanks on the streets.' Come March and April of 2020, I certainly felt like I was living in a zombie apocalypse; I remember the streets being empty as I rode my motorcycle into work at rush hour, the

---

B. B. Chiong (✉)
Department of Radiology, SBH Health System, Bronx, NY, USA

CUNY School of Medicine, New York, NY, USA
e-mail: bchiong@sbhny.org

S. B. Epstein
Department of Radiology, SBH Health System, Bronx, NY, USA

R. Rehmani
Neuro and Musculoskeletal Imaging, Department of Radiology, SBH Health System, Bronx, NY, USA

© The Author(s), under exclusive license to Springer Nature Switzerland AG 2022
R. Shabsigh (ed.), *Health Crisis Management in Acute Care Hospitals*, https://doi.org/10.1007/978-3-030-95806-0_13

neighbors not allowing me to use the apartment elevator as they literally fled the city. Things in New York City went from bad to worse from there onwards."

In the following sections, after a brief perspective of radiology, my colleagues and I describe our response to the crisis and the lessons learned at the SBH Health System Radiology Department.

The History of Medical Imaging

It would be difficult to imagine the practice of medicine in the year 2020 without a functioning radiology department. Though hard to quantify, there has been a steady decrease in the reliance on physical examination and an increase in reliance on medical imaging, which in turn continues to further devalue physical examination [1–3].

The origin of medical imaging can be traced as far back as November 1895 when Wilhelm Roentgen discovered X-rays and imaged the bones of his wife's hands [4]. Less than a year later in 1896, the technology was already in use to find bullets in wounded soldiers. In subsequent decades, radiography became essential for medical diagnoses, especially in military medicine where it was used to evaluate battlefield injuries.

With the digitalization of technology, tomography per se has been replaced by CAT (computerized axial tomography) or CT (computed tomography) scans. Popular legend has it that money from The Beatles went into making the first CT scans [5]. The Beatles were signed to EMI (electrical and musical industries), which was a record company as well as an electronics company, with a branch involved in medical research. Godfrey Hounsfield, who worked for EMI, developed the technology behind CT and was responsible for the first commercially available CT scanner in 1972. This technology would ultimately garner Hounsfield the Nobel Prize.

While the science behind using sound for detecting unseen structures dates to 1794 – Italian physicist Lazzaro Spallanzani and his work with bats [6] – commercially available ultrasound for medical imaging dates to 1963 [7]. However, it is only in the past 10 years or so that there has been a push toward using point-of-care ultrasound (POCUS) by non-radiologists as a primary diagnostic modality, especially for the lungs, and this was found to be required in this pandemic.

Magnetic resonance imaging (MRI) is a relatively recent development in diagnostic imaging, not reaching widespread availability until the 1980s [8]. Similar to ultrasound, MRI does not emit ionizing radiation but instead utilizes a combination of radiofrequency energy and strong magnetic fields to acquire images with superior tissue contrast compared to CT. However, MRI was unlikely to be useful in the COVID-19 pandemic since scans generally take an order of magnitude longer to perform than CT scans and are much more susceptible to motion artifacts, such as from breathing. These issues make MRI almost useless for evaluating lung pathology. Similarly, nuclear medicine imaging, which is based on the distribution of radionuclides within the body and is now widely used for diagnosis and progression of the disease, will also be of limited use in the COVID-19 crisis. Nuclear medicine studies take much longer to perform than CT and radiography, sometimes needing up to 4 hours of imaging with some protocols needing multiple days to complete. To evaluate patients quickly and efficiently in a respiratory predominant disease such as COVID-19, radiographs and CT would be the cornerstone of any diagnostic radiology response as they are the most utilized modalities for evaluating lungs. Moreover, physical examinations have to be kept at a minimum to reduce exposure, and thus radiological exams are preferred to better track disease progress in-patients.

Organization of a Modern-Day Radiology Department

At minimum, it would be expected that a radiology department has capabilities to perform plain radiographs, CT, MRI, nuclear medicine, and ultrasound. Each modality requires a trained technologist to perform the imaging and a medical doctor to interpret the imaging. Radiology therefore has unique needs in terms of space, equipment, and personnel. Similar to the needs of a laboratory, radiology requires very specialized equipment and machines. Unlike the laboratory, the radiology space needs to be designed so that patient can be accommodated in the department.

Radiology technologists must be located onsite to operate the imaging machines when required. The radiology physicians may be located physically in the department; however, thanks to modern picture archiving and communication systems (PACS) and radiology information systems (RIS), radiology imaging can be interpreted remotely by radiologists located anywhere in the world as long as there is an adequate Internet connection.

The Initial Response: Psyche Shift, Protect, and Plan

> Every battle is won even before it is fought. *Sun* Tzu

Paradigm Shift to Accept the New Pandemic Reality

Radiology is at the epicenter of any healthcare practice and is centrally connected to various departments such as emergency medicine, internal medicine, family practice, surgery, obstetrics and gynecology, geriatrics, ophthalmology, ear nose and throat surgery, dermatology, dental surgery, oral and maxillofacial surgery, and other clinical departments. The following is a review of a patient's journey to the radiology department on a typical day:

> After the patient enters hospital premises, the first direct contact the patient has with a healthcare provider is at the time of registration, which may involve sitting in the waiting

room with other patients and their family. From there, the patient is directed to the radiology front desk where they check in and get screened for the exam. The third contact with a healthcare provider happens when the patient undergoes an in-person interview to be consented for the test which may need contrast injection. This requires close contact with a physician provider in a small room. Given that there is a very diverse community in the Bronx, this often requires the use of a telephonic speech translation service which prolongs the contact with the healthcare provider.

In a pandemic, this process would constitute a "super spreader event." After realizing that the pandemic was actualizing, conducting this process – even with personal protective equipment (PPE) – was deemed an unnecessary risk to the patients and healthcare providers, and there followed an urgent need to restructure processes and procedures and plan for the immediate future.

The initial response of the radiology department at SBH Health System was to put on hold all nonurgent outpatient radiological tests. This required the physician radiologists to go through the schedule and determine what could be postponed and what could not. Often there were gray areas such as follow-up for cancer screenings. Difficult choices had to be made to weigh the risk of cancers becoming worse against the risk of disease transmission.

Protecting Staff and Patients Early on

First and foremost, the healthcare staff and the community in general were educated about the importance of PPE and social distancing. Employees were trained via mandatory online education courses on the correct use of PPE. PPE shortage was recognized early on, and a central stockpile and controlled supervised distribution of all PPE center were established. Every avenue for acquiring PPE was leveraged, and this led to some situations where PPE came through grassroots organizations, placing N95s from construction and beauty supply directly into the hands of the hospital employees. All employees were trained in the proper sanitization techniques to prolong the use of their PPE, and social distancing and mandatory universal mask requirement, while on hospital premises, were initiated to prevent community spread. A universal mask protocol was initiated with the use of only disposable masks, discouraging the use of nonstandardized personal masks. While this was the initial policy, there was a dire shortage of masks at the height of the pandemic, and any hospital staff who could sew, assemble, or 3D print masks with filters did so. Necessity became the mother of invention.

Patient and community awareness was also equally important to prevent the spread of the disease. Regular updates were broadcast on television and the radio, and throughout the hospital, information was posted in-patient areas with tips on how to minimize transmission of the virus. Triple screening protocols were initiated at the time of entry into the hospital, at registration, and at the time of radiology front desk check-in.

Early Testing and Isolation/Quarantine

Essential workers, including employees in the field of healthcare, are at higher risk of developing severe COVID-19 [9]. It was therefore crucial that SBH Health System put organizational practices and policies in place to support their employees. Employees had to be trained and instructed to immediately self-report any exposure to COVID-19-positive patients, symptoms such as fever or those related to upper or lower respiratory tract infections, and any recent travel history to the employee health service. Tests for COVID-19 were initially very difficult to come by and were heavily rationed. During this time, one of the radiologists, who was experiencing symptoms but was unable to be tested, chose to self-quarantine. At the same time, another SBH Health System radiologist was unable to work due to an already scheduled surgery, leaving only two of the four full-time radiologists available during the early days of the pandemic. These two radiologists did their best to only rarely be in the same room together, for fear of taking out the entire in-house radiology department. The night and weekend interpretation of radiology exams was covered by teleradiology services. Because outpatient imaging was essentially nonexistent for many private practice facilities during the pandemic, the teleradiology company was easily able to cover image interpretation using radiologists who could read/work from their homes.

Anxiety, Assurance, and Recognition

It is essential to acknowledge the anxiety that patients, employees, and communities can face in a massive health crisis such as COVID-19. At SBH, due to the nature of the work in healthcare, many suffered from stress and anxiety due to long shifts, personal risk of infection, and fear of transmission to friends and family, as well as loss of colleagues and patients [10]. The SBH Health System offered a mental health hotline which was available around the clock to help staff deal with anxiety, bereavements, and any other form of support required for their mental well-being. The psychiatry and chaplain services also provided a significant amount of help to anybody struggling to cope with the stress of the pandemic.

Considerations for Managing the COVID-19 Crisis

Dynamic Reorganization of Resources and Processes

Diagnostic radiology is generally thought of as the common form of radiology, the acquisition of imaging to aid and establish diagnoses. Just as important are the physicians who use those imaging modalities to perform procedures, referred to as interventional radiologists. Common interventional radiology procedures include biopsies, percutaneous drainage, vascular access, angiography, embolization, thrombolysis, and thrombectomy.

In response to COVID-19, the operating rooms (OR) had limited capacity. For many common surgical patients, interventional radiology (IR) can be an alternative treatment, for example, appendicitis can be treated with antibiotics, and a CT-guided percutaneous drainage can be used to get rid of any associated abscess. Instead of going to the OR for cholecystitis, a patient can be referred to IR for a cholecystostomy tube insertion which would drain the gallbladder of infected bile. Many of the skills of an interventional radiologist are unique, and these skills were extremely valuable during the pandemic; IR became responsible for placing IV access lines (central lines, midlines, peripherally inserted central catheter (PICC), dialysis catheters) and thus supplemented the hospital staff. The use of portable imaging such as radiography and Doppler, not only for in-patients but also in the ER, should be and was encouraged. Furthermore, adoption of online platforms should be considered for any teaching activities of medical students and residents, or conferences, to minimize interruptions to learning.

Communication

Regular and timely communication via updates on internal social media platforms, with open suggestion boxes for ideas, was used at SBH Health System. Email volumes were high during the pandemic, and therefore, a weekly summary letter to highlight key decisions and issues could prove more efficient. Daily updates from leadership and administrative meetings were useful to avoid any misunderstandings, and such measures helped to maintain transparency within the workplace, build trust, and boost morale within the team. It helped foster a spirit of "we are in it together" and promoted recognition of the importance of radiologists in response to this crisis. A recent survey of radiologists in China found that the crisis strengthened most respondents' belief that their professional contribution was important and cemented relationships with colleagues [11]. This indicated that radiology teams faced the crisis in a cohesive manner, central to any form of successful response to a pandemic of such magnitude as COVID-19.

How to Organize When Facing the Unknown

In the early days of the pandemic, it was obvious the SBH Health System was entering unprecedented times. The pandemic changed practices so rapidly and comprehensively that "unprecedented" quickly became a qualifier for almost everything done. It is often said that when facing an unknown challenge, we rarely rise to the level of the challenge but instead fall back on our training; this was the case for the response to COVID-19 in the radiology department. While it was at first poorly understood how COVID-19 was transmitted and what made it so deadly, there was already an understanding in the radiology department regarding how to work with other transmissible diseases. Therefore, the overall response was built upon previous experiences and the department defaulted to similar levels of precautions.

From the experience of SBH Health System and working in the City of New York, the most remarkable thing about facing the pandemic was how quickly information was disseminated about best practices. Communications within departments, among departments, and ultimately among other hospitals allowed for quick evolution of protocols on how to best proceed with the care of patients while protecting the radiology teams [12]. And while there was a two-edged sword to having such open lines of communication – in that sometimes, erroneous information was easily spread – ultimately information evolved with a trend toward improvement of practices within radiology.

Psychiatric Support

The pandemic severely affected the mental health of hospital staff worldwide leading to anxiety, depression, and stress [13]. This was no different at SBH Health System where radiologists shared a substantial burden and saw a huge impact on their work and personal lives [11]. This impact was exaggerated in COVID-19 "hot regions" such as in the Bronx, NYC.

Clear communication and education were key to promoting resilience in radiology teams. A survey of Chinese radiologist demonstrated that knowledge of COVID-19, knowledge of COVID-19 protective measures, and availability of adequate protective materials were independent influencing factors for resilience [14]. Investment in professional training of all involved personnel was advocated, along with regular two-way open communication within teams, to allow recognition and acknowledgment of the psychological impacts. Such measures are also important to aid in preserving the radiologists' well-being after the crisis when the backlog of unseen non-COVID-19 patients is released, and an alternate but still substantial burden then falls on the radiology department.

What Worked Well and What Didn't: A Reflective Practice

It's an odd quirk of human nature that when faced with dangerous and harrowing times, it is the strong sense of community that people most often feel. For instance, during World War 2 and the bombing of London known as the Blitz, it was projected that up to four million civilians might have psychiatric breakdowns. Instead, it was noted that psychiatric admissions decreased, and Londoners came together in ways that strengthened their community bonds [15]. Similarly, in the aftermath of the

9/11 attacks, violent crime and psychiatric admissions decreased in New York City [15].

In that way, there was a sense of pride and almost nostalgia for certain aspects of how the response to the COVID-19 pandemic occurred. Because there was a feeling of community, it was possible to focus on continuous problem-solving without resorting to tribalism and silo working that could sometimes interfere with the seamless functioning of a hospital. Although it was difficult to keep up with the escalating demands for resources during the pandemic, the radiology team managed as best as was possible.

Reflecting on what could have been improved, the effectiveness of communication is one such area. Although within the hospital information was internally well-communicated, there were no established channels of communication among hospitals. In the future, a laudable aim that could help overcome future crises is the implementation of a more universal electronic medical record (EMR) which could better link multiple hospital systems together. In combination with the growing power and prevalence of artificial intelligence (AI), having patient clinical course and treatment data, which can be analyzed and processed in real time by AI, will be crucial in battling such challenges.

References

1. Smith-Bindman R, Miglioretti DL, Larson EB. Rising use of diagnostic medical imaging in a large integrated health system. Health Aff (Millwood). 2008;27(6):1491–502.
2. Colli A, Prati D, Fraquelli M, Segato S, Vescovi PP, Colombo F, et al. The use of a pocket-sized ultrasound device improves physical examination: results of an in- and outpatient cohort study. PLoS One. 2015;10(3):e0122181.
3. Smith-Bindman R, Kwan ML, Marlow EC, Theis MK, Bolch W, Cheng SY, et al. Trends in use of medical imaging in US Health Care Systems and in Ontario, Canada, 2000–2016. JAMA. 2019;322(9):843–56.
4. Kaye GWC. Wilhelm Conrad Röntgen: and the early history of the roentgen rays. Nature. 1934;133(3362):511–3.
5. Alexander RE, Gunderman RB. EMI and the first CT scanner. J Am Coll Radiol. 2010;7(10):778–81.
6. Kaproth-Joslin KA, Nicola R, Dogra VS. The history of US: from bats and boats to the bedside and beyond: RSNA centennial article. Radiographics. 2015;35(3):960–70.
7. Campbell S. A short history of sonography in obstetrics and gynaecology. Facts Views Vis Obgyn. 2013;5(3):213–29.
8. Edelman RR. The history of MR imaging as seen through the pages of radiology. Radiology. 2014;273(2 Suppl):S181–200.
9. Mutambudzi M, Niedwiedz C, Macdonald EB, Leyland A, Mair F, Anderson J, et al. Occupation and risk of severe COVID-19-19: prospective cohort study of 120 075 UK Biobank participants. Occup Environ Med. 2020;78:307.
10. Mehta S, Machado F, Kwizera A, Papazian L, Moss M, Azoulay E, et al. COVID-19-19: a heavy toll on health-care workers. Lancet Respir Med. 2021;9(3):226–8.
11. Coppola F, Faggioni L, Neri E, Grassi R, Miele V. Impact of the COVID-19-19 outbreak on the profession and psychological wellbeing of radiologists: a nationwide online survey. Insights Imaging. 2021;12:23.

12. Ding J, Fu H, Liu Y, Gao J, Li Z, Zhao X, et al. Prevention and control measures in radiology department for COVID-19-19. Eur Radiol. 2020;30(7):3603–8. https://doi.org/10.1007/s00330-020-06850-5. Epub 2020 Apr 16. PMID: 32300968; PMCID: PMC7160611.
13. Hassamal S, Dong F, Hassamal S, Lee C, Ogunyemi D, Neeki MM. The psychological impact of COVID-19 on hospital staff. West J Emerg Med. 2021;22(2):346–52.
14. Huang L, Wang Y, Liu J, Ye P, Cheng B, Xu H, et al. Factors associated with resilience among medical staff in radiology departments during the outbreak of 2019 novel coronavirus disease (COVID-19): a cross-sectional study. Med Sci Monit. 2020;29(26):e925669. https://doi.org/10.12659/MSM.925669. PMID: 32468998; PMCID: PMC7282347.
15. Junger S. Tribe: on homecoming and belonging. London: Harper Collins; 2017. p. 192.

Chapter 14
Supply Chain, Material Management, and Finance

Marilyn L. G. Gates, Louis M. Santomauro, Steven M. Beltis, Patricio F. Villacreses, Ricardo Negron, Mark Sollazzo, Don Hester, Steven Berger, and Mary Grochowski

The SBH Health System Supply Shain

SBH Health System is a safety net hospital whose principal purpose is to provide care to indigent and low-income populations in an area where care is otherwise limited. A significant percentage of the population served are immigrants (documented and undocumented), homeless, and underinsured individuals who have little access to the larger academic centers within the city of New York and the five boroughs. As a result, the hospital operates on challenged finances, and, while it is a nonprofit hospital, its operating budget comes from state funding and grants.

The hospital is certified for 422 beds; however, prior to the COVID-19 crisis, it operated a total of 210 general medical, surgical and ICU beds. Other beds were designated for special purposes such as psychiatry and others. During the surge of

---

M. L. G. Gates (✉)
Value Analysis, SBH Health System, Premier/Nexera, Bronx, NY, USA
e-mail: mgates@sbhny.org

L. M. Santomauro · D. Hester
Supply Chain, SBH Health System, Bronx, NY, USA

S. M. Beltis
Purchasing Department, SBH Health System, Bronx, NY, USA

P. F. Villacreses
Supply Chain, SBH Health System, Bronx, NY, USA

R. Negron · S. Berger
SBH Health System, Bronx, NY, USA

M. Sollazzo
Materials Management, SBH Health System, Bronx, NY, USA

M. Grochowski
Department of Finance, SBH Health System, Bronx, NY, USA

© The Author(s), under exclusive license to Springer Nature Switzerland AG 2022
R. Shabsigh (ed.), *Health Crisis Management in Acute Care Hospitals*, https://doi.org/10.1007/978-3-030-95806-0_14

the COVID-19 pandemic in April 2020, the hospital's general medical, surgical, and ICU beds capacity increased by 70%. At the same time, it was able to increase capacity to care for severely ill patients on ventilators by >500%. The system includes an acute care hospital, an ambulatory care center (outpatient clinics), and other facilities in addition to one of the area's only kidney dialysis centers. Prior to the onset of the first and greatest surge of critically ill patients, the hospital was in the final stages of building and opening a wellness center that would serve pediatric and women's health as well as services designed to promote health and fitness in the local population, by providing easy access to fitness classes and equipment and a culinary educational kitchen where attendees would learn and practice healthy preparation of locally purchased farm-to-table foods.

Supply chain and materials management for the hospital comes from an embedded team of subject matter experts contractually provided by an outsourced vendor, Nexera, originally a consultation and management company that was part of the Greater New York Hospital Association (GNYHA). It is a small team consisting of three buyers and five directors, all of whom are employees of SBH Health System: the vice president of supply chain, directors of purchasing, data management, capital purchases, storeroom, and materials management. Additionally, Nexera provides the director of operating room (OR) materials management and the director of value analysis who is a former neurosurgeon. The embedded team is sponsored by the chief financial officer (CFO) of the hospital and maintains a direct line with that office.

Prior to the COVID-19 pandemic, the SBH Health System supply chain operated on a variation of "just-in-time" ordering, where each area was evaluated for items that were in general use, and from this, an operating level was established for each item. These items were then ordered and replenished as they approached a preestablished and critical level. This system is one of the many ways that a supply chain can operate; keep supplies available for use and work to eliminate waste which can occur when too many items are ordered and expire prior to use. This method of operation also avoids overstocking in limited space.

SBH Health System was built over 150 years ago; space is very limited in certain areas and storeroom space is at a premium. Prior to the pandemic surge, delivery of a large number of supplies required careful planning to allow for the accommodation of these new items. As a result, storage of some items spilled over to certain commandeered spaces. To say that storage was tight would have been an understatement.

The buyers at SBH Health System take requisitions for products from all departments. Each buyer specializes in a particular set of departments within the hospital, creating a core of highly specialized knowledge to meet the demands of those specific departments. They enter items into a database and order from the hospitals distributor who then distributes products from a large number of medical supply manufacturers, usually with discounted access. The buyers then apply pricing and add the desired quantities needed, against the quantities that items are supplied in. On an average day, the buyers source about 12,000 items per day (including items that are in boxes, cases, or by each).

The Pandemic Begins

In December of 2019, SBH Health System and the rest of the world first became aware of the potential for a worldwide pandemic when a virus from the coronavirus family, best known for causing respiratory illnesses, started to spread throughout communities. Not long after that, the first cases were identified in New York City, and, though quarantined, healthcare workers recognized how quickly the situation was starting to spiral out of control. Numerous meetings were held and decisions made to determine what was needed to protect frontline workers from exposure and what additional supplies would be required to provide care to the large numbers of critically ill patients. It was known that this disease could develop rapidly and move from mild or no symptoms to death within days, meaning that hospitals quickly had to prepare for larger numbers of critically ill patients, many of whom may require high levels of critical care.

SBH Health System was fortunate to have a former neurosurgeon (Dr. Marilyn Gates) on the supply chain team who had previously been a critical care nurse, and by utilizing the expertise and experience of this surgeon, the hospital was able to position the supply chain department slightly ahead of the curve. The team began to have an eye toward what was on the horizon, how the virus was moving, and what challenges other hospitals and healthcare workers were being faced with.

Daily Meetings

At the same time that the first case in NYC was identified, the SBH Health System supply chain members began to conduct daily team meetings. The purpose was to bring the team together, discuss the current situation and the predictions for the future, identify needs, and develop a spreadsheet that listed items identified to be critical for the care of patients and the protection of the staff. The supply chain team members kept a daily log of the "in-house" inventory of each of these items, who the supplier was, any orders that were outstanding, and daily use of these items. Additionally, the team was able to identify items that were not currently in short supply but that were soon predicted to become scarce. The main effort of the team was to determine what levels and types of PPE were required (see Sidebar 14.1).

The team worked with other departments of the hospital to develop a plan for various levels of PPE that would be required for each group of healthcare workers and support staff. Once a directive was established, the team worked with the executive and infectious disease teams to develop a daily allotment of PPE to each area including a backup supply of high-use items, like gloves, gowns, and face masks. Initially, these were handed out to department directors or their designees from the storeroom. Later, as the team and the hospital became more familiar with the day-to-day changes, PPE supplies were delivered to each area by storeroom personnel and replenished when a simple PPE request sheet was completed and forwarded to the storeroom.

> **Sidebar 14.1 Identifying Levels of PPE and Other Relevant Decisions**
> *Factors to be considered when determining PPE should include:*
> - Will high-level isolation gowns be provided to every person in the hospital or only in certain areas?
> - Does everyone require a face shield?
> - Are there other options available that will provide face coverage without a separate face shield, i.e., a mask with shield, as might be seen in the operating room?
> - Who are our primary suppliers?
> - Do we have secondary and tertiary sources?
> - Are we familiar with the specifications that are applied to call a gown a level 1, 2, 3, or 4?
> - Will there be a specific need for a particular level in a specialized area?
> - How many gowns will be used per healthcare worker per day?
> - What is the average daily number of staff (in all departments) that are expected to populate the hospital each day?

The director of data management crafted several spreadsheets that were used on a daily basis to track fundamental values: daily counts of PPE that were currently in-house, "burn rates" – how much of an item was used each day – dates those supplies were ordered and associated delivery dates, and the daily census and distribution of COVID-19 patients with their level of illness and associated equipment needs.

Surveys and Meetings

As the pandemic progressed, it became clear that the government stockpile – that many people believed would help hospitals source critical items – was now nonexistent. Government agencies like the FEMA (Federal Emergency Management Agency) and local and state governments started putting together surveys in an attempt to gather as much information as possible as to what equipment was being used and in what quantities, who was using them, and where these items were being sourced from. The supply chain was a vital resource in providing this information. Each survey asked essentially the same questions related to face shields or N-95 masks (respirator masks that were designed to filter out 95% of particulate matter including larger viruses), gowns, and gloves. As time went on, the surveys became more specific and included ventilators and tracheostomy tubes (a tube that is surgically placed in the airway to allow for long-term respiratory support), high-efficiency particulate air (HEPA) filters usage, and bilevel positive airway pressure (BiPap) equipment. As a result of these surveys, SBH Health System was luckily able to secure ventilators and needed tubing, as well as some deliveries of isolation gowns and gloves.

Because of the detail each survey required, accurate completion required additional time and sometimes required counting or explaining decision-making processes and accessibility of the items to patients and staff. While the team understood the purpose of the surveys, the time required to complete them was significant, with at least one member of the team being away for the better part of each day, and it also required at least two sets of eyes to ascertain the accuracy; SBH Health System participated in the completion of 5–10 surveys each day. Each survey came with its own warning of the consequences of *not* completing the survey or completing it inaccurately; failing to answer questions accurately could prevent the hospital from receiving equipment or supplies from governmental agencies or from obtaining access to donated equipment. Samples of the surveys are not currently available for publication.

The Group Purchasing Organization

In addition to the surveys, the supply chain team at SBH Health System was now part of a larger group purchasing organization (GPO) called Premier. A group purchasing organization is one that brings together a number of medical suppliers and manufacturers under one umbrella and allows for the hospital, which is contracted to them, to access supplies at a discount that would be unavailable if the hospital attempted to secure the same supply from another source. This is generally done using a "tier system" which is based on volume, the higher the volume, the higher the tier and the greater the discount. Large GPO's also offer greater access to healthcare information, and Premier worked to do just that.

Early in February 2020, the Premier leadership, now functioning remotely, held daily COVID-19 calls designed to bring all members together and share critical information about supplies and where the best sourcing could be obtained. They developed a portfolio of vendors who could supply items deemed essential though which had previously been of marginal use. For example, when extubating (removing the endotracheal tube or "breathing tube"), a patient will usually cough following the tube removal. The increased secretions present in their airway, as a result of being extubated, would become aerosolized, due to the cough, and healthcare workers subsequently exposed to these particles, likely containing active virus. In pre-COVID-19 days, a mask and appropriate distancing from the patient would provide adequate protection. However, the currently known properties of COVID-19 include an ability to live on inanimate surfaces for long periods of time, increasing the risk of exposure [1, 2]. Premier located vendors or manufacturers that could supply barriers like vinyl curtains or plexiglass three-sided boxes, allowing team members to safely remove the tube and contain secretions away from any of the providers.

In addition to the daily COVID-19 calls, there were a series of additional calls: calls which team members could join to discuss the sourcing of PPE, calls to discuss allocations available, calls to discuss overseas vendors, CDC predictions and guidelines, mental health issues of healthcare providers, and calls to develop solutions for the very high number of decedents that were filling hospital morgues beyond capacity – to name a few. The vice president (VP) of purchasing dealt with many of those calls, team members dialing in when possible. He also fielded calls from the NYC Mayor's office, the office of the governor, liaisons, volunteers, and people who simply wanted to help. As with the surveys, this was a monumental task and took hours, often with calls overlapping with meetings.

The VP of purchasing also played an integral part of discussions happening in all areas of the hospital as they were challenged with the pandemic; teams were meeting to discuss plans for expanding resources, developing visitor policies, building a second morgue, closing operating rooms, and reconfiguring the endoscopy suite or postanesthesia care units (PACU) into patient care areas, updating supplies or developing lists of needs.

Sourcing Under Pressure

Regardless of whether or not a hospital is dealing with a healthcare crisis, there are a number of fundamental items every hospital must have on hand to provide safe and effective patient care. The supply chain is responsible for following trends: interacting with departments, determining how much of each item is needed, and also responding to emergency or "one-time" needs. The latter can entail several team members stopping the usual ebb and flow of their daily work to find an item that is unique or in sudden demand. They must identify the item, its specifications, its function, where it can be obtained, and how quickly it can be shipped or delivered. The team members, with the exception of the director of value analysis, don't have a clinical background, and in the case that the requested item is unavailable through the usual supplier, a clinically appropriate substitute may be chosen though must be vetted by someone with knowledge of the product and its use.

In pandemic mode, the director of the supply chain would meet with the team to discuss anticipated needs. She followed patterns of spread of the disease, death, and recovery rates, how area hospitals were faring, and she developed a list of items that would be essential for patient care, estimated the use of PPE, and anticipated shortages. She reviewed every mask and gown offered, which met with both specifications and were approved by the National Institute of Occupational Safety and Health (NIOSH) and the Centers for Disease Control and Prevention (CDC), and frequently helped the team determine which of the offerings of several suppliers should be considered, as well as the volume that should be ordered and in stock. The average daily order of items was significantly increased by eightfold during the pandemic surge (see Fig. 14.1).

Fig. 14.1 The effect of the surge of COVID-19 pandemic on the hospital's need for supplies is illustrated here with the comparison of the same month during the peak of the pandemic (April 2020) with the same time of the year, 1 year later (April 2021)

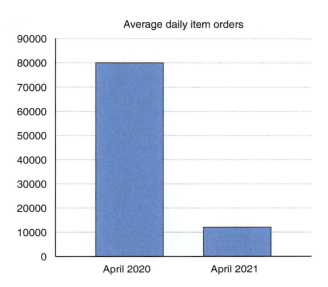

Managing a Shortage of Supplies

One of the first items to be in short supply was face shields. The director worked with the team to develop a solution – an "in-house" crafted face shield – using supplies readily available: eggcrate mattress foam, clear vinyl sheets (used for separating parts of a bound report), and bias tape (donated from a local fabric manufacturer), and the help of a team of 3-D printing enthusiasts was enlisted, headed by the emergency physician Dr. Mina Ataalla, to make headgear to hold the shields in place. Hospital engineers volunteered to punch holes in the vinyl at specified places to allow the reuse of the headpiece with new vinyl. When there were spare moments, every member of the team participated in crafting the shields, and, ultimately, this task was taken over by the dental residents who stepped up to help during the crisis.

The next shortage was HEPA filters. For a short while, these could not be obtained from any source since every hospital treating COVID-19 patients was using them in extraordinary numbers. The team therefore developed a plan in case of a complete HEPA shortage: the plan detailed purchasing the filtering material in bulk, cutting it down to size based on the currently used filters, and subsequently breaking down the used filters, sterilizing the containers, and refilling them with newly created filters. Luckily, before that plan was put into action, HEPA filters slowly became available, and, with the help of respiratory therapy and anesthesia/critical care and a few practice modifications, the HEPA crisis was averted.

Allocations and Back Orders

"Allocations" and "back orders" became dreaded terms during the pandemic, and they had a tremendous impact on supplies of PPE. Material shortages, as a result of factories closing, continue to be a reality for many of the usual items required for the day-to-day operation.

Allocations

An allocation is a specified amount of an item that is set aside for use by a particular hospital; a hospital therefore *might* be able to receive a requested item, but there are a number of "ifs" attached. In the case that a hospital uses a large volume of material supplies, is good at paying on time, and is generally a good customer, it will likely be rewarded by being pushed to the head of the queue. If the hospital requesting the material is smaller, uses less volume, or hasn't developed a significant relationship with the supplier, it will likely be pushed down the line. An allocation can also be based on the use of an item over the 3 months prior. In the 3 months prior to the highest COVID-19 surge, the use of certain critical items at the SBH Health System was either nil or negligible, as needs were quite different in the pre-COVID-19 Bronx, and the SBH Health System found itself at the end of, or not on a list for allocation at all, several times. This created another supply chain challenge of how and where to source items that were needed immediately and in large quantities. Due to shipping delays, unavailability of raw materials, factory slowdowns or closing, and the continued pandemic on an international scale, this is predicted to continue for some time and will likely affect significant items that the SBH Health System needs to source.

Back Orders

Everyone working in the supply chain is familiar with back orders, but COVID-19 brought with it a whole new understanding of the concept. Under normal circumstances, a back order means that the supplier is likely to have a product available in the future and will give the purchaser an estimated date. During the pandemic, many items went on back order, anticipated supply dates passed, and these back orders persisted. In some cases, companies suddenly stopped supplying the products at all. Generally, if an order has been on back order for more than 3 months, it is not going to be available in the future. Despite being on the tail end of the first pandemic surge, challenges still exist in obtaining goods as some companies, for example, may have discontinued a specific product on contract and reissued a product that appears to be nearly identical but at a higher price. A continual effort is made to find substitutes for basic items that are either no longer available, on undetermined backlog or have been discontinued and repackaged at significantly higher prices.

The Ongoing Challenges in Obtaining Resources to Cope with Increasing Patient Volume

Despite the competition for items, the SBH Health System supply chain team continued to fight for resources. Information shared at the daily meeting was crucial in identifying which team members would try to source critical items on the "needed" list and items that were predicted to become rare but necessary, and the VP would continue to field calls and continue to work on the access to PPE.

The team established a threshold of 30 days' supply based on current inventory that was on the premises and current "burn rates" (usage) and figured-in the historical times from order to delivery to maintain enough availability of most items for a hospital that had increased its general medical, surgical, and ICU bed capacity by 70% and increased its critical care capacity by >500% within a matter of a few weeks.

While the focus remained on obtaining supplies, the team had additional responsibilities. While COVID-19 and its effect on the frontline workers and hospitals in the area were of paramount importance, the team also had to determine what items were needed to open up units that had been closed for some time – hospital beds (virtually unobtainable at that time due to the demand), overbed tables, chairs, lamps, daily personal care items, intravenous (IV) poles, etc. For each, the task was to decide which items were essential and then look at the demands on each item and match that to what was available. Thinking "outside-the-box" became a significant part of everyday (see Sidebar 14.2): For example, when the team could not find a hospital bed, they began to look at stretchers, other types of beds, and mattress combinations, did the substitute have a control that allowed it to move up and down? Could the head of the bed be rolled up or electrically elevated? Did the bed have wheels? Was there a mattress included? What material was the mattress was made of? Could it be cleaned properly and withstand abuse? Every single challenge that arose during the pandemic required a multifaceted approach in order to solve it.

> **Sidebar 14.2 Outside-the-Box Thinking at Its Finest**
> *It was noted that the cleaning supplies used in the terminal cleaning of each operating room (OR) were eroding the finish on the operating room lights, and chips and bits of metal were noted to be on the OR tables. Immediately the call went out for the OR lights to be replaced, but that takes time, quotes, research, and then actual installation. The next call was for purchasing to find a mobile light source strong enough for the OR; however, no solutions could be found. OR lights are featured on several television programs, and bright lighting is used on Broadway. Broadway was closed and there wasn't much filming being done. Using the "6 degrees" of association, the team found someone who had a relative that was in the Broadway theater business, called in a favor, spoke with several film companies and lighting teams on Broadway, and came up with a source. That is "outside-the-box" at its finest.*

The Importance of the Chief Financial Officer and International Sourcing

The CFO

As mentioned, the SBH Health System purchasing team is an embedded team of consultants under contract to the hospital who share the responsibility for all purchasing and materials management, contract management, and have a concurrent objective to find items of excellent quality and preferred cost, with a promise to never compromise care. COVID-19 did not change these goals, but it did put savings on a different plane. Each embedded team under contract to a hospital has an executive sponsor, an individual on the executive team with whom there is a stronger relationship and is considered the team's direct upline at the hospital level: at the SBH Health System, that is the CFO.

The CFO at any hospital is someone who oversees all monies going in and out, manages and sets the budgets, and is concerned with controlling cash flow and spending. At a safety net hospital with a budget that is essentially dependent on state funding, those responsibilities are tremendous. Not only is the CFO responsible for keeping the hospital operating by providing the necessary equipment to allow for healthcare providers to give excellent care to all patients, but the CFO also has to manage the replacement costs of items that are broken or have gone well beyond their expected lifespan. The VP of purchasing and the CFO speak frequently throughout the day to share information about anticipated expenses, emergency expenditures, potential substitutes, and cost-saving measures. The pandemic significantly impacted the relationship between the CFO and VP, increasing and improving communication at this senior level in order to help tackle the expanded needs that accompanied the high influx of patients, the need for equipment previously unessential to hospital operation, and the high cost and limited availability of PPE.

Securing Resources, International Sourcing, and the Importance of Relationships

One of the greatest challenges during the pandemic was obtaining isolation gowns, procedure masks (double-layer masks with ear loops), N-95 masks, face shields, booties, gloves (sterile and non-sterile), eye protection, hand sanitizers, and caps to cover the hair. Competition was high for these supplies since every hospital in the world was in need. As previously discussed, some hospitals were given allocations of these items, but the amount received depended on the type of customer the hospital was and what they had used in the 3 months prior, and then 20–40% was taken off the allocated amount. A hospital in full pandemic mode cannot operate on three cases of 100 isolation gowns for the month.

The instance of "gray markets" started to increase, cold callers demanding huge sums of money upfront even though they didn't have any product at the time of the call. Distributors and GPOs warned daily of these gray markets: companies and individuals who were advertising that they had CDC and NIOSH certified products that met US specifications but who had no samples, or alternatively were showing a sample that met the specifications, but the supplied product was markedly inferior to the samples. Some suppliers in the United States were offering a single isolation gown for $17; normal pricing of these gowns, depending on the level of isolation that is required, would usually sell for between $1 and 5 for high end isolation gowns impermeable against chemotherapy medications.

The team at SBH Health System was fortunate to find a company that was owned and operated by a local couple who had expanded from their fashion design company to become an import-export business. They had contacts, recommendations, an ability to source in Southeast Asia and Turkey, and a good grasp on shipping, customs paperwork, trucking from the port to warehousing, and delivery. Over several calls and meetings, it was confirmed that this was a reputable organization that had the necessary international contacts to be able to provide bespoke PPE from factories in SE Asia. As a result of the relationship and reliability of the supplier, SBH Health System was extremely fortunate to be one of only a few hospitals in the region that never ran out of any critical item and always had enough PPE to supply the entire staff at all times. This significant achievement was a reflection of the strong relationship that existed between the VP and CFO, built on trust and confidence, enabling them to execute these crucial decisions.

Additional Storage Space

Another facet that required close collaboration between the VP and CFO was finding additional storage space for supplies. The state government had begun ordering hospitals in New York to keep 90 days of supplies on hand, and despite reorganizing the entire storeroom and commandeering additional space wherever it could be found (including hallways, walkways, and floor to ceiling), there was no more room. SBH was struggling to find space for 30 days' worth, and the trucks and ships kept arriving.

Fortunately, some members of the purchasing team had experience in other areas than their immediate jobs, including operation of a warehouse and managing large volumes of product in and out. These members became engaged in searching for additional storage space, and this was narrowed down to a warehouse. The warehouse needed to be close enough so that items could be moved from hospital to warehouse and back at a reasonable cost and within a reasonable period. It also needed to be safe, insurable, under some surveillance, close to port, and with room to expand. The most experienced member of the team took on the responsibility of viewing all potential spaces and negotiated pricing which, because of the state mandate and the pandemic, was well outside the fair market value. With the trust of the CFO, the team obtained warehouse storage in nearby Newark, NJ.

However, despite the extra storage space, the storeroom and storage areas within the hospital that are associated with materials management are small, and the space has only marginally improved because the demand remains high. As a result, many of the items from storage must be brought in in advance of need. Items are moved from one place to another on wooden pallets. As an example, a pallet may hold 1000's of non-sterile gloves in packages of 100–250 single gloves per box. These do not stack (at the hospital) and take up significant floor space, so the storeroom unfortunately continues to look like a war room.

Reflection on Lessons Learned During the COVID-19 Pandemic

The challenges brought about by the crisis and solutions created to address them gave rise to valuable learned lessons for future management of the supply change in health crisis times (see Table 14.1).

Table 14.1 Challenges and solutions for the supply chain and material management during a health crisis

Challenge	Solutions	Comment
Change from "just-in-time ordering" to "ordering for sustained high consumption with short supplies"	Change supply chain operations to crisis mode with daily meetings with data-driven materials management, real-time inventory, adjustment of critical thresholds, accurate consumption rates, predictor calculations, prioritization, suppliers' evaluation, calculating risks and margins of errors, establishing mitigation strategies and alternatives, etc.	Data management includes several spreadsheets or dashboards that track fundamental values: daily counts of supplies currently in-house, "burn rates," dates those supplies are ordered along with associated delivery dates, and the daily census, distribution, and associated needs
Limited on-site storage space	Efficient management of on-site storage and acquisition of off-site storage with easy access	Close coordination must be done daily for coordination of on-site storage, off-site storage, movement from site to site, distribution to end users, delivery of new supplies, labeling and access, attention to expiration and near-expiration dates, and others
Responding to governmental crisis surveys in a timely and accurate fashion	Assignment of one team member to receive and fill out the responses and another team member to review and edit to assure accuracy	Compliance with timeliness and accuracy of responses to governmental crisis surveys will assure continued support of the hospital by the various governmental agencies

Table 14.1 (continued)

Challenge	Solutions	Comment
Shortage of supplies	Finding alternative suppliers and products. Outside-the-box creative solutions of improvised products	Keeping active communications with frontline product users creates the foundation of improvised solutions in time of crisis and shortage
Allocations and back orders	Keeping contacts and even contracts with alternative suppliers to activate in case conventional suppliers fall short	Alternative suppliers may include local, national, and/or international sources. They may be private and/or governmental
High consumption rates of certain supplies	Interactive communications with clinical and administrative leaders to warn about potential shortage and help in the creation of conservation policies	Supply chain participation and representation in daily clinical and administrative meetings is very important during a crisis, for example, participation in the critical care committee, bed management committee, etc.

Conclusions

A pandemic of the proportion experienced by hospitals all over the world created a disruption in the supply chain to a degree not fully anticipated and one that had not been seen in recent history. It created shortages of equipment essential in ensuring that healthcare workers could work in a safe environment and deprived many of equipment that was deemed essential to the saving of lives. It overwhelmed hospital morgues, caused post-traumatic stress disorder and depression in those who were most forward in the frontlines, and broke families, businesses, and lives. Yet, behind the lines, when there was so much despair and angst, supply chain members in every hospital continued to work feverishly around the clock to find the items that were so badly needed.

At SBH Health System, purchasing and supply chain team members were very fortunate to have an extraordinary team of dedicated subject matter experts who had no difficulty rolling up their sleeves and digging in. They were resourceful even in the face of potentially apparent failures. For them, failure was not an option, and a good day was when they found a solution to a seemingly unsolvable problem. They made face shields when none could be sourced. They tried out samples for every conceivable source. They did endless searches, prepared a nightmare of Excel spreadsheets, responded to surveys, attended mandatory calls (albeit maybe just one team member who was also multitasking), and managed to outfit an entirely new structure for health and wellness for opening in November 2020. In spite of this, they never ran out of any critical items.

> If you believe your actions may lead to the survival of one person, use that to drive your approach to the day and you will be successful.

References

1. Chin AWH, Chu JTS, Perera MRA, Hui KPY, Yen HL, Chan MCW, Peiris M, Poon LLM. Stability of SARS-CoV-2 in different environmental conditions. Lancet Microbe. 2020;1(1):e10. https://doi.org/10.1016/S2666-5247(20)30003-3. Epub 2020 Apr 2. PMID: 32835322; PMCID: PMC7214863.
2. Harbourt DE, Haddow AD, Piper AE, Bloomfield H, Kearney BJ, Fetterer D, Gibson K, Minogue T. Modeling the stability of severe acute respiratory syndrome coronavirus 2 (SARS-CoV-2) on skin, currency, and clothing. PLoS Negl Trop Dis. 2020;14(11):e0008831. https://doi.org/10.1371/journal.pntd.0008831. PMID: 33166294; PMCID: PMC7676723.

Chapter 15
Information Technology, Healthcare Data and Analytics, and Clinical Engineering

Jitendra Barmecha

Information Technology at the Epicenter of a Crisis

The COVID-19 surge initially placed New York City as the epicenter of the pandemic in America. It was recognized early on that information technology (IT) would play a crucial role, not only in individual hospital adaptations but also in statewide responses to the crisis. Across NYC, focused efforts to improve staff efficiency, including rapid medical screening exams for low-acuity patients, use of "SmartNotes," improved vital sign monitoring, and the creation of multiple statewide dashboards, were implemented [1]. This allowed an element of vital collaboration between state hospitals and facilitated the transfer of resources, data, and good practice to and from some of the hardest-hit hospitals like SBH Health System in the Bronx. While linking hospitals this way undoubtedly improves patient care, the following account details the SBH-specific response to the COVID-19 surge, how it responded to the unprecedented demands of the pandemic, and how the adaptations that were made have prepared SBH to work in a more integrated fashion going forward.

J. Barmecha (✉)
SBH Health System, Bronx, NY, USA

CUNY School of Medicine, New York, NY, USA
e-mail: jbarmecha@sbhny.org

© The Author(s), under exclusive license to Springer Nature Switzerland AG 2022
R. Shabsigh (ed.), *Health Crisis Management in Acute Care Hospitals*, https://doi.org/10.1007/978-3-030-95806-0_15

Virtual Command Center in a Crisis

Setting up hospital contingency plans to prepare for a patient surge and demand for clinical services required establishment of a command center or a collaborative communication platform for all the stakeholders. With a mandate to increase inpatient capacity including ICU beds by at least 50%, along with setting up and enhancing virtual care capacity, dependencies on staff communication, remote access to networks, access to medical supplies and physical space was overwhelming. A virtual command center (VCC) is an operational entity for collaborative communication to ensure business continuity, which becomes crucial during a health crisis. With the availability of virtual (audio-video) platform technologies, a 24/7 virtual command center can be established instantaneously based upon the model of an incident command system (ICS) of the Federal Emergency Management Agency (FEMA) (Fig. 15.1).

Virtual command center platforms are comprised of unified communications solutions using voice over Internet protocol (VoIP) that enable a highly secured and responsive infrastructure for effective communication. The deployment and scaling of these license-based platforms are relatively simple. At SBH Health System, CISCO WebEx virtual conferencing platform was initially activated but was later migrated to the more HIPAA-compliant collaborative tool, Microsoft Teams (MS Teams), as the need grew to include patients and caregiver access.

Based on the surge management plan of a health system, the virtual command center can be rapidly activated and deactivated, as required. The deactivation process – from 24 hours, 7 days a week, to business hours – should be gradual upon receiving input from all the stakeholders, including local health authorities.

Technology and Communication Infrastructure

Unlike other natural disaster preparedness, the COVID-19 pandemic posed a very unique and difficult environment, where communication between various parties became challenging due to social distancing rules, Caregivers faced visitation

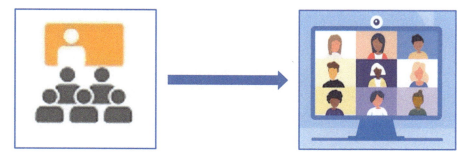

Fig. 15.1 Transition from in-person command center to virtual command center

restrictions, and this made it difficult for them to support hospitalized patients. Communication between providers (hybrid work force, increased demand, and acute shortage of clinicians) and communication between providers and patients (virtual care) were tested, and communications to stakeholders was also challenged.

MS Teams was deployed as a portable bedside communication tool to help maintain connections between patients, who didn't use a smartphone, and their caregivers. With a secure, reliable, and robust IT infrastructure, including enterprise Wi-Fi capabilities (guest and internal network), the deployment of such portable devices can be simple and scalable. Training on these devices and on using the MS Teams application is vital for successful implementation. This was carried out virtually with a dedicated team of accessible IT staff. Wi-Fi coverage was expanded by adding new access points, including cabling installation by vendors using the COVID-19 protocol, with access points to accommodate an increased capacity of in-patients.

An increased need for staff and material supply often coexists during a pandemic, and there are often continuing challenges to overcome shortages in both. Staff shortages can exist due to illness, quarantine due to COVID-19 exposure, exhaustion, or simply an incapacity to cope with the high influx of critically ill patients. These issues can be supported and often overcome by cross-training staff and managing overtime. A reliable IT infrastructure network with enterprise Wi-Fi technology can enable mobile devices (handheld and on carts) to perform virtual communication between providers and between providers and patients (Virtual Care), thereby increasing access, preserving personal protective equipment (PPE), and limiting exposure to COVID-19 infection.

Expanding IT Applications and Devices During a Pandemic

The COVID-19 pandemic resulted in increased inpatient, intensive care and emergency room bed capacity, ambulatory care and point of care lab testing, vaccinations, virtual care, and the healthcare workforce becoming either hybrid or remote workers. All these environments created a voracious demand for IT hardware and an expansion of existing and new software systems. Having a robust and reliable IT and telecommunication infrastructure with virtual servers made it easier to deploy new hardware (desktops, mobile carts, tablets, and phones) and software systems. If the new or repurposed patient care area didn't have an existing network infrastructure, either a temporary or permanent Wi-Fi access implementation was needed to access the software systems. Laying down the new cabling work for network infrastructure during the pandemic presented a complex scenario for staff who were faced with a shortage of PPE and a number of fluid infection control policies. However, despite these challenges, the projects were completed by having a hybrid model of staffing who knew hospital infection control policies and worked collaboratively with the vendors.

The creation of a drive-through or makeshift COVID-19 testing center also requires expansion of existing IT and telecommunication infrastructure. Although addition of software systems' licenses generally does not pose a problem, the procurement of hardware, e.g., servers, desktop and laptop computers, mobile tablets, Wi-Fi access points, and accessories, can be extremely challenging due to increased demand and breakdown in the supply chain during a crisis. To control and contain the spread of COVID-19 infection, technology solutions (along with processes), which screen and monitor the temperature of the staff, patients, and visitors, were implemented at the entrances of the health system. Initially, facial recognition-enabled thermal kiosks were installed at the limited entry points to the facility for healthcare workers. Nursing clinical staff had to be deployed to perform the screening questionnaire, and visitors entering the facility were screened by nursing staff and the concierge using a manual contactless thermometer. The health systems payroll swipe-in system was modified to include mandated COVID-19 screening questions, and laser thermal cameras were also installed at entry points. This evolved within 8 weeks into a more streamlined system with fewer staff required with corresponding decrease in PPE requirements.

Electronic Health Records

Since the Medicare and Medicaid electronic health records (EHR) incentive program, commonly called Meaningful Use, was implemented with the aim to promote the widespread exchange of health information, the majority of hospitals in America now use an EHR system [2, 3]. Enterprise EHR is the major software system that is impacted while increasing or repurposing bed capacity during a pandemic. EHR needs to be accessible to provide appropriate clinical care and data collection. Once the COVID-19 surge manifested, New York State mandated the expansion of inpatient bed capacity including the intensive care unit (ICU) for individual hospitals by 50%. In order to comply with the regulation, locations were identified within the facility that could be converted to accommodate these increased inpatient beds. Areas, such as ambulatory surgery, cardiac catheterization lab, the postanesthesia care unit (PACU), and the endoscopy suite, were identified due to their ability to provide additional monitored/ICU beds, and offices within the hospital were also moved to enable bed capacity. Adding new locations in the registration system, new end users, interfacing new lab systems, building clinical documentation, and adding new pharmacy and laboratory items, all requires dedicated IT staff collaborating with clinical and finance departments. A flexible change control IT policy and quick turnaround time help in deploying the EHR in the new or repurposed clinical areas.

Implementation of innovative clinical care pathways during a pandemic requires a rapid cycle build, test, train, and production methodology in the EHR with an agile project plan. As new treatment guidelines evolve during a pandemic, ordering items (medical devices, laboratory, and pharmacy items) in the computerized physician order entry system (CPOE) are built, and clinical documentation must be created and tested with multidisciplinary collaboration, before being put into production. Training of the new clinical care pathways for the end users can be done virtually using MS Teams platform.

Data Reporting and Analytics

Prior to the pandemic, the reporting and analytics workflow usually worked within a linear infrastructure with completion of data extracts occurring one at a time. This workflow enabled creation and pushing out real-time datasets and dashboards across all businesses with limited flexibility. However, during the pandemic, the need to push real-time dashboards for clinical, operational, regulatory, and financial departments becomes mission critical. As a result, moving from a standard linear development cycle to a rapid cycle using PDSA (Plan-Do-Study-Act) methodology (see Box 15.1) in collaboration with end users became the new normal. Rapid cycling of PDSA provides a structure for iterative testing of changes within a system with the aim to improve the quality of those systems. The original PDSA method [4] was subsequently adapted and is a widely accepted methodology in healthcare improvement [5].

> **Box 15.1 The Plan-Do-Study-Act methodology**
> - ***Plan***: *Close collaboration across departments, managers, and frontline staff, affording data analysts a better understanding of the rapidly evolving workflows, datasets, and reporting requirements.*
> - ***Do***: *Create and update reporting streams and dashboards as outlined in the planning sessions.*
> - ***Study***: *Continually review and validate data output, with respect to workflows. Test hypotheses developed in the planning stages comparing past, present, and future views.*
> - ***Act***: *Refine data models to reflect what is learned as the output is reviewed and studied. Use feedback to determine what modifications are needed.*

In response to the initial surge during the early part of the pandemic, IT applications, devices, and patient locations (patient beds) were added for capacity management, and these required configuration changes within the EHR. Careful planning is critical, along with updates to all the reporting streams, in order to capture all necessary data elements. For example, those reports pulling data from new and/or updated documents, flowsheets, newly added patient locations, or medication cabinets, all required updates, validation, and proper quality control. Without the involvement of frontline staff, those most familiar with workflows, systems, and any new changes within the department, this process of rapid reiteration would not have been possible. Data analysts working closely with the relevant end users along all aspects of the PDSA process brought efficiencies and speed to the process of honing into the required reporting streams.

Table 15.1 Common features of a communication and collaboration tool

Communication	Collaboration
Email	Electronic whiteboard
Text messaging	Application sharing
Audio calls or conferences	Shared office solutions
Video calls of conferences	Group calendars
	Project management
	Storage
	Integration with other apps
	Screen sharing

Communication and Collaboration Tools

The secured communication and collaboration tools (Table 15.1), along with remote access to the hospital network, play a very important role in business continuity during a pandemic. MS Teams provided the critical infrastructure that allowed communication and collaboration amongst staff, between individuals, specific teams, and even across the entire organization. The tools are practically a virtual workspace that ensure everyone is involved and include messaging, video calling, file sharing, storage, calendar, and other integration features. During the pandemic, the telecommuting policies were enhanced to accommodate hybrid and remote working staff so that they could continue to perform their duties. End user training using a learning management platform is critical to the success of the deployment and adoption of these tools.

Virtual Care Platform

The pandemic resulted in an increased demand on the healthcare ecosystem managing COVID-19 patients; an increased need for isolation/quarantine of patients, the caregivers, and the staff; and additional measures to protect the healthcare workforce and preserve PPE. The pandemic also resulted in a citywide lockdown with partial closure of the public transportation or mass transit systems. During such time, the use of telehealth and digital technology capabilities allowing virtual care and remote patient monitoring (RPM) skyrocketed several folds. Virtual care helps provide necessary care to patients while minimizing the transmission risk of COVID-19 to healthcare workers and other patients. The use of RPM and engaging patients around their virtual care have previously been used and appear to be accepted by patients for management of a range of chronic diseases and episodic care after discharge from hospital [6–8]. The implementation of virtual care, which includes telehealth, remote patient monitoring, e-consults, and tele-ICU, requires comprehensive strategies and multidisciplinary collaboration between clinical, operational, and finance staff. The virtual care platform chosen should be integrated with the enterprise electronic health record through patient portals for scheduling, virtual visits, and clinical documentation. Telephonic calls can be an alternative solution for patients who do not have smartphones or broadband access. Tele-ICU or e-ICU, with central monitoring capabilities, enables a colocated team of critical care clinicians to remotely monitor patients in the ICU regardless of their location. ICU clinicians based in a telehealth e-ICU hub are supported by high-definition cameras, patient monitoring solutions, and real-time data visualization tools in order to provide effective care. Similarly, hospital at home, post-discharge patients from the emergency room, or in-patients can be monitored remotely via RPM platforms. The role of digital door and virtual waiting rooms has also expanded through virtual care platforms to improve efficiency and maintain patient engagement.

IT Infrastructure for Rapid Cycle Quality Assurance and Performance Improvement During a Health Crisis

Close collaboration between application or system analysts, data analysts, and key leaders within the organization is critical in the expansion of the morbidity and mortality dashboards to better describe and inform the organization of patterns and trends related to the pandemic. Utilizing the rapid cycle PDSA methodology process was a critical component in designing, redesigning, incorporating, and implementing the necessary data elements into the datasets to ensure high-quality reports to the end user, depicting the clear picture of pandemic progression. How the data is captured, how it should be sliced, and what data elements and filters are required to provide clarity and meaning to the data visualizations were of the utmost importance. As an example, determining whether COVID-19 status should be reported for mortality, based upon the current visit (visit specific) or all visits (medical record number/MRN specific) (Figs. 15.2 and 15.3). Real-time outcome dashboards are

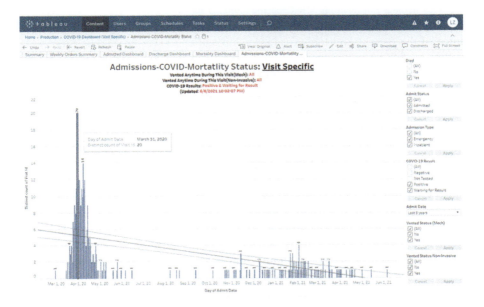

Fig. 15.2 Example of reporting visit-specific mortality status

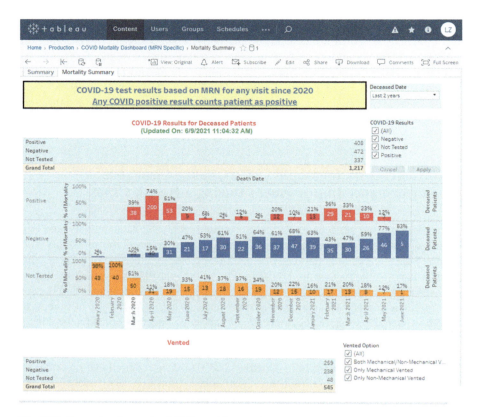

Fig. 15.3 Example of reporting MRN-specific mortality status

some of the most useful tools for leadership and end users to validate processes, update workflows, and keep track of progress. Several dashboards are presented below to show examples of data visualization for the management of the various aspects of a health crisis and a pandemic (Figs. 15.2, 15.3, 15.4, 15.5, 15.6, 15.7, 15.8, 15.9, and 15.10).

Enhanced Information Security

Data and network security, as well as data integrity, are critical back-office components to providing quality healthcare. During the pandemic, when remote work and virtual care (telehealth) became the primary methods of caring for patients and performing other healthcare support services, having the utmost confidence in the safety of the infrastructure providing those services could not have been more important. The shift to electronic and remote working seen during the pandemic created many potential security and privacy risks that generated anxiety among

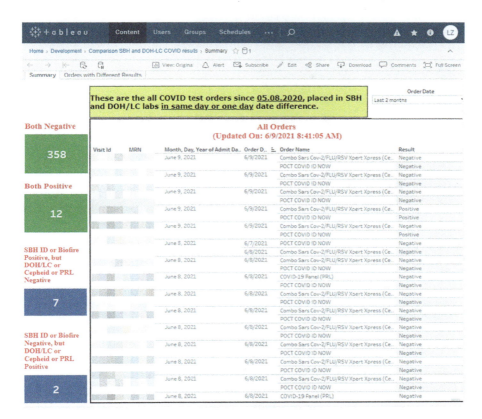

Fig. 15.4 Comparison of COVID-19 tests between health system and external laboratories: validation between specific COVID-19 lab tests was critical in deciding how tests are ordered for optimal operations

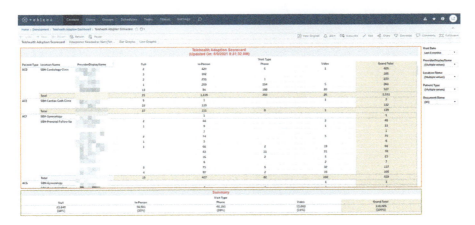

Fig. 15.5 The virtual care scorecard dashboard was developed to keep track of progress with telehealth adoption from both provider and patient perspectives

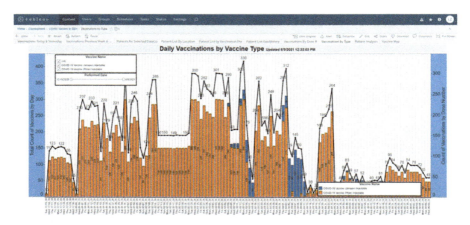

Fig. 15.6 The COVID-19 vaccine at the health system dashboard was not only critical in reconciling vaccinations as the vaccination program progressed through the ever-changing DOH criterion but was a way to quantify overall vaccinations along with demographics

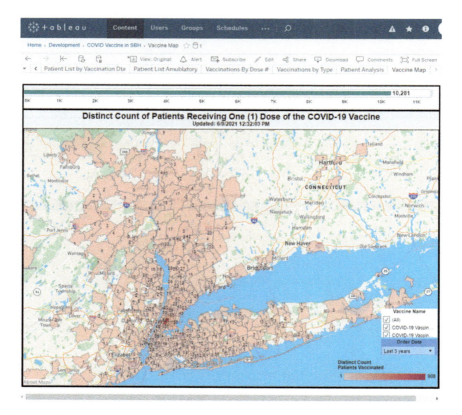

Fig. 15.7 The map displays the count of patients receiving one dose of the COVID-19 vaccine. The dashboard was not very helpful in understanding the progress of vaccination in the immediate and distant areas around SBH, NYC

15 Information Technology, Healthcare Data and Analytics, and Clinical Engineering 251

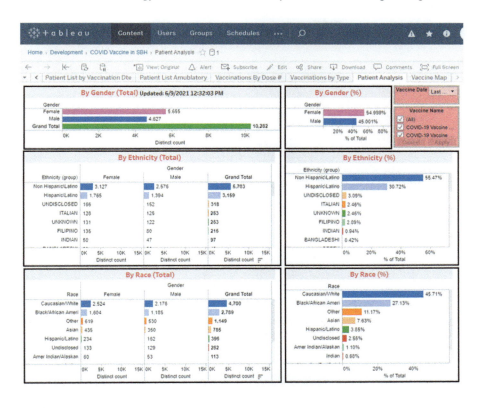

Fig. 15.8 The COVID-19 vaccination subgroups dashboard clarified the impact and progress of vaccination in the various ethnic and racial groups

patients and medical workers who were afraid of losing control over sensitive medical information, which was stored on servers or clouds [9]. Regulations such as the Health Insurance Portability and Accountability Act of 1996 (HIPAA) have been put in place to ensure national standards of strong protection of medical records [10].

Data protection rests with every user that accesses a certified EHR. Mandatory yearly training modules (on learning management system- LMS) can be designed to keep the protection of the network and patient data foremost in the minds of the end user. Periodic updates from the IT department provide end users with a high-level view and rating of the end user and technology devices used to provide patient care. It is important for end users to understand the health system's current security posture and general ratings from the security analysts or vendors in order to feel part of the process. End users using personal mobile devices to access hospital communication require additional mobile device management services.

While the IT department uses most of the current industry agnostic data protection best practices of encryption, firewalls, password, update management, least

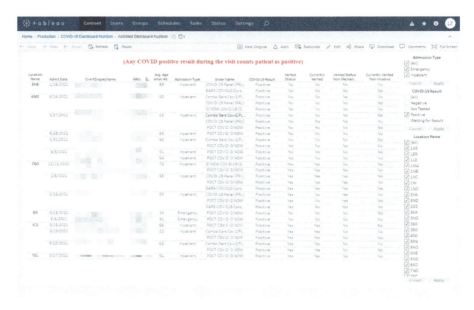

Fig. 15.9 The admitted nutrition dashboard was developed to provide the nutrition department with valuable information regarding their patients' key measures

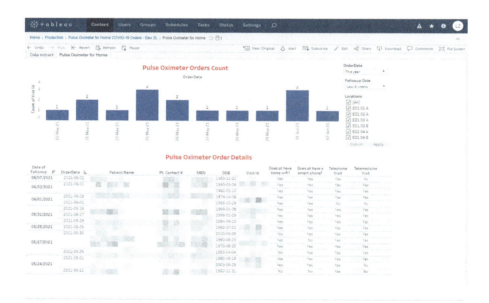

Fig. 15.10 The pulse oximeter orders dashboard for emergency department patients

privilege, and multifactor authentication (MFA) when possible, there must be an ongoing assessment of system access rules and polices to make sure nothing is missed. The IT infrastructure and information security division ensure all network infrastructure and systems are secured during a pandemic when the vulnerability of the healthcare sector to cyberattacks is at an all-time high.

The most likely scenario of patient data intrusion will take place by an attacker attempting to freeze or hold their data hostage in hopes of a ransom payment by the institution. IT and security resources are focused on the probable with an eye on the possible. Protecting the hospital from the most likely intrusion events is the primary goal.

Clinical Engineering: Patient Care Monitoring Solutions

COVID-19 is a respiratory viral illness where patients require continuous monitoring of vital signs, invasive hemodynamic monitoring, and sometimes ventilator support. As a result of capacity management, the number of inpatient beds was increased by 50% and ICU beds were increased by 250%, respectively. These additional beds required FDA-approved patient monitoring solutions and associated accessories. Since there was a robust, reliable, and flexible IT infrastructure, the expansion of the patient care monitoring solution was seamless. The existing vendor's integrated platform and medical devices were chosen for the project under speed to value methodology. The project was completed within 90 days (under budget) instead of the projected 180 days, as a result of extensive collaboration between the vendor, IT, clinical engineering, and the nursing department.

The supply chain for all IT hardware, medical devices, parts, and accessories procurement was totally disrupted due to underproduction, increased demand, and logistics disruption; short-term rental for medical devices could be an alternative in such circumstances. Creation of a checklist (Fig. 15.11) of devices, parts, and

Item	Serial Number	Model	Vendor	Units	Total	Current Inventory	Under Repair	Burn rate / week
Information Technology								
Desktops								
Laptops								
Mobile Carts								
Webcams								
Speakers								
Electrical Cords								
Phones								
Servers								
Scanners								
Label Printers								
Clinical Engineering								
Pulse Oximeters								
Beside Monitors								
BP Cables								
Pulse Oximeters Cables								
EKG Cables								
Arterial Gas cables								

Fig. 15.11 IT and clinical engineering checklist for devices and accessories

accessories, along with their burn rate, is highly recommended for proactive procurement. Daily input from various stakeholders mitigated shortages and enhanced clinical care and throughput.

IT Customer and Technical Support

Help desk calls to the IT customer support and technical services team increased tremendously during the early part of the pandemic, as most of the health system's staff shifted to remote or hybrid working, conducting virtual visits, teaching, and learning. During the same period, there was an increased demand for IT and telecommunication devices deployment in inpatient units to support bed capacity management. Staff who had shifted to remote working had questions on setting up their home office, launching collaboration and communication tools, and onboarding new employees. IT customer support staff also became hybrid due to lockdowns and sickness/home quarantine. Unreliable Internet or phone connection access at home for remote workers, coupled with limited technical staff working remotely with no peer or managerial support to perform in-person assistance (elbow support), resulted in the simple tasks/service calls becoming complex. The majority of the calls were issues regarding network access and use of collaborative tools. Existing IT and analytic staff were redeployed to the help desk to field the increased volume of calls and provide any additional support required.

The technical services team had been trained on infection control policies, which previously helped immensely for break-fix hardware issues or in deploying new ones to a clinical area where caution was needed to be employed and important restrictions were in place. This was aided by the distribution of adequate PPE and sanitizers to the IT department, which facilitated the rapid response times, protecting staff themselves and potentially containing the spread of infection during the pandemic.

Overall and despite limited resources, IT customer support and technical services team responded well by rapidly deploying innovative solutions like a unified telecommunication system, remote access to networks, collaborating platforms, and the use of data and analytics to prioritize service calls. The IT and analytics team felt privileged to collaborate with the clinical and operational teams daily – both remotely and in person – and to provide the necessary technical support during the pandemic.

Contingency Plan for EHR Downtime

Downtime occurs when access to the network, IT, and telecommunication systems is interrupted, resulting in the activation of preformulated contingency plans. This can be scheduled as a systems' upgrade or unscheduled during a natural disaster.

The culture of "teamwork and patient first," along with the focus on IT infrastructure's performance, efficiency, and reliability, has been tested through prior experience with IT systems upgrades, power outages, hurricanes, and other disruptive events. Contingency plans are in place that can be adapted to the challenges of a pandemic such as COVID-19. The highest priorities are business continuity, safer patient care, and communication. Both scheduled and unscheduled downtime, based on the level of network, IT systems, and telecommunication outage, have a contingency plan, which are discussed and updated with all the stakeholders periodically. Collaboration and communication are key prior to, during, and post downtime. The contingency plan developed is departmental specific with periodic reviews, and all systems and methods of communication are taken into consideration. There are many different components in a downtime plan; the common factor is moving documentation to paper, which is scanned into a separate accessible system after the downtime is over. With the implementation and period upgrades of EHR in the past years, scheduled downtime has now prepared end users well for the contingency plan response in the event of any disaster or crisis. Remarkably during the COVID-19 pandemic surge, there was no downtime.

Reflection and Key Lessons Learned from Adaptation to the COVID-19 Crisis

There are many important lessons learned during the pandemic, both on a personal and professional level, for the members of the IT department at SBH. Transparency, effective collaboration, decisive leadership, clear communication, being resilient, humility, responsiveness, dependable supply-chain infrastructure, adaptability, and being innovative are some of the key traits required to respond to a pandemic. Daily assessments must occur to quickly redeploy staff, improve cross-training, and increase the par level of devices and accessories for both additional clinical areas and employees working from home.

On a positive note, the pandemic potentiated the digital transformation journey (Fig. 15.12).

In healthcare, electronic health record (clinical and financial) systems have become equally as important as the technology infrastructure. Agile project planning, along with collaborative team efforts, can quickly respond to enhanced patient capacity and assist clinical innovations during a pandemic. Several workflows can be done remotely through accessing to the network and on a collaborative platform. The staff can be equally productive whether on-site or working hybrid as long as appropriate systems and tools are accessible. Virtual care and remote work are the new normal in the workplace and will continue to play an important role in the healthcare delivery services.

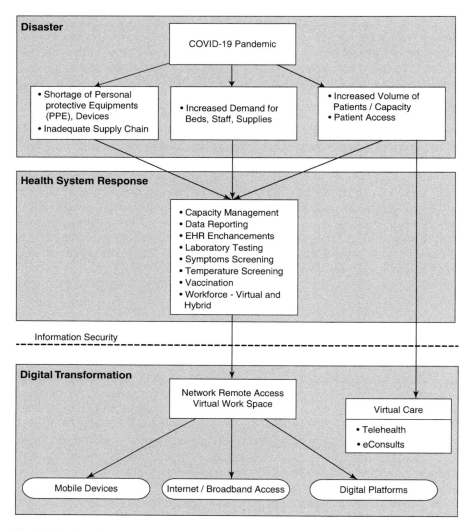

Fig. 15.12 A health system's response to a disaster/pandemic through digital transformation

What Would Be Done Differently Next Time? How and Why?

As touched upon earlier, close collaboration and communication are critical factors when working in highly technological and integrated environments. As the pandemic forced working at least 6 feet apart, if not from home, it took a moment to readjust and find the footing and the right tools to stay connected. It was with the extensive, phased rollout of a collaborating tool – such as MS Teams – that allowed the bridging of these gaps. While the organizational deployment came rather early in the pandemic, this type of infrastructure and the ease of cross-connecting with peers within and across departments were invaluable and could have been deployed earlier. Additionally, it is imperative that both IT, the analytics department, and end users are abreast of current affairs at an organizational as well a global level. This will give a better understanding of how current data streams might be affected by expected changes. To that end, predictive analytics, robotic process automation, the use of machine learning, and augmented intelligence could have provided better insights and outcomes.

Summary and Conclusions

SBH Health System and its IT, Healthcare Analytics, and Clinical Engineering departments have relied on people, processes, and technologies that have been built over many years and which can respond to any crisis or disruptive event. This combination of disaster preparedness, crisis management, reliable infrastructure, workflow processes innovation, and competent, committed staff – along with their collaboration – has allowed us to play a central role in supporting the organization's response to the COVID-19 pandemic. Work must continue to enable the department to build upon lessons learned from this pandemic and create templates for future crises.

References

1. Salway RJ, Silvestri D, Wei EK, Bouton M. Using information technology to improve COVID-19 care at New York City health + hospitals. Health Aff (Millwood). 2020;39(9):1601–4. https://doi.org/10.1377/hlthaff.2020.00930.
2. Furukawa MF, Patel V, Charles D, Swain M, Mostashari F. Hospital electronic health information exchange grew substantially in 2008-12. Health Aff (Millwood). 2013;32(8):1346–54. https://doi.org/10.1377/hlthaff.2013.0010.
3. Furukawa MF, King J, Patel V, Hsiao CJ, Adler-Milstein J, Jha AK. Despite substantial progress in EHR adoption, health information exchange and patient engagement remain low in office settings. Health Aff (Millwood). 2014;33(9):1672–9. https://doi.org/10.1377/hlthaff.2014.0445.
4. Deming WE. Out of the crisis, 1986. Cambridge, MA: Massachusetts Institute of Technology Center for Advanced Engineering Study xiii; 1991. p. 507.
5. Speroff T, O'Connor GT. Study designs for PDSA quality improvement research. Qual Manag Health Care. 2004;13(1):17–32. https://doi.org/10.1097/00019514-200401000-00002.
6. Sohn A, Speier W, Lan E, Aoki K, Fonarow G, Ong M, et al. Assessment of heart failure patients' interest in mobile health apps for self-care: survey study. JMIR Cardio. 2019;3(2):e14332. https://doi.org/10.2196/14332.
7. Walker PP, Pompilio PP, Zanaboni P, Bergmo TS, Prikk K, Malinovschi A, et al. Telemonitoring in chronic obstructive pulmonary disease (CHROMED). A randomized clinical trial. Am J Respir Crit Care Med. 2018;198(5):620–8. https://doi.org/10.1164/rccm.201712-2404OC.

8. Walker RC, Tong A, Howard K, Palmer SC. Patient expectations and experiences of remote monitoring for chronic diseases: systematic review and thematic synthesis of qualitative studies. Int J Med Inform. 2019;124:78–85. https://doi.org/10.1016/j.ijmedinf.2019.01.013.
9. Fabian B, Ermakova T, Junghanns P. Collaborative and secure sharing of healthcare data in multi-clouds. Inf Syst. 2015;48:132–50.
10. U.S. Department of Health & Human Services, Health Information Privacy, HIPAA for Professionals. https://www.hhs.gov/hipaa/for-professionals/index.html. Accessed 26 Sept 2021.

Chapter 16
Medical Students and the Medical School

Nancy Sohler, Lisa Auerbach, and Erica S. Friedman

Educational Setting

The City University of New York School of Medicine (CUNY School of Medicine) is an accelerated BS-MD program in New York City (NYC) with a dual mission: to increase the number of physicians from groups traditionally underrepresented in the medical profession and to encourage graduates to practice primary care medicine in medically underserved communities in New York [1]. The CUNY School of Medicine is part of the City University of New York and is located at the City College of New York campus. The City University of New York is the largest public university in the country and a demonstrated social mobility university [2].

The CUNY School of Medicine was founded in 1973 as the Sophie Davis School of Biomedical Education, a 5-year undergraduate program located in NYC's Harlem neighborhood that offered a bachelor's degree, during which the students also completed the coursework of the first 2 years of medical school. Graduates from Sophie Davis were matched to cooperating medical schools for their clerkship years before entering residency. The mission of the program, together with its relatively low tuition, attracted a diverse student body [3].

Today, the CUNY School of Medicine offers both preclinical training and clerkships largely through its partnership with SBH Health System, a community teaching hospital located in the Bronx, New York, that has a healthcare mission parallel to the CUNY School of Medicine educational mission. The CUNY School of Medicine also has clinical partnerships with Staten Island University Hospital and other hospitals throughout the NYC area. The CUNY School of Medicine program remains an accelerated program, now expanded to 7 years, that encourages seamless

---

N. Sohler (✉) · L. Auerbach · E. S. Friedman
CUNY School of Medicine, New York, NY, USA
e-mail: nsohler@med.cuny.edu

© The Author(s), under exclusive license to Springer Nature
Switzerland AG 2022
R. Shabsigh (ed.), *Health Crisis Management in Acute Care Hospitals*,
https://doi.org/10.1007/978-3-030-95806-0_16

educational transitions that avoid many of the hurdles, which have previously led to race/ethnicity disparities in access to medical education [4].

The CUNY School of Medicine's curriculum is unique in many ways beyond its 7-year structure, reflecting its commitment to serving underserved communities and training future physicians to offer comprehensive medical care that includes activities to address aspects of the local community that inhibit health and well-being. The curriculum prepares students to take not only the role of clinicians but also the roles of community health promoters, researchers, and agents of change [5]. These latter three roles, essentially omitted from traditional medical education until recently, are introduced to CUNY School of Medicine students in a series of courses that begin in the undergraduate years and include curricula in humanities, social sciences, and community health, which are taught in parallel with the basic sciences. Several of these courses include faculty from the other schools of the City College of New York, giving students opportunities to learn from and study with people from a range of academic disciplines.

Clinical training at the CUNY School of Medicine also prepares students for the expanded roles of physicians as envisioned by its model. Students take a lifestyle medicine course that teaches them the importance of lifestyle on health and wellness, including diet, exercise, and sleep. Students are placed in a clinical setting early in the program, often in Federally Qualified Health Centers throughout the city. In these outpatient settings, students are trained as health coaches and contribute to the work of the health centers in this capacity. In the clerkship years, the CUNY School of Medicine embraces its mission by increased exposure to primary care practice. More than half of the clerkships are in primary care, including an extended (8-week) clerkship in family medicine.

As described below, many of the curricular changes that the CUNY School of Medicine adopted because of the coronavirus disease 2019 (COVID-19) pandemic have served to strengthen the CUNY School of Medicine's mission, curricular focus in social medicine, and its partnership with the surrounding NYC community.

Curricular Changes and Innovations in Response to COVID-19

The COVID-19 pandemic stretched the limits of the US healthcare system and forced the largest changes to the medical education system that most can remember [6], and its impact is still evolving [7]. Colleges and universities, including medical schools across the United States, abruptly closed in March of 2020, suspending in-person classes and exams, and hands-on training [8]. Educators, relying on Internet-based communication forums, were forced to transition class format, content, and schedules with little time for preparation. Many of these changes are illustrated from the CUNY School of Medicine experience that includes both undergraduate and preclinical curriculum, as well as clerkships. It is important to note that the curricular changes in the CUNY School of Medicine were developed in the context of NYC, the epicenter of the first wave of COVID-19 in the United States. This occurred alongside the co-occurring surge of police brutality that magnified the long-standing history of racism across the United States, and the resultant community outrage. These crises created significant hardships for students, faculty, and staff, and the curricular adjustments were consistent with the mission of training physicians to address healthcare needs with a social justice lens.

The changes made to medical school curricula are described in three main areas: the teaching environment, service learning, and the clinical curriculum. Later, a discussion is presented on how COVID-19 impacted student graduation requirements, and finally, there is a discussion about the consideration of wellness.

> Although not the nation's first pandemic, COVID-19 overwhelmed hospital systems and challenged the medical schools that rely on these systems to educate our future physicians.

Teaching Environment

Prior to COVID-19 shutdowns, preclinical training in medical schools across the country typically relied at least in part on lecture-based classroom teaching. This component of education was quickly transformed to fully online formats. To do this, all faculty and students were given the virtual meeting platform, Zoom [9]; those without computers were provided laptops; and those without adequate Internet coverage were provided tablets with hotspots. This quick transition was possible at the CUNY School of Medicine and other schools because of the trend to incorporate the use of new technologies to enhance medical education, implement self-directed learning, and promote life-long learning techniques that allow for individualized instruction and asynchronous learning [10]. However, prior to COVID-19 shutdowns, medical students still met in person for a substantial part of their training that was based on small-group interactions, laboratory sessions, patient simulations, and instruction with standardized patients. Transitioning these interactive instructional sessions to online formats was more difficult.

Problem-based learning (PBL) is a pedagogical practice that is commonly used in medical schools striving to incorporate system-based courses, self-directed student research, and teamwork by using case studies that require progressively complex decision-making skills of a group of students (Fig. 16.1). It targets higher-order learning and engages students in ways that result in better long-term retention of content than traditional, lecture-based courses [11]. While there are resources that allow medical schools to share PBL cases, the CUNY School of Medicine has developed its own cases for its preclinical curriculum to ensure students gain a deep understanding of social, economic, and political determinants of health outcomes and healthcare access and practice recognizing and speaking comfortably about how these determinants impact health equity and patient outcomes. The major challenge to transitioning this approach to the virtual

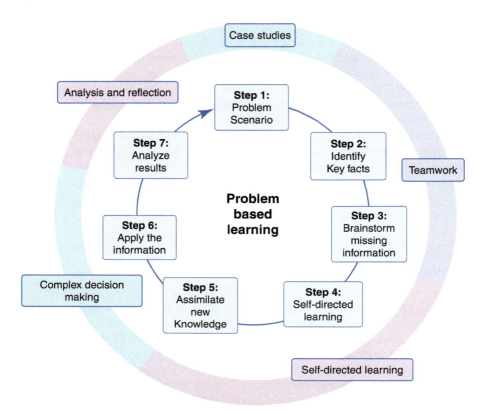

Fig. 16.1 Steps involved in problem-based learning for medical students at the City University of New York School of Medicine (COSM). The process is centered around the use of medical case studies to promote the development of complex decision-making skills

arena was its reliance on student interactions during class sessions. Encouraging balanced student discussions during PBL sessions is particularly critical in schools that include a strong focus on social medicine, which often touches on sensitive and controversial issues. Since students were frequently reluctant to use their cameras and microphones from home where other members of their household were also living and working during the pandemic, students became increasingly reliant on chat features or jam boards. Interestingly, these features improved participation in the PBL group from in-person sessions, by providing a means for the quieter students to engage. Overall, there is promise for ongoing utilization of online PBLs [12].

Virtual laboratories, simulations, and instruction with standardized patients were also developed and shared by medical schools across the country [13, 14], and this allowed students to meet course and program learning objectives. However, prior to the pandemic, these teaching modalities provided more than simply the exchange of information and development of critical thinking skills; these interactive practices helped to fulfill the necessary social connection, community building, and socialization in learning that are only possible with in-person interactions [6]. During the COVID-19 shutdown, this social connection was lost, and the impact this will have for the cohorts affected by these changes is still unknown, but the immediate impact on the students was clearly evident [15]. The CUNY School of Medicine initiated several mechanisms to encourage student-faculty and student-student interactions within virtual platforms to attempt to mitigate this problem. For example, monthly class-wide support sessions were initiated and attended by all of the deans and faculty. These sessions gave students time to share their concerns about their education, difficulties with focusing and studying, and, often times, other more personal experiences of social isolation, fear, and anxiety. Students later noted that these sessions succeeded in fostering a sense of community and a space to support one another and the faculty.

> Technology was already incorporated into much of pre-clerkship medical education before the pandemic. The quick expansion of these platforms allowed schools to continue to educate students during the early pandemic.

Service Learning

Service learning, or value-added education, is a required component of medical school education. Traditionally, medical schools were structured with the premise that substantive learner contributions to healthcare or education can only begin in the last year of medical school, or, maybe more realistically, during residency. However educational experts increasingly are advocating for developing value-added medical education earlier [16]. Value-added educational experiences, such as experiential roles that have the potential to positively impact individuals and population health outcomes, cost of care, or other processes within the healthcare system, can enhance student knowledge, attitudes, and skills in the clinical or health systems sciences and can be applied even in the undergraduate and preclinical curriculum. Learner roles could include patient navigators, clinical care extenders, patient advocates, and resource managers.

COVID-19 shutdowns presented challenges for offering service learning opportunities, but medical schools overcame them in novel ways. For example, students engaged in online public and community welfare activities [17, 18], healthcare delivery through telehealth technologies [19] (see clinical curriculum section below) or even assisting patients with scheduling appointments, workforce assistance in the form of providing childcare and other activities that allowed providers to spend more time in the clinics, and medical education by piloting new education materials and providing increased student feedback and evaluation [20].

The CUNY School of Medicine requires that all students complete a six-credit service-learning course in the summer before their third undergraduate year. Typically, students are placed in a clinical or social service setting and asked to work with a mentor to contribute to an ongoing initiative at their setting and present a report summarizing their work. The projects often involve collecting a needs assessment or program evaluation data from patients, analyzing these data, and making suggestions based on the lessons learned from these data. Students apply the knowledge from previous population health and epidemiology training, as well as their training in-patient interviewing and communication skills and interprofessional collaborations in clinical settings. Successful completion of this course is a critical bridge between undergraduate and medical school, training the CUNY School of Medicine students to be active participants in their education outside of the classroom as well as in the classroom. Clearly during the COVID-19 shutdown, students could not participate in service learning activities in the clinic or social service agencies. Further, most of the service learning teaching sites across the city were unable to host medical students during the first few months of the pandemic because clinical and social service settings were either closed or inundated with patient care activities. Thus, the CUNY School of Medicine took this opportunity to develop a new program, which will continue as an elective service learning opportunity.

The CUNY School of Medicine partnered with a health and science charter high school in the Bronx and developed a program to allow medical students to work with high school students to explore how COVID-19 had impacted their local communities. This program gave high school students a unique opportunity to learn about community health assessments, social determinants of health, and simple research methodologies. It also gave the CUNY School of Medicine students a chance to be role models for high school students in a few brief interactions, hopefully encouraging them to seek further education in medicine or other sciences. The CUNY School of Medicine then used what they learned about the students and their high school programs to develop a brief curriculum in community and population health. These curricula were then shared with the high school, and several of the CUNY School of Medicine students are working this summer to help implement aspects in a summer program.

> Mission driven schools like CUNY School of Medicine had to innovate to continue to offer a curriculum that meets the mission. CUNY School of Medicine pivoted a service learning program from clinical and social service clinics into a program to engage with students at a local high school.

Clinical Curriculum

The impact on the clinical part of medical school curriculum was more dramatic and perhaps more consequential for the long term. Across the country, and particularly in large urban areas like NYC, training hospitals quickly were overwhelmed with patients who were sick with COVID-19. Clinicians did not have time to engage in medical student training and could not spare the limited personal protective equipment (PPE) that would be needed to engage medical student trainees safely. Thus, onsite clinical training was suspended both for students in their required clerkships and students in their clinical electives.

The required clerkships are typically in the third year of medical school. This is when medical students have an opportunity to observe and participate in-patient care within each specialty, both developing clinical competencies and choosing a career path. Finding strategies within the virtual environment to help students develop clinical competencies was easier than giving students sufficient exposure to understand each specialty. Clerkship students attended didactic sessions with clinical teams via virtual platforms relying on online patient cases and virtual chart reviews to practice clinical reasoning and meet required clinical experiences. Some schools held virtual patient rounds, which have the potential to be a lasting component of clerkship education, as its flexibility might allow for increased teaching time [21, 22]. In virtual patient rounds using virtual platforms medical students follow hospitalized patients but do not participate in actual patient care.

Telemedicine provided opportunities for students to have in person interactions with patients. The structure was in place to allow for this even before COVID-19, and there was a growing trend toward integrating telemedicine-based lectures, clinical cases, and case studies into medical school curricula [23, 24]. Prior to COVID-19, 25% of medical school programs included telemedicine training in the pre-clerkship education and even more in clerkships [23]. It is not surprising that many success stories of COVID-19 transitions included expanded reliance on telemedicine for training and clinical care [19, 20]. This included medical students interviewing patients during routine outpatient telemedicine visits, conducting and documenting follow-up with patients on laboratory and other test results, assisting with patient education for homebound geriatric patients, and engaging as connectors between family members, who were not allowed to visit inpatient relatives, and their busy frontline physicians. It is likely that this will be an enduring transformation in medicine and education [20].

The clinical training years typically also include electives, which allow students to engage in clinical care or research either at their home institution or elsewhere while applying and interviewing for residency. Away electives or audition rotations are strongly suggested for some specialties, and give students experiences with different hospitals, faculty, and patient populations, but were discouraged during COVID-19 [25]. The lack of away electives created hardships for both the students' ability to explore and apply to residencies in some specialties and for the residency programs' ability to make complete and fair decisions using established processes [26]. However, the true impact of away electives on the residency match is unclear [27], making this COVID-19 adjustment another that will require longer-term evaluation to truly understand its impact on medical education.

With these changes, many medical schools across the country made temporary adjustments to both required and elective clerkships. Several required clerkships were truncated. Clerkship schedules were adjusted to delay the required direct patient experiences, so that students across years might have the longest in-person clinical training allowed by the pandemic restrictions.

The removal of students from clinical sites was unanticipated and a challenge to the students' ability to finish required experiences in time to apply for residency and graduate on time.

Graduation and Residency

Not only were medical schools and clinical sites closed, but the organization that created and administered medical school standardized exams – including those required for medical school graduation and licensure, the National Board of Medical Examiners (NBME) – also closed numerous testing centers across the country and suspended use of the customized and standardized exams. This impacted both the availability of licensing exams and assessments needed in medical schools, creating delays in student academic progression that lasted until late summer 2020. Medical schools experimented with open book exams and with creating their own in-house summative exams with variable results [28], but the lack of licensing exams created enormous hardship for students [29]. Many schools that previously required students to pass the United States Medical Licensing Exam (USMLE) Step 1 exam prior to entering clerkships paused that rule in order for students to progress while waiting to pass the USMLE Step 1. Additionally, across the country, students were allowed to graduate without completing the USMLE Step 2 clinical skills exam, previously required for licensure. In January of 2021, the Federation of State Medical Boards and NBME announced that this clinical skills exam would be discontinued permanently.

The loss of the clinical skills exam requirement is likely to remain a controversial result of the pandemic on medical education. This exam was first required in 2004, and it led to medical school development of more sophisticated clinical curricula to ensure students met these clinical competencies [30–32]. While there was debate about this exam prior to COVID-19, some educators worry that the cancellation of this exam will reverse the positive trends in strengthening clinical skills training in medical schools [33]. Other clinical skills educators greet this change with a sense of optimism; clinical skills teaching can be broadened rather than focusing on training students to pass an exam that was based on unrealistically brief patient interactions. Objective structured clinical examination cases can be more flexible to include pre- and post-encounter activities, which is critical to ensuring broad application of social medicine practice.

The impact of the COVID-19 pandemic on the healthcare workforce was so extreme that not only were standardized exam processes modified but also state physician licensing boards across the country relaxed their requirements. Medical students were allowed to participate in healthcare activities normally not allowed until they received their licenses [28]. Medical schools revised graduation requirements by temporarily truncating clerkship experiences and eliminating one or more required electives to allow students more flexibility in their educational timeline. Many medical schools, including the CUNY School of Medicine, graduated students 2 months early so that they could contribute to caring for COVID-19 patients during the crisis. There are numerous examples of how these newly graduated physicians became frontline caregivers in NYC and across the country [34, 35].

In the meantime, the deadline to apply to residency programs and the resulting match were delayed with the intention of giving students extra time, if needed, to complete clerkships and electives that would support their applications and to secure important letters of recommendation. As with the rest of medical education, residency interviews across the country were held in the virtual environment. For some students, this allowed them to apply to more programs, because the time and cost of travel was eliminated. However, there was concern that this advantage was not equally experienced across student groups [36]. Data so far have demonstrated that the 2021 residency match results were similar to previous years, but further explorations of outcomes are clearly warranted [37].

> The NBME relies on commercial test centers to deliver licensing exams. The closure of these test centers put an enormous level of stress on individual students.

Wellness Needs

The COVID-19 pandemic created upheaval in lifestyle, work, personal interactions, and worldview for many people. For medical students, it had the added impact of abruptly changing how they saw their future as agents of change in a healthcare system that seemed so inadequately prepared to meet its responsibilities to patients and communities. When training was suspended, medical students struggled to find ways to help their mentors manage the crisis in the clinical sites that were formerly their educational homes. They watched their mentors suffer substantial loss and face illness and uncertainty, while they also suffered similar tragedies. Structural racism in the healthcare system and throughout the community was magnified by COVID-19 through increasing disparities in health outcomes, access to care, ability to quarantine, and extreme financial hardships, all of which forced medical students to find ways to address these challenges even before completing their education.

Medical schools, including the CUNY School of Medicine, responded by adjusting curricular schedules to be mindful of the needs of medical students to care for their families during the crisis, spend more time investing in self-care activities, and find ways to volunteer in their communities. Attendance and on-camera participation were modified to allow students a degree of flexibility. Medical school faculty worked with student groups to facilitate volunteer activities that gave students learning opportunities, as well as opportunities to engage with the healthcare workforce that behaved so heroically during the crisis [38].

At the CUNY School of Medicine, new wellness activities and virtual check-in meetings were also adopted for the entire community; virtual mindfulness and yoga classes were offered, and virtual social events were held to keep the school community connected including movie nights and community dialogues to reaffirm the values as leaders of healthcare change. An annual event, "Lives of Courage," [39] was initiated to promote conversations with healthcare leaders who have advocated for social justice and health equity and provided inspiration for the meaningful impact that physicians can have in their communities. Weekly emails were also sent that informed the CUNY School of Medicine community about virtual wellness events throughout the City College of New York and NYC. Virtual, and when possible physical, vision boards were established so that students could share feelings, thoughts, and strategies to successfully manage stress. These wellness activities were essentially community building strategies that also served to remind students of why they chose to pursue a career in medicine and population health and help them to envision hopeful roles for their future as healthcare leaders and agents of change.

> The pandemic created opportunities for schools like CUNY School of Medicine to develop new programs around wellness that will continue into the future.

Research and Community Service Activities

While medical education activities during the pandemic allowed students to learn, practice skills, and contribute to the healthcare crisis, medical students across the country searched for ways to contribute outside of their required educational experiences. Numerous papers have been published by medical student teams reporting on student volunteer activities at call centers, PPE donation drives, food drives, and many other venues [40]. In fact, the publication of these activities itself is a productive use of medical student time and service to the healthcare system, as it encourages others to engage in similar, positive activities [41, 42]. The research and community service activities that allowed students to contribute to the healthcare system as volunteers are described below.

New Research Synthesis

One particularly useful activity that allowed medical students to assist clinical teams safely was identification and synthesization of research publications regarding COVID-19. During the pandemic, the medical research community responded rapidly by producing a surge of COVID-19-related peer-reviewed publications. The number of manuscripts submitted increased at least twofold, and the time to publication after submission of a manuscript decreased by about 50% [43, 44]. Further, preprints, which are not peer-reviewed and often do not have rigorous oversight in terms of scientific rigor and accuracy, have received increased attention as the number skyrocketed during the pandemic. Distinguishing preprint and peer-reviewed materials was often challenging, as was filtering published opinion pieces from evidence-based reports. These trends made it difficult for clinicians to practice evidence-based medicine during the pandemic; there simply was not enough time to care for the overload of patients as well as to monitor the growing and evolving literature. Thus, medical students across the country helped to keep busy clinicians informed [45, 46].

At the CUNY School of Medicine, undergraduate and medical students worked together to develop a database of COVID-19-related publications and update it on a weekly basis, and they also provided an annotated bibliography that SBH Health System physicians could use as an up-to-date resource. Each week, the CUNY School of Medicine librarian identified new peer-reviewed articles based on data-based research from PubMed, MEDLINE, and SCOPUS. A team of students, who had taken at least one semester of epidemiology and biostatistics, read these articles, indexed them into broad categories, and briefly synthesized the findings into a weekly COVID-19 new literature summary. Advanced students, and, at times, faculty mentors, helped newer students understand more sophisticated research methodologies that they had not yet explored in coursework or research experiences, allowing students to gain new skills while participating in this activity.

Harvard Medical School took this project a step further by developing a COVID-19 educational curriculum by medical students for medical students. This project was similar to the service-learning course adopted by the CUNY School of Medicine to use a training opportunity both to provide students with community service and to solidify skills and knowledge but drew from the evolving COVID-19 research to develop an internationally renowned resource [18]. So far, this eight-module curriculum has been translated into 27 different languages and has been accessed by people from more than 100 countries across the globe.

These volunteer projects present considerations for medical school curricula going forward. Perhaps training in evidence-based medicine should take on a more action-oriented approach, helping both medical students and their teaching faculty keep on top of the most recent medical literature, locate changes in publication trends in specific fields that might impact on practice patterns, and prepare training materials for the next cohort of students.

COVID-19 Patient Chart Reviews

When the number of hospitalized patients began to decrease, students were able to assist with other research activities as well. For example, at SBH Health System, physicians partnered with CUNY School of Medicine faculty to develop a database to explore clinical, social, behavioral, and economic risk factors and outcomes of the first wave of COVID-19 patients in the Bronx, the initial epicenter of cases in NYC. Using secure Internet connections, students were trained to conduct electronic health record reviews from home. This database will be de-identified and shared with SBH Health System/CUNY School of Medicine faculty for research with medical residents and students.

In fact, medical students across the country were able to contribute to understanding the COVID-19 pandemic through exploration of the growing databases of electronic health records from COVID-19 patients [47]. In some cases, medical students were able to conduct prospective analyses by following patients after discharge and interviewing them and their families on the phone. Without medical student input, many of these clinical epidemiological studies could not have taken place. In the United Kingdom, medical students were called upon to substitute for physician investigators who were pulled off clinical research onto emergency clinical service [48]. These opportunities not only provided useful activities for clinician-researchers in training but also helped medical students gain appreciation for the role of data and research in medicine.

Community Service

Medical students also engaged in community-based service in response to COVID-19 pandemic needs. Numerous publications have already summarized in more detail the broad array of extracurricular activities that medical students engaged in during the pandemic shutdown, which allowed them to make contributions to the healthcare system as their faculty planned educational transitions [17]. These activities ranged from telemedicine assistance (see descriptions related to clinical training) to food shopping for busy physicians who needed help caring for family members while caring for COVID-19 patients. It is important to note that these volunteer activities are wide-ranging and reflect the variation in the type of activities that medical students were comfortable engaging in during the pandemic [49]. While policy makers, educators, and some medical students themselves carefully defined learners as nonessential clinic personnel who deserved protected status, some students expressed a desire to be seen as adult learners, capable of self-direction and independent decision-making [26, 50]. Volunteer activities provided opportunities for those students to interact with communities in the ways that were comfortable to them.

Three areas that are particularly important to review and consider applying in ongoing medical education are contact tracing, patient navigation in testing sites [51], and recruitment to vaccination sites [52]. All three activities are necessary public health activities that require patient contact. The shortage of resources and trained personnel for these activities across the country provided opportunities for medical and public health trainees to step in once they could do so safely. Now medical educators are beginning to consider how to make scaling up medical student volunteers in these and other public health emergency activities more efficient. Perhaps a stronger focus on public health activities and community health and social medicine perspectives within the medical curriculum would facilitate this [53].

> COVID-19 and health disparities inspired students around the country to engage in research and community service. The long-term impact of this research and this service may help the country in its mission to improve nation-wide health equity.

Conclusions: Long-Term Impact and Reflections

In the previous sections, the impact of the COVID-19 pandemic on medical school education was broadly described through the lens of the community of educators at the CUNY School of Medicine an urban, public medical school dedicated to its unique social mission. Four areas that are likely to be lasting are highlighted below.

First, medical schools across the country successfully transitioned their curricula to online formats at each educational stage, including undergraduate information exchanges, problem-based case discussions, laboratory and anatomy classwork, standardized patient interactions, and clinical simulations. Even training involving patients took place at least partially in the virtual environment. It is expected that the use of new technologies to facilitate online and digital medical education will expand, hopefully resulting in more flexibility in medical education that can broaden its content and expand educational sites geographically [14, 54]. In the meantime, to ensure the healthcare and medical education systems are not vulnerable to similar crises in the future, medical schools are more likely than ever to adopt a hybrid environment, blending traditional teaching methods with these newly developing technologies, and lean heavily on small group education, more easily accommodated by online education. At the CUNY School of Medicine, benefit was found from the ongoing use of large group sessions, perhaps not for lectures but for community building. Nevertheless, like other medical schools, the socialization component of education may be the most important use of in person group sessions in the future.

Second, medical schools like the CUNY School of Medicine, whose clinical campus is geographically separate from the medical school, have seen benefits from developing a virtual community of educators and administrators across sites. Many academic medical center organizations held weekly or biweekly virtual meetings during the pandemic to share resources and to brainstorm solutions to common problems [55]. This use of the virtual environment has, in many ways, improved collaborative teaching and research across clinical and other community-based sites.

Third, student evaluation of medical school curriculum is critical across medical schools and by the accrediting body, the Liaison Committee on Medical Education. During the beginning of the COVID-19 pandemic, the students at the CUNY School of Medicine struggled tremendously, and school administrators and faculty sought mechanisms to provide forums for discussion and support. Because the classes are relatively small, class-wide meetings could be held in the virtual platforms, in which students felt safe to report on which of the educational changes were working and which were still lacking. This forum for real-time student feedback and immediate faculty responses was found to be helpful for the community to build trust during the most challenging of times, and we intend to maintain these interactions in the same format going forward.

Finally, and most importantly, to make useful contributions during the COVID-19 crisis, medical students across the country relied on skills and training that fell outside of the bioscience curriculum [17, 55]. Students found ways to fill in gaps in the healthcare system by providing for the emotional and social needs of patients and their families. They drew from education and experiences in medical activism and community health needs assessments that developed from their understanding of the social determinants of health and healthcare needs. The students of the CUNY School of Medicine benefitted from its unique educational mission and partnership with SBH Health System as they faced the COVID-19 pandemic. At the same time, the lessons learned from watching this extraordinary cohort will help medical educators ensure the healthcare system will be better prepared for the next pandemic.

References

1. City College of New York. CSOM. https://www.ccny.cuny.edu/csom. Accessed 23 July 2021.
2. Reber S, Sinclair C. Opportunity engines: middle-class mobility in higher education. Brookings Report. May 2020. https://vtechworks.lib.vt.edu/bitstream/handle/10919/98982/OpportunityEnginesFinal.pdf?sequence=1&isAllowed=y. Accessed 28 June 2021.
3. Roman SA Jr, McGanney ML. The Sophie Davis School of Biomedical Education: the first 20 years of a unique BS-MD program. Acad Med. 1994;69(3):224–30.
4. Roman SA Jr. Addressing the urban pipeline challenge for the physician workforce: the Sophie Davis model. Acad Med. 2004;79(12):1175–83.
5. Geiger HJ. Sophie Davis School of Biomedical Education at City College of New York prepares primary care physicians for practice in underserved inner-city areas. Public Health Rep. 1980;96(1):32–7.
6. Rose S. Medical student education in the time of COVID-19. JAMA. 2020;323(21):2131–2.
7. Byrnes YM, Civantos AM, Go BC, McWilliams TL, Rajasekaran K. Effect of the COVID-19 pandemic on medical student career perceptions: a national survey study. Med Educ Online. 2020;25(1):1798088.
8. Association of American Medical Colleges. 2020, March 17. Important guidance for medical students on clinical rotations during the coronavirus (COVID-19) outbreak. https://www.aamc.org/news-insights/press-releases/important-guidance-medical-students-clinical-rotations-during-coronavirus-COVID-19-outbreak. Retrieved 13 July 2021.
9. ZOOM. Zoom for education. https://explore.zoom.us/education?_ga=2.262429004.179602944.1626201355-1196185239.1610734526. Accessed 13 July 2021.
10. Bernard RR, McNeil SG, Cook DA, Agarwal KL, Singhal GR. Preparing for the changing role of instructional technologies in medical education. Acad Med. 2011;86(4):435–9.
11. Wood DF. Problem based learning. BMJ. 2003;326:328–30.
12. O'Donoghue O, Kasselman L, Ayala G, Shelov SP, Ragolia L. Best practices learned from online problem-based learning help prepare students for global health care challenges of the future. BMC Med Educ. https://doi.org/10.21203/rs.3.rs-518716/v1.
13. American Medical Association. 2020, November 4. COVID-19 resources for medical educators. https://www.ama-assn.org/delivering-care/public-health/COVID-19-resources-medical-educators. Accessed 13 July 2021.
14. Mukhopadhyay S, Booth AL, Calkins SM, Doxtader EE, Fine SW, Gardner JM, et al. Leveraging technology for remote learning in the era of COVID-19 and social distancing. Arch Pathol Lab Med. 2020;144(9):1027–36.

15. Ferrel MN, Ryan JJ. The impact of COVID-19 on medical education. Cureus. 2020;12(3):e7492. https://doi.org/10.7759/cureus.7492.
16. Gonzalo J, Dekhtyar M, Hawkins RE, Wolpaw DR. How can medical students add value? Identifying roles, barriers, and strategies to advance the value of undergraduate medical education to patient care and the health system. Acad Med. 2017;92(9):1294–301.
17. Long N, Wolpaw DR, Boothe D, Caldwell C, Dillon P, Gottshall L, et al. Contributions of health professions students to health system needs during the COVID-19 pandemic: potential strategies and process for U.S. medical schools. Acad Med. 2020;95(11):1679–86.
18. Soled D, Goel S, Barry D, Erfani P, Joseph N, Kochis M, et al. Medical student mobilization during a crisis: lessons from a COVID-19 medical student response team. Acad Med. 2020;95(9):1384–7.
19. Iancu AM, Kemp MT, Alam HB. Unmuting medical students' education: utilizing telemedicine during the COVID-19 pandemic and beyond. J Med Internet Res. 2020;22(7):e19667.
20. Rolak S, Keefe AM, Davidson EL, Aryal P, Parajuli S. Impacts and challenges of United States medical students during the COVID-19 pandemic. World J Clin Cases. 2020;8(15):3136–41.
21. Sukumar S, Zakaria A, Lai CJ, Sakumoto M, Khanna R, Choi N. Designing and implementing a novel virtual rounds curriculum for medical students' internal medicine clerkship during the COVID-19 pandemic. MedEdPORTAL. 2021;17:11106. https://doi.org/10.15766/mep_2374-8265.11106.
22. Calhoun KE, Yale LA, Whipple ME, Allen SM, Wood DE, Tatum RP. The impact of COVID-19 on medical student surgical education: implementing extreme pandemic response measures in a widely distributed surgical clerkship experience. Am J Surg. 2020;220(1):44–7.
23. Waseh S, Dicker A. Telemedicine and undergraduate medical education: lessons in capacity building. JMIR Med Educ. 2018;5(1):e12515. https://doi.org/10.2196/12515.
24. Wijesooriya NR, Mishra V, Brand PLP, Rubin BK. COVID-19 and telehealth, education, and research adaptations. Paediatr Respir Rev. 2020;35:38–42.
25. Association of American Medical Colleges. 2021, April 14. Medical student away rotations for remainder of 2020–21 and 2021–22 academic year. https://www.aamc.org/what-we-do/mission-areas/medical-education/away-rotations-interviews-2020-21-residency-cycle. Accessed 13 July 2021.
26. Papapanou M, Routsi E, Tsamakis K, Fotis L, Marinos G, Lidoriki I, et al. Medical education challenges and innovations during COVID-19 pandemic. Postgr Med J. Published Online First: 29 March 2021. https://doi.org/10.1136/postgradmedj-2021-140032.
27. Griffith M, DeMasi SC, McGrath AJ, Love JN, Moll J, Santen A. Time to reevaluate the away rotation: improving return on investment for students and schools. Acad Med. 2019;94(4):496–500.
28. Fuller R, Joynes V, Cooper J, Boursicot K, Roberts T. Could COVID-19 be our 'there is no alternative' (TINA) opportunity to enhance assessment? Med Teach. 2020;42(7):781–6.
29. Borsheim B, Ledford C, Zitelny E, Zhao C, Blizzard J, Hu Y. Preparation for the United States medical licensing Examinations in the Face of COVID-19. Med Sci Educ. 2020;16:1–6. https://doi.org/10.1007/s40670-020-01011-1.
30. Association of American Medical Colleges. Number of Medical Schools Requiring Final SP/OSCE Examination. https://www.aamc.org/data-reports/curriculum-reports/interactive-data/sp/osce-final-examinations-us-medical-schools. Accessed 12 May 2021.
31. Barzansky B, Etzel SI. Educational programs in US medical schools, 2003-2004. JAMA. 2004;292(9):1025–31. https://doi.org/10.1001/jama.292.9.1025.
32. Gilliland WR, La Rochelle J, Hawkins R, Dillon GF, Mechaber AJ, Dyrbye L, et al. Changes in clinical skills education resulting from the introduction of the USMLE step 2 clinical skills (CS) examination. Med Teach. 2008;30(3):325–7. https://doi.org/10.1080/01421590801953026.
33. Baker TK. The end of step 2 CS should be the beginning of a new approach to clinical skills assessment. Acad Med. 2021; Volume Publish Ahead of Print-Issue. https://doi.org/10.1097/ACM.0000000000004187.

34. Miller DG, Pierson L, Doernberg S. The role of medical students during the COVID-19 pandemic. Ann Intern Med. 2020;173:145–6. https://doi.org/10.7326/M20-1281.
35. Pravder HD, Langdon-Embry L, Hernandez RJ, Berbari N, et al. Experiences of early graduate medical students working in New York hospitals during the COVID-19 pandemic: a mixed methods study. BMC Med Educ 2021;21:118. https://doi.org/10.1186/s12909-021-02543-9.
36. Hammoud MM, Standiford T, Carmody JB. Potential implications of COVID-19 for the 2020-2021 residency application cycle. JAMA. 2020;324(1):29–30. https://doi.org/10.1001/jama.2020.8911.
37. American Medical Association. 2021, March 23. 2021 match hits record highs despite pandemic's disruptions. https://www.ama-assn.org/residents-students/match/2021-match-hits-record-highs-despite-pandemic-s-disruptions. Accessed 13 July 2021.
38. Hueston WJ, Petty EM. The impact of the COVID-19 pandemic on medical student education in Wisconsin. WMJ. 2020;119(2):80–2.
39. City College of New York. CUNY Med Hosts Lives of Courage: doctors who are changing the world. https://www.ccny.cuny.edu/csom/dr-kamini-doobay-discusses-healthcare-and-social-justice. Accessed 23 July 2021.
40. Baecher-Lind L, Fleming AC, Bhargava R, Cox SM, Everett EN, Graziano SC, et al. Medical education and safety as co-priorities in the coronavirus disease 2019 (COVID-19) era: we can do both. Obstet Gynecol. 2020;136(4):830–4.
41. Coffey CS, MacDonald BV, Shahrvini B, Baxter SL, Lander L. Student perspectives on remote medical education in clinical core clerkships during the COVID-19 pandemic. Med Sci Educ. 2020;14:1–8. https://doi.org/10.1007/s40670-020-01114.
42. Theoret C, Ming X. Our education, our concerns: the impact on medical student education of COVID-19. Med Educ. 2020;54(7):591–2.
43. Else H. COVID-19 in papers: a torrent of science. Nature. 2020;588:553.
44. Park JJH, Mogg R, Smith GE, Nakimuli-Mpungu E, Jehan F, Rayner CR, et al. How COVID-19 has fundamentally changed clinical research in global health. Lancet Global Health. 2021;9:e711–20.
45. Boscamp JR, Duffy CP, Barsky C, Stanton BF. Medical students on the virtual front line: a literature review elective to provide COVID-19 clinical teams with essential information. Acad Med. 2021;96(7):1002–4. https://doi.org/10.1097/ACM.0000000000004070.
46. Boodman C, Lee S, Bullard J. Idle medical students review emerging COVID-19 research. Med Educ Online. 2020;25:1770562.
47. Alshak M, Li HA, Wehmeyer GT. Medical students as essential frontline researchers during the COVID-19 pandemic. Acad Med. 2021;96(7):964–6.
48. Rainbow S, Dorji T. Impact of COVID-19 on medical students in the United Kingdom. Germs. 2020;10(3):240–3. https://doi.org/10.18683/germs.2020.1210.
49. Harries AJ, Lee C, Jones L, Rodriguez RM, Davis JA, Boyson-Osborn M, et al. Effects of the COVID-19 pandemic on medical students: a multicenter quantitative study. BMC Med Educ 2021;21:14. https://doi.org/10.1186/s12909-020-02462-1.
50. Menon A, Klein EJ, Kollars K, Kleinhenz ALW. Medical students are not essential workers: examining institutional responsibility during the COVID-19 pandemic. Acad Med. 2020;95(8):1149–51.
51. Koetter P, Pelton M, Gonzalo J, Du P, Exten C, Bogale K, et al. Implementation and process of a COVID-19 contact tracing initiative: leveraging health professional students to extend the workforce during a pandemic. Am J Infect Control. 2020;48(12):1451–6. https://doi.org/10.1016/j.ajic.2020.08.012.
52. Albert Einstein College of Medicine. Einstein Students Join COVID-19 Vaccination Effort. https://einsteinmed.org/features/2509/einstein-students-join-COVID-19-19-vaccination-effort/. Accessed July 13 2021.

53. Association of American Medical Colleges. 2020, July 21. Back to Clinic and Back to Campus-July 2020 Conversations. https://www.aamc.org/what-we-do/mission-areas/medical-education/back-clinic-and-back-campus-july-2020-conversations. Accessed July 13 2021.
54. Spielman AI, Sunavala-Dossabhoy G. Pandemics and education: a historical review. J Dent Educ. 2021;85(6):741–6.
55. Sklar DP. COVID-19: lessons from the disaster that can improve health professions education. Acad Med. 2020;95(11):1631–3.

Chapter 17
Dynamic Decision-Making and Effective Communications

Ridwan Shabsigh, Eric C. Appelbaum, and Robert D. Karpinos

The Lead Up to the Crisis at SBH Health System

The Ebola outbreak in 2014 created extreme conditions that resulted in high-level action plans, rapid mandatory education, drills for donning and doffing enhanced personal protective equipment (PPE), creation of new isolation rooms, and additional precautions for suspected cases including decontamination tents. Although the Ebola virus carried a very high mortality rate [1], there were thankfully very few mortalities associated with this virus in the United States.

When news of COVID-19 first broke in the United States, many believed that this was just another "exercise" where the medical community would be called upon to develop action plans, identify resources, and prepare for the worst; no one anticipated the degree of devastation that COVID-19 would bring. After all, SARS and MERS were also coronaviruses, and they were easily contained with minimal impact in the United States.

R. Shabsigh (✉)
Department of Surgery, SBH Health System, Bronx, NY, USA

Department of Urology, Weill Cornell Medical College of Cornell University, New York, NY, USA

CUNY School of Medicine, New York, NY, USA
e-mail: rshabsigh@sbhny.org

E. C. Appelbaum
SBH Health System, Bronx, NY, USA

R. D. Karpinos
Perioperative Services and Department of Anesthesiology, SBH Health System, Bronx, NY, USA

CUNY School of Medicine, New York, NY, USA

© The Author(s), under exclusive license to Springer Nature Switzerland AG 2022
R. Shabsigh (ed.), *Health Crisis Management in Acute Care Hospitals*, https://doi.org/10.1007/978-3-030-95806-0_17

In early 2020, the COVID-19 crisis became very "real" in New York City (NYC) and its five boroughs. Within days of the first reported case, hospitals and healthcare systems, both large and small, became overwhelmed. NYC and the Bronx were among the early epicenters and the hardest hit with what several months later would become known simply as the "surge."

SBH Health System is a small, freestanding community hospital system that serves as a safety net for an underserved population that is largely dependent on government programs. Despite financial challenges, the system remains mission driven with a culture of clinical collaboration and service to the community. All the chairs and chiefs provide direct patient care, and many clinical leaders provide additional administrative service. When the initial impact of COVID-19 was recognized, the senior leadership at SBH huddled with administrative and clinical leaders and began planning what would soon be the largest imaginable expansion of clinical services.

Strategic Decisions Made Early on in the Pandemic

Being a small center had many advantages for SBH; a flat hierarchy and a culture of collaboration meant that information pathways were well-defined and the dissemination of information was clear and flowed freely. Direction came at regular intervals and was easy to anticipate. Consensus was reached rapidly, and whatever silos that had existed previously were swept away. The systems and approach to crisis management employed by SBH are easily applicable to any system, large or small.

Once it became evident that the COVID-19 pandemic was spreading to the NYC area, the hospital leadership made several strategic decisions that later proved to be significant in determining the successful outcome of the hospital's functioning during the surge of the pandemic. Table 17.1 illustrates a list of these strategic decisions, their implementation, and impact. The strategic decisions that were made for health crisis management at the acute care hospital, SBH Health System, included the following: centralizing the overall management of the response to the crisis, striking a healthy balance of macro- and micromanagement, recognizing that critical care is the pillar of the clinical response, planning for utmost efficiency to address limitations and shortages of human and material resources, and constantly learning and improving. Within these, SBH prioritized the two top goals of serving large numbers of severely ill patients and protecting the healthcare workers.

Readiness in a Crisis

The real test for a hospital's ability to tackle a healthcare crisis is in the time of crisis itself. While training, drills, and simulations are highly valuable for the preparation of hospital systems, nothing replaces an actual crisis in testing the ability of a hospital. Under normal circumstances, most hospital systems will be functioning adequately. It takes years of focused continuous effort to develop the "readiness" to tackle such crises. To be prepared for a health crisis requires a comprehensive effort from all departments and ranks throughout the healthcare system to adapt facilities,

Table 17.1 Strategic decisions, implementation, and impact

Decision	Implementation	Impact
Serving rapidly increasing numbers of patients with high severity of illness	Setting up a crisis response team Establishing an emergency operations plan Establishing a crisis surge plan	Effective expansion of hospital bed capacity by >50% in a short time with the ultimate ability to serve unprecedented large numbers of patients with long hospitalization
Protecting the healthcare workers	Setting up virtual infrastructure for communications, meetings, and tele-ICU Provision of PPEs ahead of CDC and governmental agency requirements	Maintenance of services Relatively low number of infected healthcare workers
Centralizing the management of the response to the crisis	Setting up command center Creation of data dashboards Establishing communications processes	The ability to manage the big picture of the crisis internally and externally Executing an organized recovery after the crisis surge
Striking a healthy balance between macro- and micromanagement	Empowering clinical leaders Involvement of the frontline workers	Dynamic decision-making Creative solutions Flexible response High morale
Recognizing that critical care will be the pillar of clinical response to an infectious (viral) crisis	Unifying critical care under one leadership and structure Hospital-wide critical care committee responsible for all critical care affairs	Effective expansion of critical care and ICU by >500% caring for unprecedented large numbers of ventilated patients with multi-organ failure
Recognizing the need for high efficiency because of limitations and shortages of human and material resources	Daily float pool Cross-training Conservation Utilization guidelines Team to coordinate transfers	Meeting the majority of the huge demands of the crisis surge Avoiding ending up as an "overwhelmed hospital"
Seeing the challenge of the crisis as an opportunity to learn and improve	Collecting "lessons learned" from the entire hospital with openness and transparency	Implementation of multiple major improvement projects after the crisis, transforming the hospital to a vastly improved crisis-ready state

Top goals for a hospital in a health crisis
In a highly infectious health crisis, a hospital system should prioritize:
   1. Serving the rapidly increasing numbers of patients with high severity illness
   2. Protecting its own healthcare workforce

equipment, skills, systems supply chains, management processes, finances, and the overall culture of the hospital. Each of these entities requires a specific process, which can be focused into accessible checklists to ensure its readiness and implementation of plans when a crisis unfolds (Table 17.2). Periodic review and reflective

Table 17.2 An example checklist to ensure the hospital's readiness in the face of a crisis

Entity	Ready	Not ready
Physical facilities	Ability to expand overall patient capacity by ≥50% and sustain expansion for at least 3–6 months	Limited or no ability to expand and/or sustain expansion
Clinical staff	Ability to staff and sustain expansion of overall capacity and critical care capacity	Limited or no ability to staff and/or sustain expansion
Clinical departments	Well-organized clinical departments with strong leadership	Disorganized departments with ineffective leadership
Critical care	Ability to expand critical care capacity by ≥200% with all that is needed, physicians, nurses, therapists, ventilators, dialysis, equipment, supplies, medications, and other necessities	Limited or no ability to expand and/or sustain expansion and/or long stay
Emergency medicine	High-reliability emergency department	Weakness in triage, initial diagnosis and treatment, and multitasking
Infection control department	Active structure for prevention/reduction of hospital-acquired infections Ability to protect all staff, especially clinical staff, and all frontline staff	Weaknesses in infection prevention and employee health
Informatics	Ability to provide information technology solutions for expanded operations Ability to provide timely and accurate technological support for dynamic decision-making	Poor ability to produce actionable real-time data
Engineering	Creative solutions for unexpected problems Flexibility and agility in improvisations	Weakness in the management of outsourced vendors and consultants
Supply chain	Realistic practical contingency plans for expanded needs for equipment and supplies	No contingency plans or contingency plans that are merely theoretical
Other supportive departments	Ability to support and sustain expansion of frontline services	Limited or no ability to support and/or sustain expansion
Finance	Efficiency and wise spending Ability to apply for crisis aid	Unfocused spending
Senior management	Effective goal-setting vision-inspiring servant leadership with transparency and fairness	Unclear vision Secretive Favoritism
Values and culture	Unified genuine focus on "patient first" and strong culture of collaboration	Disparate values Working in silos Tribalism

practice at all levels, using this or similar tables as a guide, may help with the assessment of preparedness, gap analysis, and setting improvement tasks and timelines prior to and during crisis. An empowered multidisciplinary committee for crisis preparation is a great forum to coordinate such activities.

While all hospitals are required to have a so-called "disaster plan," some may treat this, especially under normal circumstances, as a tick-box exercise. One of the big lessons learned from the COVID-19 crisis is that *the surge can happen quickly and escalate rapidly with little warning,* catching hospitals unprepared. It only took a period of 3 weeks from the beginning of the pandemic for it to reach its peak. Such a short period leaves little time for preparation, especially if there is no plan in place for crisis management. Another lesson learned from the COVID-19 surge is that *warnings and predictions by governmental health agencies and other entities may not be accurate.* In NYC, the peak of the surge occurred in actuality 3–4 weeks earlier, with more severity than many predictive modeling announcements and warnings suggested.

Dynamic Decision-Making During a Crisis

Dynamic decision-making is a decision-making process in an evolving environment, either due to external factors or as a function of choices made previously that can affect the environment [2]. Decision-making has to be quick, timely, and flexible to allow for agile adjustments in response to conditions that are also fluid and changing frequently – such as the pandemic – and the decision-makers need to be aware that they may not be able to control all the factors influencing the situation. Establishment of a clear mechanism (Fig. 17.1) and a reliable structure for dynamic

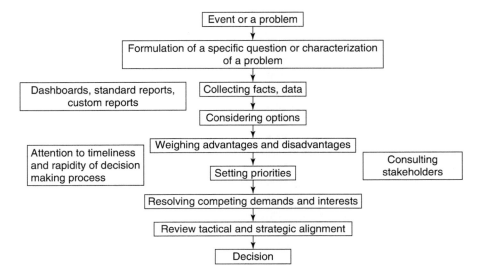

Fig. 17.1 The dynamic decision-making mechanism

Table 17.3 The main features of the dynamic decision-making process

Feature	Requirements	Focus	Benefits	Risks
Multiple simultaneous or closely timed decisions	Comprehensive large amounts of data about multiple parts of the situation Multiple stakeholders	Top goals Changing priorities	Ability to address a multifactorial crisis	Missing important factors Unawareness of overwhelmed decision-making capacity
Dynamic decisions are frequently interrelated and interdependent	Continuous process of understanding the positives and negatives of every decision	Clear principles and mechanism of resolving competing decision demands Complete representation of the different stakeholders	Incremental steady successes toward reaching the top goals	Miscalculating priorities
Rapid, timely, almost real-time	Availability of data and stakeholders all the time with uninterrupted communications	Updated data Access to stakeholders, team leaders, and experts Effective communications	Appropriately timed rapid responses to a rapidly changing situation	Small or no opportunity or time to analyze the results of past decisions and draw lessons for improvement

decision-making is vital in the preparation of a hospital system for navigating a health crisis. There also needs to be widespread awareness of already established mechanisms and transparency in the decision-making process. The structure needs to be in place prior to the crisis, and periodic training, drills, and simulations should be undertaken to ensure preparedness for all involved, when facing a crisis.

There are three main features to dynamic decision-making (Table 17.3). Firstly, dynamic decision-making frequently involves making multiple simultaneous or closely timed decisions. This requires that an infrastructure be in place so that all relevant up-to-date data from multiple sources can reach the decision-makers. In addition, decision-makers need to have regular access to the multiple stakeholders that may be affected by the decisions and the various situations and problems for which decisions need to be made. Stakeholders may be internal and/or external to the hospital and can include the various clinical department directors, nonclinical leaders, and regulatory bodies as well as financial stakeholders. While the focus should remain on the strategic priorities, which in the case of an infectious pandemic would be to "serve large numbers of severely ill patients and protect the healthcare workers," dynamic decision-makers must keep in mind that the tactical priorities may change. A risk of dynamic decision-making, especially in a very intense crisis, is exceeding the decision-making capacity and overwhelming the decision-makers. Keeping updated checklists and decision dashboards will help mitigate such risks. Only if a hospital health system establishes a comprehensive process for dynamic decision-making will it be able to successfully tackle the multifaceted challenges of a health crisis. However, there remains a real risk that important factors may be overlooked.

Secondly, dynamic decisions are frequently interrelated and interdependent, and therefore, continually understanding and weighing up the advantages and disadvantages of decisions is necessary. Checklists and self-discipline may help decision-makers to consistently question the pros and cons of their choices and decisions. Competing demands and interests, no matter how well negotiated, will always leave some level of conflict in their wake. Clarity of the priorities must be maintained, in addition to a "sold fair" mechanism of resolving competing demands and interests. However, the risk of miscalculating priorities exists. This risk can be mitigated by assuring complete representation of all stakeholders and parties of interest and reassuring them that their voices and interests will be heard. Another risk mitigator is inherent in decision-makers' openness to quickly recognize and correct any wrong decisions.

Finally, dynamic decision-making must be rapid and timely, almost in real time [3]. To enable this, the decision-makers need to be equipped with up-to-date data, as well as open lines of communications with the stakeholders and relevant experts. However, the need for quick decisions brings with it the risk that there may be little or no opportunity to analyze the consequences of past decisions and draw lessons from them. To minimize this risk, an archive of accurate summary documentation, such as meeting minutes and decision communications, should be maintained, with a member of the decision-making team given responsibility of detailed documenting and in essence becoming the "historian" for the crisis.

The rapid nature of decision-making may result in some of the more common principles to be overlooked. For instance, the principle of "do no harm," which is the bedrock of healthcare, should always remain the primary focus of the decision-making team. Other such principles, such as "choose the least risky among multiple risky options" and "the enemy of the good is the perfect," could be very useful in ensuring that the decisions made are patient-centric and in everyone's best interest and are made in a timely fashion. While consumed in making decisions about issues small and big, especially during a healthcare crisis, it is vital that decision-makers ensure the alignment of their tactical and strategic decisions (Box 17.1).

Macromanagement Versus Micromanagement: Where Is the Balance?

To introspect on the managerial effectiveness for an organization or a hospital is healthy and requires careful review, especially under normal circumstances, to be in a good stead during times of crisis. At the organizational level, most hospitals tend to be macromanaged or prefer a balanced managerial style [4, 5] (Table 17.4). However, management styles may vary at the department and/or team levels,

Table 17.4 Various management styles

	Focus	Requirements	Advantages/benefits	Disadvantages/risks
Macromanagement	Big picture and strategy	Overall knowledge of vision and goals and command of teams and resources	Promotion of ownership at multiple levels and ranks	Potential failure of complex, detail-intensive processes
Micromanagement	Details and tactics	Large, centralized management	Assurance of completion of tasks with high value in selected high-stake items	Suppression of creativity and initiative Keeping teams and leaders weak and indecisive
Balanced management	Focus on big picture and knowledge of details with alignment of strategy and tactics	Trust and empowerment of teams and leaders at all ranks High-reliability organization	High efficiency Strong morale	Failure at strategy and/or tactics if balance is not right

Table 17.5 Macro- and micromanagement choices in a healthcare crisis

What should be macromanaged	What should be micromanaged
Frontline clinical operations, such as admissions, rounding, triage, diagnostics, and therapies	Essential disposables in short supply, such as PPEs, virus testing kits, certain medications
Critical care and intensive care units	Essential tasks that have many internal and external hurdles, such as hospital-to-hospital transfers
Specialized structured functions, such as the laboratory, blood bank, and pharmacy	Existential high-stake problems, such as high liability events and lawsuits

depending on specific requirements, circumstances, and the individual leaders at those levels. Generally, leaders tend to shift toward micromanagement in high-stake situations, such as a health crisis [6]. Remarkably during a crisis, there is a substantial need for a more balanced approach to management, with the senior management remaining on the side of macromanagement [7].

During a crisis, the value of the tireless efforts over the years of setting up well-organized departments and teams, empowering leaders and healthcare workers at all ranks, upholding values and collaborative culture, and shaping up a high-reliability organization becomes clear. The senior management will be well advised to resist the temptation of micromanagement during a crisis, especially at its peak (Table 17.5) [8].

Table 17.6 Communication dos and don'ts, especially during a health crisis

Do	Don't
Frequent communications	Write long, difficult-to-read emails
Give honest clear messages	Argue back and forth by email or text
Relay good and bad news transparently	Send mixed or unclear messages
Spread empathy and positivity	
Be careful with "CC" and "reply to all"	

Effective Communication of the Decisions

Effective communication is extremely important in healthcare and in hospital systems, and inadequate communication is often the root cause for many problems. While essential under normal circumstances, effective communication becomes a survival necessity in a crisis and is vital to successfully navigate it. For communication to be effective in a crisis, it has to be clear, simple, frequent, and actionable. It has to be framed in a manner which is easily internalized by the intended audience and should prefer candor and transparency over "sugarcoating" facts (Table 17.6).

Furthermore, choosing an appropriate medium for communication assures higher efficiency and adoption. To overcome a crisis, such as COVID-19, communication also needs to occur at multiple levels between individuals, communities, organization, regulatory bodies, emergency services, and the government. A robust infrastructure and communication channels developed prior to the crisis are essential to ensure a quick and appropriate response to evolving challenges (Box 17.2) [9].

Box 17.1. Case Study 1: Illustrating Dynamic Decision-Making and the Value of Flexibility and Agility During a Crisis
The experience at SBH Health System during the COVID-19 pandemic in new York City serves as a good case study. The unprecedented nature of COVID-19 was one of the primary problems faced by hospitals all over the world. The course of disease remained unknown, and consequently, the workflow for patients had not been established. Knowing the course of a disease is very important for resource allocation and expansion planning. There were many examples of the unknown with the pandemic, such as severity upon arrival to the emergency department, percentage of patients requiring admission, percentage of admitted patients requiring critical care, percentage of patients requiring mechanical ventilation, percentage of patients requiring hemodialysis, length of hospitalization, mortality rate, and others. This situation required the hospital to be flexible and agile on the job and also to make decisions dynamically. The different scenarios for the disease course and the consequent patient workflow are illustrated in the figures

Below:

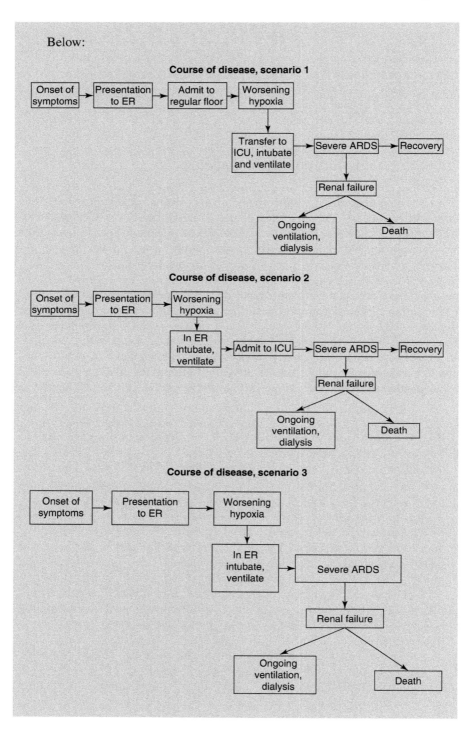

Box 17.1. (Cont.) Depending on the rapidly changing scenarios, the clinical leaders in collaboration with the command center made frequent timely decisions on disposition of patients and the subsequent workflows. There were flexibility and agility in the decision-making and practicality in its implementation. Decisions were adjusted and changed on a daily basis, and sometimes even more frequently, to meet the changing situations, such as the severity of the disease or requirement for critical care and recovery or mortality events.

Box 17.2. Case Study 2: Reorganizing Hospital Resources – Employing the "Fair Process" Model
The following is an illustrative case study of dynamic decision-making and effective communications during a health crisis. This was the case of the management of the operating rooms and the perioperative services during the COVID-19 crisis, giving examples of decision mechanisms, the processes involved, and communication channels used.

Shutting down the engine. The ports of entry to most acute inpatient healthcare facilities include the emergency department (ED), labor and delivery units, and the operating room (OR). During the pandemic the workflow, focus, and function of these portals needed to change. Although case volume for the labor and delivery unit is not something that can be adjusted internally, the need for new or different yet necessary safety policies may create unfamiliar operational stresses and strains. The ED, by its very nature, is susceptible to becoming overwhelmed rapidly in the face of massive increases in-patient inflow. The OR, often viewed as the revenue engine of the hospital, must remain available for emergency surgery, while truly elective procedures can be deferred. Postponing elective procedures can free up resources, such as space, supplies, and staff, that could be repurposed.

SBH Health System saw its first COVID-19 patient in march of 2020. Within days, a state of emergency had been declared by the governor of NY state. The predicted peak for new COVID-19 cases was just weeks away, and new executive orders were being released daily. As the general system prepared to accept the wave of patients, the perioperative leadership prepared to maintain essential services and divert any remaining resources to the front line. The chair of surgery, the chair of anesthesiology, and perioperative nursing leadership were quite comfortable collaborating on OR management, perioperative program development, and individual case management. As part of the initial response to the pandemic, the perioperative team was called upon to do the unthinkable – Develop a plan to effectively shut down the elective service line, leaving only emergency surgical services intact. Recognizing that this action could easily create confusion, mistrust, resistance, and resentment, the team focused on developing a plan.

The perioperative leaders recognized the advantages of a "fair process" model, which includes the three "E's": Explaining, engaging, and setting expectations for the reorganization.

"*Fair process* is a decision-making approach that addresses basic human need to be valued and respected. When people feel a decision affecting them was made fairly, they trust and cooperate. They share ideas and willingly go beyond the call of duty." [10]

To employ the fair process model, the perioperative leadership would call upon all the stakeholders from all of the service lines, to participate in the reorganization and provide perspective, integrate ideas, and implement the final plan. To initiate this process, it was necessary to meet face-to-face with the stakeholders to "explain" the need and reasons for the changes. Each surgical division (surgical specialty, such as general surgery, orthopedics, neurosurgery, etc.) chief was apprised of the rapidly approaching crisis and the need to allocate and reallocate physical space, material supplies, and human resources. This explanation included the source of the direction, defined the crisis team, identified the necessary roles and the prescribed flow of information, and acknowledged the anticipation of further potential governmental mandates.

The next essential element of fair process is "engagement" – And to create engagement, each stakeholder needs to be immersed in the process development and decision-making. Therefore, each stakeholder was asked to provide specific criteria and to set the definitions of emergency and nonemergency surgery, by recognizing the unique impact delaying surgery may have for their specific patients. Each stakeholder was also asked to identify potential areas for reallocation where their unique skill sets could be best utilized.

Finally, to set expectations – It is required that stakeholders are informed about how and when to expect information updates, compliance requirements, and the anticipated duration of the new processes. This allows for additional clarity and removes the opportunity for misunderstanding, misinterpretation, and manipulation. This was a bit more challenging as, at the time, it was unclear when the surge would pass or what the "new normal" would look like. Based on the available data, an expectation was set of a 6-week pause for elective surgical services. However, it was made very clear that this was based on current information and two alternative end point scenarios were discussed with each chief:

A. Should the crisis conditions abate early, elective services could resume sooner.
B. Should crisis conditions persist, an extension of the "pause in service" would be executed, as dictated by local and current conditions.

The fair process model was successful. Armed with good understanding, having participated in the plan development, and setting expectations, the surgical division chiefs were requested to engage the service lines as owners of the new process and to disseminate the information to their divisions.

To support the surgical division chiefs, face-to-face meetings were followed by a carefully constructed joint communication from the leaders of the perioperative service line to the entire service, announcing the details of the plan that had been collaboratively constructed. This initial communication was then followed by several video conferences, each projecting, clarifying, and bolstering the same message. Sending the same message multiple times in multiple formats through multiple avenues to all levels of the system made it clear and uniform, as well as easy to understand and rely upon in times of uncertainty. As with any process, irrespective of it being trivial or temporary, there have to be opportunities to raise issues candidly to alleviate fears and concerns. This was done in open forum meetings or via video conferencing or even by telephone conference. While individual concerns do need to be addressed and generous time should be made available to address individual needs and concerns, group meetings should be well choreographed to avoid diverting the process to individual concerns, which can be addressed more thoroughly off-line.

Conclusion

The ability of a hospital system to successfully overcome a crisis, such as the COVID-19 pandemic, requires a leadership who can dynamically make decisions and an infrastructure which ensures its rapid implementation. A balanced management style, characterized by a healthy mix of macro- and micromanagement, high efficiency, and a strong morale, is always useful but especially when managing a crisis. It is also essential that effective communication channels exist, allowing clear actionable messages to be communicated and responded to, quickly and appropriately. Finally, the key to success seems to be in the preparation that the organization should undertake to build systems and processes in absence of crises, which places it in a better position to overcome them.

References

1. Gulland A. Ebola mortality is highest among babies, finds study. BMJ. 2015;350:h1718.
2. Gonzalez C, Fakhari P, Busemeyer J. Dynamic decision-making: learning processes and new research directions. Hum Factors. 2017;59(5):713–21.
3. Brehmer B. Dynamic decision-making: human control of complex systems. Acta Psychol. 1992;81(3):211–41.
4. Nicholls J. Leadership in organisations: meta, macro and micro. Eur Manag J. 1988;6(1):16–25.

5. Liccione WJ. Balanced management: a key component of managerial effectiveness. Perform Improv. 2005;44(2):32–8.
6. Delgado O, Strauss EM, Ortega MA. Micromanagement: when to avoid it and how to use it effectively. Am J Health Syst Pharm. 2015;72(10):772–6.
7. Mitroff II. Crisis management: cutting through the confusion. Sloan Manag Rev. 1988;29(2):15.
8. Bundy J, Pfarrer MD, Short CE, Coombs WT. Crises and crisis management: integration, interpretation, and research development. J Manag. 2016;43(6):1661–92.
9. Reynolds B, Quinn CS. Effective communication during an influenza pandemic: the value of using a crisis and emergency risk communication framework. Health Promot Pract. 2008;9(4 Suppl):13S–7S.
10. Kim WC, Mauborgne R. Fair process: managing in the knowledge economy. Harv Bus Rev. 1997;75(4):65–75.

Chapter 18
Collaborative Culture and Lean Daily Management

David Perlstein, Daniel P. Lombardi, and Ridwan Shabsigh

Introduction

Planning, preparing for, and managing a health crisis requires significant resources on a financial, human, and managerial level. Hospitals worldwide face financial challenges on a daily basis resulting from limited revenue, high operating costs, and tight budgets, and these challenges can create difficulties in assuring the necessary resources when responding to a health crisis. Just as important as securing financial resources – if not more – are the nonfinancial resources such as the role management have in setting vision and values, establishing a specific workplace culture and providing leadership to the healthcare workers. These nonfinancial resources may end up being more influential in the outcome of a health crisis.

The COVID-19 pandemic is a powerful reminder that we live in a highly complex and unpredictable world. It also presented a multitude of novel and acute challenges that have resulted in an opportunity for healthcare leaders to better position and transform their organizations in case of future surprises. COVID-19 brought with it four key challenges to the healthcare sector: a demand to cope with huge patient volume, an urgent need to protect the physical and mental health of frontline staff, significant financial loss as elective procedures and routine care were disrupted, and a need for real-time redesign of care models for patients [1]. Effective

---

D. Perlstein (✉) · D. P. Lombardi
SBH Health System, Bronx, NY, USA
e-mail: dperlstein@sbhny.org

R. Shabsigh
Department of Surgery, SBH Health System, Bronx, NY, USA

Department of Urology, Weill Cornell Medical College of Cornell University, New York, NY, USA

CUNY School of Medicine, New York, NY, USA

© The Author(s), under exclusive license to Springer Nature Switzerland AG 2022
R. Shabsigh (ed.), *Health Crisis Management in Acute Care Hospitals*,
https://doi.org/10.1007/978-3-030-95806-0_18

collaboration and communication can help arm healthcare organizations with tools to aid management and therefore aid in timely recovery from such a crisis.

In this chapter, the unique experience of SBH Health System – a safety-net hospital – during the COVID-19 pandemic will be discussed, highlighting how the nonnegotiable focus on "patient interest first" and the development of a strong collaborative culture contributed substantially to its success in managing this huge health crisis surge. In addition to cultivating the workforce around certain values, the process and adoption of lean daily management (LDM) will also be presented. Both the cultivation of values and LDM were essential in bringing the hospital system closer to crisis preparedness. As an important reflection post pandemic surge, lessons will be drawn from the double pursuit of both the right institutional culture and the right corporate operations.

Workplace Values and Culture in an Acute Care Hospital

The COVID-19 Experience at SBH and How Culture Influenced the Successes

COVID-19 gave rise to the most challenging period in the collective careers of many health professionals at SBH. Arriving from the already ravaged capital city of Wuhan in China and parts of Europe to New York City in late 2019, it was first in early March 2020 that SBH began to admit patients suspected and later confirmed to be infected with what was known as COVID-19. SBH was presented with exponential increases in-patient volume and severity, and when the intensity started to subside slowly in May 2020, staff and the surrounding community had been severely tested, with many workers having lost friends and family to the virus. Considering the chronically tightly resourced SBH facility, which is located in the poorest congressional district in the United States, SBH performed incredibly well and saved many more lives than were lost. Why was SBH successful? Why did so many of the SBH staff trust their leadership and show up to work committed and willing to perform any jobs required to save lives? Why, during the peak of the pandemic, did employees from various departments volunteer to help move those decedents being held in a refrigerated truck into another truck, which could accommodate three times the volume? Why did staff from a dental department voluntarily agree to manage and perform COVID-19 testing in a tent placed in a parking lot? Why did highly trained specialists, nurses, and other clinicians from one field agree to cross-training to perform tasks and roles not otherwise considered during normal times? Why did those who could not clinically serve, voluntarily serve administratively to support patients' families and colleagues emotionally and physically? The answer to all those questions had to include two nonexclusive possibilities: SBH either has extraordinary staff or SBH has the right culture. In reality, the answer was simple: "SBH has both."

The Constitution of SBH Health System Staff and Patients

SBH Health System is comprised of a large ambulatory network and is an urban safety-net hospital located in the Bronx, New York. The hospital has been in continuous operation since 1866 and has transformed itself many times over to bend to the needs of the ever-changing community. SBH patients are multicultural, primarily Black and Hispanic, and are predominantly living in poverty, but this is by no means homogeneous with respect to the country of origin or year of immigration. SBH staff are also multicultural, a reflection of both the community and also its status as a teaching hospital. This creates challenges for an organization needing to deliver a unified and shared vision and mission since perspectives and experiences are not always identical. Luckily these challenges are not insurmountable.

Building a Culture

The culture at SBH did not suddenly appear; it was collectively molded, took many years to create, and continues to evolve. The current chief executive officer/president Dr. David Perlstein joined the staff of St. Barnabas Hospital in 1999 as a general pediatrician and director of ambulatory care. His immediate sense was that the staff were dedicated to their patients and that patients were receiving appropriate and high-quality care. However, what was missing was an overall vision for the hospital with a focus on how SBH could differentiate itself from other providers in the Bronx and beyond. A couple of years after Dr. Perlstein's predecessor (a practicing pulmonologist) took the reins, it was clear to see how he had redefined the culture and the organization around increased patient and community centeredness. Occurring simultaneously was a period of transition in the Medicaid program in New York and a shift towards focusing on value over volume, along with the implementation of a mandatory Medicaid managed care system. This led to an increase in choices for patients over their preferred providers and services and provided an incentive for SBH to prove to payers that they were a step above neighboring facilities.

The immediate focus was to work on continuous improvement more consistently throughout the institution. SBH implemented new educational programs covering process improvement and created institutional goals around preventing errors and hospital-acquired infections and conditions. As a part of this program, SBH also worked on becoming more transparent as an organization, sharing its failures, highlighting risks and opportunities, and celebrating its successes. This served as a foundation for what was to come and primed the culture engine. In 2008, SBH engaged the Baptist Health Leadership Team to help advance the hospital, focusing on improving satisfaction ratings and collectively building a new culture around patient and staff satisfaction. Within a few years, the consistent focus on "patient interest first" permeated the entire organization at all ranks. This was manifested in multiple actions and operations, including but not limited to: hiring and cultivating new healthcare workers, aligning individuals and groups, deep rooting of performance improvement, taking quality assurance out of formality and into sincerity, and upholding patient safety above all.

The Journey to Patient-Centered Excellence: Creating a Pathway

Focusing the hospital workforce at all levels and ranks on "patient first" and patient-centered excellence took coordinated efforts and projects. Some of these were conducted in parallel in order for the benefit from synergistic impact to be felt, mutually enhancing the processes. Others were implemented sequentially and in a phased manner to allow maturation and broad adoption. Some examples include the daily safety call, "safety Friday," the "just culture" initiative, the performance improvement fair, and LDM. LDM particularly is believed to have had a significant positive impact on the preparation of the hospital for the COVID-19 crisis.

Lean Daily Management

During a health crisis, an acute care hospital will be in urgent need for a solid pre-established framework for operations, effective communication processes, and a culture of focus on problem-solving adopted by all ranks. LDM is a recognized method known to both achieve and sustain such essential needs [2–4]. The following includes a brief general description of LDM and a case study of the implementation of LDM at SBH Health System, its contribution to the COVID-19 preparedness and management, and lessons learned about the role of LDM in health crisis planning and management.

What Is LDM?

LDM is an organizational management method that has proven its effectiveness and high value in many industries, especially in healthcare. It is a structured, daily process of collecting data and evaluating performance metrics, which subsequently drives appropriate behaviors and actions, creates operations, and culminates in a culture where the workers desire to not only seek but also solve the organization's problems. The ultimate goal is to turn an organization's workforce into focused problem-solvers, with room for continuous daily improvement. LDM is anchored on the quadruple aim (see Box 18.1). Alongside promoting a culture of continuous improvement, the goal is to implement processes that are value-added from the perspective of the patient and eliminate those that are not. By aligning staff and workers around a shared vision, the willingness to change, by identifying the root cause of problems and making corrections to improve processes, will be greater and more profitable.

> **Box 18.1. LDM – Quadruple Aim**
> 1. Better health outcome
> 2. Better care experience
> 3. Lower cost (least waste)
> 4. More joy for those providing the care and those receiving the care

There are several defined steps to the LDM process [2]:

1. Create targets by identifying goals and metrics linked to the quadruple aim.
2. Gather and collect data on a daily basis.
3. Analyze immediate past performance.
4. Implement actions to solve problems and address their causes.
5. Review processes to assure sustainability of solutions and sharing of learned lessons.

LDM is performed by the daily joint engagement of three constituencies of healthcare workers: frontline staff, managers, and executives. The frontline staff should be engaged for the selection of goals and metrics and for reviewing, presenting, and problem-solving. Managers make sure that the data is collected, analyzed, and ready to be presented. Executives interact with the frontline staff and the managers and facilitate problem-solving, assuring removal of hurdles and resistance [2]. The focus is on the process, not the people (see Box 18.2).

> **Box 18.2. The Benefits of LDM**
> - Creates an organization of focused problem-solvers
> - Establishes a framework for effective, efficient, and safe operations
> - Instigates a culture change towards more open communications
> - Provides an agile bottom-up approach to quality and performance improvement
> - Frontline engagement and empowerment
> - Improves managers' accountability
> - Supports executives as servant leaders

Case Study: LDM, SBH Health System, and the COVID-19 Health Crisis

The Beginning Three years before the COVID-19 crisis, SBH executive leadership made the strategic decision to bring LDM into SBH. At that time, the goals were to add the missing bottom-up approach to safety and quality to the already established top-down approach. Prior to LDM, there were certain safety measures, processes, and programs at SBH at the managerial and executive levels. An example is the 15-minute daily safety call, which occurred throughout the entire organization; here, a medical director would engage managers and directors who would then report operational and quality/safety events from the last 24 hours. SBH also adopted "just culture," another tool and method of managing people based on behavioral choices and evaluation of the overall system design. Moreover, the third process named "patient safety Friday" was developed to aid and assist managers on the Joint Commission, New York State Department of Health, and the Centers for Medicare & Medicaid Services (CMS) standards and directives. Missing from these top-down initiatives was a bottom-up plan. This bottom-up initiative was needed to engage frontline staff and create a "learning organization." Prior to LDM, learning mostly came from managers, directors, and executive staff and was based on data or outcomes. LDM contributed by providing input to compliment some of the top-down approach processes with a bottom-up approach in order to create sustainable, reliable improvement, and systems. In lieu of replacing one approach with another, LDM was instead a second and complimentary approach. With this in place, the entire organization started moving in one direction, as far as performance improvement and safety was concerned, with guidance from the LDM quadruple aim.

The Change LDM was practiced at SBH during the 3 years leading up to the COVID-19 crisis and resulted in two major changes: one in the frontline staff and the other in the executive staff. Firstly, frontline staff were introduced to some executives whom they typically did not have interactions with. Furthermore, they developed confidence when speaking with the executive team members and felt comfortable to voice safety concerns, any barriers or shout-outs, or even expressing recognition of exceptional team members' work. LDM daily rounding became a central place for communication, not only related to metrics but also to daily work. LDM shifted the thinking of frontline staff from focusing on "finishing the daily work" to *how* they could actually make that work *better*. On the executive side, it was a great learning experience for them to hear directly from and interact with frontline staff. The value of this learning was especially significant for nonclinical executives.

One of the features of LDM was the series of short daily meetings. This scripted design accomplished a few important things: (1) it allowed for a constant level of communication where executives and frontline staff were able to effectively communicate in a short period of time, (2) it allowed for the exchange of high-yield information, and (3) it allowed for comments on safety concerns or barriers to the work. The brevity also created a sense that these meetings were an integrated part of everyday and not an additional activity outside of daily operations. Another advantageous feature of LDM was the frequency of meetings; daily collection and analysis of data, then subsequent discussion of how to solve problems and improve, gave overall flexibility to make adjustments and changes within a short time span. The dynamic nature created by this framework allowed for a potential change of focus, even on a daily basis, ensuring that the workforce stayed active, alert, and focused. The overall impact of LDM was transformational for the workforce and the executive leadership. Although this incremental gradual transformation was probably not felt by everyone, its benefits became much clearer when the COVID-19 health crisis occurred.

Maturing as an LDM Organization After its phased introduction to SBH, LDM became an established method of management in many departments. This in turn transformed the way healthcare workers looked at their work; it wasn't just a job, it was about doing a *better* job with feeling of engagement, satisfaction, and appreciation. At the executive level, LDM created a true "collaborative servant leadership." LDM engaged the executive team to work through frontline staff barriers, of which were identified by the frontline staff during rounds. Barriers included both operational and safety barriers, which could hinder daily work. The executive team became more efficient in timely communication, follow-through, and correctly identifying barriers.

Contributions of LDM to COVID-19 Preparedness During and immediately after the COVID-19 crisis, several questions arose about whether LDM had actually helped in crisis preparation, and if so, how. On reflection, it was concluded that LDM had significantly helped to create a better prepared organization for a health crisis. The first reason for this was the framework and culture it contributed. The framework ensured a way to do things "right" and "better," every day. The culture changes helped shift towards a more open, structured, and communicative environment. The second reason supporting the success of LDM was the change in structure to the executive team, with executive team members becoming more involved in the "every day" by doing daily rounds with the frontline staff and communicating more frequently. By doing so, they developed a deeper understanding of the day-to-day operations they usually weren't involved in (Box 18.3).

Box 18.3. Contributions of LDM to Health Crisis Preparedness
- Framework for effective, efficient, and safe operations
- Frequent communications that transcend all ranks
- Culture shift to problem-solving, improvement, and safety
- Structure for engaged executive interactions

Examples of the Benefits of an LDM-Trained Organization During the COVID-19 Surge Crisis in Spring 2020 The standard LDM was suspended in March 2020 during the peak of the pandemic, and SBH instead took the existing framework, communication mode, culture, and structure and shifted to a different platform of communication where executive team, departments, divisions, teams, and work groups would speak each and every day, sometimes several times a day if necessary. Practical discussions were held on what was and was not working, what barriers existed preventing the hospital from overcoming the crisis, and how to manage the crisis as best as pragmatically possible.

LDM After the COVID-19 Crisis and Lessons Learned In the recovery stages following the surge of the COVID-19 crisis, LDM was resumed, however, with new methods and improvements in place. One of the main innovations was the virtual platform. On reflection, several lessons can be learned from the crisis.

What worked was having senior staff present with frontline staff each and every day. What also worked was talking about barriers, assigning executive team members to manage certain barriers, open communication, and the chance to engage the entire hospital community and educate them, allowing for a continual exchange of ideas and opportunities. Another lesson learned is that inclusion of co-leads from the various departments is essential to assure continuity of engagement.

Reinforcement, however, was needed to ensure some LDM practices. For example, one of the most important components of LDM, in order to make progress on certain metrics, is gathering data regarding the lack of progress of a certain metric. A big focus of LDM after COVID-19 would, therefore, be to expect a daily deep dive to understand any lack of progress of a metric and to hold each other more accountable in making sure reasons for this are addressed.

LDM for Planning and Preparation for a Future Health Crisis

Planning in lieu of a crisis is critical to survival of a healthcare system. Fitting the LDM quadruple aim into crisis planning and preparation may present an opportunity for a more prominent role of LDM in health crisis preparedness and management in the future, providing a platform for a paradigm shift towards operational preparedness instead of focusing purely on quality and safety. In this sense, the change has a greater focus on the immediate future instead of the immediate past.

Summary

The nonnegotiable focus on "patient first" and a collaborative culture can contribute substantially to the success of a healthcare system in managing a health crisis such as the COVID-19 pandemic. Using a recognized method such as LDM to achieve the necessary framework and encourage better communication processes is highly advantageous under normal operating circumstances but could be deemed a necessity both during and after a healthcare crisis situation. Not only does such a method allow the hospital to track goals on a daily basis but ensure that any corrective actions taken are being sustained. LDM is known to have been implemented as a management strategy at a number of institutions following the COVID-19 pandemic [5] to help optimize every aspect of the patients' process flow and allow for improvements, which ultimately create more value for the patient. However, competent leadership and workforce flexibility are paramount to the success of LDM, since an implementation gap may exist between strategy and execution [6]. Despite the enormous suffering, the pandemic has brought with it fruitful lessons learned, which may allow healthcare institutions around the world to be better prepared in the face of a future crisis.

References

1. Begun JW, Jiang J. Health care management during COVID-19: insights from complexity science. NEMJ Catalyst. 2020; https://catalyst.nejm.org/doi/full/10.1056/CAT.20.0541.
2. With permission from Greater Baltimore Medical Center HealthCare System: https://www.gbmc.org/gbmc-lean-daily-management-explained.
3. Eamranond PP, Bhukhen A, DiPalma D, Kunuakaphun S, Burke T, Rodis J, Grey M. Interprofessional, multitiered daily rounding management in a high-acuity hospital. Int J Health Care Qual Assur. 2020 (ahead-of-print). https://doi.org/10.1108/IJHCQA-09-2019-0158. PMID: 32918544.
4. Po J, Rundall TG, Shortell SM, Blodgett JC. Lean management and U.S. public hospital performance: results from a national survey. J Healthc Manag. 2019;64(6):363–79. https://doi.org/10.1097/JHM-D-18-00163. PMID: 31725563.
5. Pellini F, Di Filippo G, Mirandola S, Deguidi G, Filippi E, Pollini GP. Effects of lean thinking and emerging technologies on breast cancer patients' therapeutic process during COVID-19 pandemic: a case-control matched study. Front Surg. 2021; https://doi.org/10.3389/fsurg.2021.582980.
6. Van Rossum L, Aij KH, Simons FE, van der Eng N, ten Have WD. Lean healthcare from a change management perspective: the role of leadership and workforce flexibility in an operating theatre. J Health Organ Manag. 2016;30(3):475–93. https://doi.org/10.1108/JHOM-06-2014-0090.

Chapter 19
Soft Skills, Emotional and Social Intelligence, and Resilience

Lizica C. Troneci and Ridwan Shabsigh

The Psychological Burden of COVID-19 on Healthcare Workers

Global response to the COVID-19 pandemic has exposed inherent weaknesses in our preparedness and response. The health systems have been grossly overwhelmed by the pandemic [1]. In the United States, the COVID-19 pandemic encountered an already flawed healthcare system, fraught with inequalities in insurance coverage as well as economic, racial, and ethnic disparities, providers' financial losses, and a deep crisis in public health. Changes had to be implemented in a matter of hours or days as the illness affected increasing numbers of people. The pandemic created an additional physical and emotional burden, which was superimposed on an already hectic and loaded work schedule. The lack of medical knowledge about the COVID-19 illness, coupled with the initially limited availability of personal protective equipment (PPE) and the rapidly advancing rate of death, further stretched the tired and burned-out healthcare workers (HCWs).

From an individual HCW's perspective, the COVID-19 pandemic has imposed additional hardships on professional and personal levels. High rates of death and infection, limited information about COVID-19 illness and management, rapid

---

L. C. Troneci (✉)
Department of Psychiatry, SBH Health System, Bronx, NY, USA

CUNY School of Medicine, New York, NY, USA
e-mail: ltroneci@sbhny.org

R. Shabsigh
Department of Surgery, SBH Health System, Bronx, NY, USA

Department of Urology, Weill Cornell Medical College of Cornell University, New York, NY, USA

CUNY School of Medicine, New York, NY, USA

© The Author(s), under exclusive license to Springer Nature Switzerland AG 2022
R. Shabsigh (ed.), *Health Crisis Management in Acute Care Hospitals*, https://doi.org/10.1007/978-3-030-95806-0_19

changes in work-related processes, and long hours impacted the HCWs' physical and psychological wellness in the work environment. At home, HCWs were faced with fear of contaminating family, loss of friends or relatives, homeschooling children, and of course also simply taking care of themselves. Some HCWs were burdened by having to make difficult decisions about patient end-of-life aspects and rationing limited resources among growing numbers of critically ill patients.

Even under non-pandemic working conditions, HCWs experience stressful daily situations, witnessing death and pain, overcrowded hospitals, and present with high rates of burnout with up to 33% of critical care nurses and 45% of critical care physicians experiencing burnout syndrome, and even higher numbers reporting at least one of the classic symptoms of burnout including emotional exhaustion [2]. Research conducted by Guo et al. on a sample of 1,805 HCWs in eight hospitals in China during May 15th to May 31st 2020, showed high incidence of depression (56.4%), anxiety (45.2%), and insomnia (79%) [3]. From June to September 2020, Mental Health America (MHA) conducted a survey of 1,119 HCWs to assess their experiences during the COVID-19 pandemic [4]. Stress was the most commonly reported feeling (92.76%), followed by anxiety (86.06%), frustration (76.94%), and burnout (75.96%). When asked about emotional support, HCWs reported family as the number one resource (56.66%), followed by supervisor (15.28%) and support groups (live, virtual, or social media 5.09%) following same level co-workers (38.43%). Mount Sinai Hospital in NYC conducted a survey to assess the psychological impact of the COVID-19 pandemic on HCWs. Data was collected between April 14, 2020, and May 11, 2020, which corresponded with the peak and the beginning of the downward slope of the pandemic in NYC, and included 1,005 HCWs who screened positive for COVID-related symptoms of mental illness. The most common reported symptoms were of major depressive disorder (MDD, 26.6%), followed by generalized anxiety disorder (GAD, 25%) and post-traumatic stress disorder (PTSD, 23.3%) [5]. In response to trauma and adversity, human beings' resort to resilience (how one copes) can affect the individual's well-being, the well-being of family, colleagues, community, and, in the case of HCWs, their patients (Box 19.1).

Coping with the Crisis

Resilience

Resilience is the capacity to respond to stress in a healthy way such that goals are achieved at minimal psychological and physical cost. Resilience helps to reduce burnout, increases compassion, and reconnects one with the joy of practicing medicine and taking care of sick people [6]. The COVID-19 pandemic confirmed what prior research has shown, with HCWs experiencing similar problems during the previous pandemics (2003 SARS and 2014 Ebola virus) and that the mental health of HCWs during such periods is of paramount importance.

HCWs experienced serious emotional and psychological problems during the COVID-19 pandemic. Many of them were exposed to traumatic and destructive situations to which some have responded by developing anxiety and depression, while others have recovered. Due to the very rapid increase in workload (high volume of sick patients) and the fast pace of changes (workflows, management of illness, coverage) during the initial days/weeks, the HCWs had to resort to their existent "reservoirs" of psychological and physical resilience [7].

In a non-pandemic noncrisis environment, resilience can be measured by using tools such as the following: the Brief Resilience Scale (BRS), Survey of Perceived Organizational Support (SPOS) brief form, Satisfaction with Life Scale (SWLS), or Positive and Negative Affect Schedule (PANAS) [7]. The results can then inform the type of interventions a healthcare system can implement to maximize the healthcare worker's well-being. For example, identification of insomnia as a symptom can inform a hospital administrator of an intervention geared towards enhancing HCWs' access to sleep, by creating sleeping arrangements in the hospital, coordinating backup, and shifting schedule changes.

There was no time to formally assess or measure the resilience of HCWs during the surge of COVID-19 patients at SBH. Instead, the planned and implemented interventions were built on knowledge and experience from prior research conducted into resilience during major outbreaks and disasters.

Emotional and Social Intelligence

Emotional intelligence, or EI, defines a person's ability to sense the feelings of those around them, their own feelings, and to respond appropriately. Social intelligence emphasizes awareness of others. The five key attributes of people with emotional intelligence are the following: self-awareness, self-regulation, motivation, empathy, and social skills [8]. Emotional intelligence is apparent in the healthcare environment on both an individual and institutional level in managing stress and stressful situations, working as a team member, or managing a team, and delivering bad news to patients and families, to name just a few [9]. EI is considered a primary and fundamental leadership and managerial competency and represents the basis for the development of "soft" skills (interpersonal and communication skills) which are essential for frontline and managerial staff. Healthcare leaders with a high degree of EI are better equipped to recognize and assess the psychological and emotional status of HCWs and respond rapidly and appropriately to signs of deterioration in worker well-being.

During a pandemic, emotional self-awareness, a component of emotional intelligence, is vital in assisting a healthcare leader understand how one feels and how one can effectively support self and others [10]. A health crisis, like the COVID-19 pandemic, tests the healthcare leaders' emotional intelligence and their ability to lead through uncertain times. It allows them to manage their colleagues' anxiety and fear, to make clear and confident decisions, to manage disappointment and distrust, and to motivate and encourage others. The SBH Health System relied on its administrators and clinical leaders' EI to implement several different strategies during the surge of the crisis.

> **Box 19.1 Personal Memories from a Psychiatrist and Administrator**
> "No experience and even prior knowledge of pandemics would have prepared us, personally and professionally, for the events in NYC in early 2020. The first COVID-19 case in NYC was announced by Governor Cuomo on March 1st, 2020. Our hospital began preparations for the surge of COVID-19-infected patients. From a psychiatrist and department administrator perspective, my priorities became keeping our team and our psychiatric patients safe from infection. As the number of positive cases increased, our outpatient team of providers mounted a huge effort to expeditiously implement telehealth. On March 22, 2020, Governor Cuomo issued the "New York State on PAUSE" order. It was also around that time that the number of infected patients started to grow every day, while the number of psychiatric patients in need for hospitalization started to decrease. The fear of infection prevented people from calling 911 or coming to the hospital's emergency room.
>
> I recall coming to the hospital and walking to my office located on the same floor with one of the medical units, passing by my colleagues, doctors and nurses who were treating "COVID-19 patients." They looked tired, worried, and fearful. There was an eerie quietness interrupted by the operator calling "respiratory therapist to ED" or "rapid response to 2 north" (which identifies the need for patient resuscitation efforts).
>
> Almost every day in March, April, and May was marked by an enormous amount of change and new information – about the most appropriate PPE, the guidelines for staff's testing for COVID-19, guidelines for telehealth provision; guidelines on patients' testing prior to admission to the inpatient psychiatric units. Anxiety and fear had reached sky heights. When will "this" end? Why so much death? How can I protect my family? How can I protect myself?
>
> The emergency department was packed with "COVID-19 patients," and it seemed as if no other illnesses existed anymore. The psychiatry team evaluated few patients for behavioral reasons during 24 hours' shifts. The world of psychiatry was apprehensively waiting for the "mental health surge" although it became apparent that was nowhere in sight, at least not immediately. By March 23, 2020, it was evident that staff of all disciplines and from all departments, clinical and nonclinical, needed emotional support."

Strategies to Address Stress and Trauma During the COVID-19 "Peak" Weeks

The COVID-19 crisis continued for many weeks and months, but the peak period in NYC, and more specifically at the SBH Health System, occurred over approximately 4 weeks in March and April 2020. These can be divided into week 1 (March 16–22), week 2 (March 23–29), week 3 (March 30–April 5), and week 4 (April 6–12).

Week 1

Basic needs were addressed during week 1; the hospital provided free meals and extended hours for the cafeteria; sleep accommodations were created throughout the hospital; free parking in the hospital's garage was instituted; and PPE was made available incrementally to address HCWs' fear of contamination and to secure their safety. Such provisions ensured the first set of initiatives to care for and support HCWs during the crisis.

Lesson learned: The initiatives were welcomed by staff, and the timeliness of implementation was much appreciated.

During week 1, each department adjusted work schedules and created backup arrangements. The psychiatry residency program changed rotation assignments (since the behavioral health clinic closed and shifted to telemedicine) for the specialty clinics (geriatric, addiction psychiatry).

Lesson learned: Create a "change" team tasked with tracking changes and new initiatives. The team would be responsible to identify gaps in processes and HCWs in need of support and monitor responses to changes.

Week 2

During week 2, a recurring virtual meeting with all the psychiatry department's medical staff was scheduled on a weekly basis. The need for a meeting became apparent since there was such a high volume of emails and changes, which needed to be communicated and implemented in a timely fashion. The virtual meeting alleviated HCWs concerns, improved communication, and provided a united front in the face of adversity.

Lesson learned: Implement a departmental weekly virtual meeting as early as feasible in the crisis.

There was no time or need to conduct a formal assessment of the HCWs' level of stress or burnout as these were apparent by simple observation. The hospital had to focus on strategies to enhance HCWs' resilience in the face of mounting adversity and death. Plans had been made to address the surge of COVID-19 patients, but there was no formal plan/strategy to address the HCWs' escalating stress and burnout.

Lesson learned: Consider developing a strategy to address HCWs response to stress and trauma ("surge" of HCWs' emotional distress) at the same time creating a "surge" plan for patients.

Box 19.2 COVID-19 Emotional Support Line Protocol
The call number: XXXXXX.
Callers from SBH campus and SBHBH can dial ext. XXXX.
Employees calling from the outside will call XXXXXX.

- *Purpose of call* – The hotline has been established to provide emotional support to the SBH staff. The hotline is not a substitute for therapy, and the calls are expected to last for around 15 minutes.
- Should you feel that the person could/would benefit from therapy, the caller should be given referral contact staff name and contact number.
- *Confidential* – Nothing discussed during the call will be relayed to any supervisor.
- *Anonymous* – While we will be introducing ourselves, the person calling the hotline does not have to give their name or department.
- *Neutrality* – The call is a neutral, nonjudgmental zone where we are talking to the caller in a supportive manner and where we are offering information about additional sites as needed.
- *Debriefing* – After the first week of calls, we will all get together via zoom to discuss the process, any difficulties we had, and what we need going forward.
- *Repeat/frequent caller* – If the person calling the hotline is a repeat caller, consider referring to therapy.
- *Prank/test calls* – (a) Offer the caller the opportunity to make a genuine enquiry of your service, provided they are not too abusive to do so. (b) Explain the goals and areas of action of the helpline. (c) Explain that what the caller is doing is negative and unproductive, and inform the caller that they should only call if they have real issues to discuss and that they are preventing another caller from utilizing the service. Having covered all of the points above, the call can be terminated (hang up).
- *Sexual gratification calls* – Terminate the call, in a clear and respectful way. Discuss the call during our debriefing session.
- *Suicidal calls* – Suicidal callers demand special attention and handling from the helpline staff. As with all calls, maintain a calm supportive tone with caller. Try to establish caller's supports, if there is someone that they can talk to or explore the idea of contacting a specialist service after the

call, depending on the severity of the suicidal ideation; ask for their phone number, where they are calling from, and send EMS to bring them to the nearest hospital.
- *Data collection* – At the end of the call, note the time and day of the call and the general topic. This is solely for us to know how many people are utilizing the service and how we can better the service. The data collection sheet has been posted on google docs, and a link has been sent to everyone.
  - At the start of the call, introduce yourself, and let the caller know that everything discussed during this call will be confidential and that they do not have to give their name or tell you in which department they work.
  - "Hello, you are speaking to_____, and you have called the SBH Covid19 Emotional Support Line. This line is for emotional support, and everything discussed will be confidential."
  - If the person starts to ask medical questions, give them the medical question hotline number, and then ask what they can do to help them.
  - Emotions to keep in mind when on the phone with someone, they may be experiencing: Grief at the loss of their regular routine, death of family/friends/co-workers, depression, anxiety, loss of control, anger.

At the beginning of week 2, in consultation with the hospital's leadership, the department of psychiatry organized and staffed the "COVID-19 ESL" (employee support line – see Box. 19.2), which was advertised via mass email and via "Workplace" (the hospital's intranet site for communication and information). The psychiatrists, psychologists, and psychology externs, along with psychiatry residents and therapists, were trained in providing such support.

Week 3

The ESL opened on the first day of week 3 (March 30) and was available 7 days/week, 8 am–6 pm. The staff logged the calls and the type of intervention on a dedicated confidential record sheet (Fig. 19.1).

Many mental health and support resources, disseminated by various agencies, became available for distribution on individual and departmental levels (Table 19.1).

The department of psychiatry received requests for individual referrals who were referred to the SBH Health System Behavioral Health outpatient clinic. This process was derived from the managers' and leaders' emotional intelligence skills who identified the HCWs in need of mental health assistance.

Moreover, starting in week 3, HCWs support groups were developed for the most affected areas, namely, the emergency department, medical units, and ICU, which included all disciplines (Table 19.2). The support groups were scheduled to meet

Hotline Record Sheet

Day/Date of Call	Time/Length of Call	Topic(s)	Outcome	Caller's dept	Caller's Profession	Responder
Th - 4/2/2020	2:15 - 2:25	Anxiety, not sleeping	encouraged good sleep practices, taught some relaxation tech.	ICU	RN	X

Fig. 19.1 Example employee support line record sheet that was used to log information about each call that was made by members of the healthcare system during the COVID-19 pandemic

Table 19.1 Mental health and support resources distributed to departments and individuals at the SBH during the COVID-19 crisis

Resource	Type/for	Title	Contact	Info
Mental health	Crisis line/ anyone	OMH COVID-19 emotional support helpline	Call 844–863-9314	8:00 AM–10 PM, 7 days/week. NYS Office of Mental Health support line, staffed by licensed behavioral health volunteers
Mental health/ addiction	Crisis line/ anyone in NYC	New York City well	https://nycwell.cityofnewyork.us.en Text WELL to 65173* Or call 888-NYC-WELL Contact CHAT via website	Free, confidential mental health support. Speak to a counselor via phone, text, or chat, and get access to mental health and substance use disorders services in >200 languages, 24/7. Based in NYC
Mental health	Crisis line/ anyone	National Suicide Prevention Lifeline	Call 800–273-TALK	24/7 nationwide crisis and suicide hotline; in addition to English, Spanish language operators are available
Mental health/ addiction	Crisis line/ anyone	SAMHSA – Substance Abuse and Mental Health Services Administration	Call 800–662-HELP	Free, confidential, 24/7 treatment referral and information service in English and Spanish, for individuals and families facing mental health and/or substance use disorders

Table 19.2 The Healthcare Worker Support Groups at the SBH during the COVID-19 crisis

Provider Name	**Monday** Psychological Support for Medical Personnel Group	**Thursday** Psychological Support for Medical Personnel Group	**Friday** Psychological Support for Medical Personnel Group-With Grief Bereavement Addendum
A	Emergency department staff 9am and 4pm		
B		Department of medicine staff 9am and 4pm	
C			ICU -9am Ambulatory Clinic 4pm

once a week via virtual platform. The schedule and contact information were distributed via email and posted on noticeboards in accessible areas.

Week 4

Once the ESL lines were open, the waiting period started for HCWs to reach out and receive the emotional support they needed. However, the COVID-19 ESL line received only 3–5 calls every week. The HCWs support groups connected only once, and participation was limited. Meanwhile, death, uncertainty, fear, pain, anguish, and anxiety continued to be witnessed in the psychiatry department staff and throughout all staff at the SBH Health System. Emotional support was clearly needed, but the interventions were just not being utilized by the HCWs. During week 4, an in-depth assessment and reflection of the implemented support resources and interventions that were currently in place were conducted to evaluate their success and usefulness as tools to promote mental well-being of the HCWs. From this, it was clear that staff were too tired and burdened to "call a number" or to connect virtually to a support group. They needed more. They needed real-time and real-life interventions, and rapid planning was undertaken to adapt the resources to better fit these needs (Box 19.3).

Lessons learned: Create fliers with available resources and post them throughout the institution (cafeteria, nursing stations, call rooms). Use email sparsely as HCWs will not have the time to check. Assess outcome on a weekly basis. Escalate to the next type of intervention if not efficient (measured by number of calls made to employee support line or number of HCWs attending the virtual groups).

Box 19.3 A Personal Account

"After the first onsite intervention, it was clear that THIS was much more relevant and appropriate for the HCWs and that it was the "right" modality to deliver support. Personally, I recall my first round and the anxiety of having to wear full PPE (which by then was in full supply) and to walk on a "COVID-19" unit, which was much different than the inpatient psychiatric unit I was accustomed to. While everybody's faces were covered with masks and shields, their eyes were filled with tears but also with hopefulness and gratefulness. The number of COVID-19-infected patients had started to decrease; there was enough and adequate PPE; there were more treatments available for the seriously ill patients; yet the burden on HCWs' well-being was clear. During those sessions, staff shared their personal and professional experiences, along with their most intimate feelings and emotions of the current situation and the buildup from the previous peak weeks. During those intervention rounds, HCWs approached us individually, asking for help for themselves or for their family members. We shared with them the resources we had collected (provided by various agencies or private psychologists/therapists who were conducting virtual free therapeutic interventions)."

Table 19.3 Schedule for psychiatrist rounds to support healthcare workers at SBH

Unit	Morning	Afternoon	Assignment
7N/7S nursing MDs/residents	715am 830-1030am	330pm	X, MD Cell phone xxx-xxx-xxxx
6N/6S nursing MDs/residents	715am 830-1030am	330pm	Y, MD Cell phone xxx-xxx-xxxx
ED all staff	1030-1130am		Z, PhD Cell phone xxx-xxx-xxxx
ICU all staff	715am		A, PhD Cell phone xxx-xxx-xxxx
2N/2S nursing MDs/Residents	715am 830-1030am	330pm	B, MD Cell phone xxx-xxx-xxxx
3N/3S nursing MDs/Residents	715am 830-1030am	330pm	C, PhD Cell phone xxx-xxx-xxxx

Beyond the Peak Weeks

On April 22 (week 6), a group of psychiatrists and psychologists initiated the "onsite intervention" – each one was assigned to round a clinical area (medical units, ICU, emergency department) at the time of the most impact for attendance. For medical units, that time was 7:15 am (for nursing staff), 8:30 am (for other disciplines), and 3:30 pm (for nursing staff at the change of shifts), and the sessions lasted approximately 30 minutes (Table 19.3).

The model for this type of intervention, while not formal and evidence-based, focused on debriefing and reflection. Initial guidance was provided by the Center for the Study of Traumatic Stress/Uniformed Services University, in the below format (Fig. 19.2). Additional information was provided by the National Center for PTSD/US Department of Veterans Affairs [11].

Following completion of these support rounds within the clinical areas, onsite interventions were expanded to include other disciplines, such as environmental workers, dietary workers, and security officers, all of whom needed emotional support. The initial encounter with each group was always followed up by repeated sessions, which were provided at alternate hours to include the evening and night shifts, to maximize the reach of the intervention and ensure that all workers had support available.

Reflecting on HCW Well-being at the SBH Health System During the Initial Surge of the COVID-19 Crisis

The COVID-19 crisis has united HCWs from all over the world in their professional challenges, inadequate PPE, long work shifts, and, most shockingly, the abundant suffering and loss of lives. The mental health crisis that has followed the pandemic

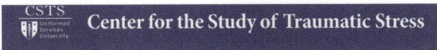

Fig. 19.2 Guidance provided by the Center for the Study of Traumatic Stress/Uniformed Services University used as a framework to assist with effective debriefing and reflective support of healthcare workers in the COVID-19 crisis at the SBH Health System. (With permission from the Center for the Study of Traumatic Stress)

will most likely be present for years. HCWs were particularly vulnerable to the initial part of the crisis since they were on the frontline for exposure to the COVID-19 illness and related impacts on well-being and mental health. It has become apparent that their well-being needs to be prioritized and addressed on a larger scale. Until this occurs, the soft skills of the administrators and leaders play a vital role in maintaining both the hospitals and the workforces' highest levels of functioning. These soft skills can be beneficial in the identification of mental health struggles and the implementation of the needed interventions to frontline workers and essential staff.

The SBH Health System, by virtue of its location and patient population, was exposed to many of such challenges triggered by the pandemic. Leadership worked to develop and implement processes "on the spur of the moment" to support HCWs challenged by the excessive burden of these new challenges. Some interventions failed or had limited benefit while others were successful and generated positive change. Through all of them, lessons were learned from experience and analyzed by reflection. While interventions were often impactful, they were constantly analyzed to provide the best support possible to an overburdened yet vital service to our communities.

Implementation of initiatives and responses to them have been reflected upon over the course of those peak weeks, and those that immediately followed, and it was helpful to generate a list of potential improvements:

1. Communication is of paramount importance – the hospital had a daily morning safety call, which included all departments, and reported on census, problems, and solutions. In hindsight, for the first 2–3 weeks, where processes/workflows/guidelines were changing even a few times per day, a psychiatry departmental daily call would have been beneficial to address concerns and alleviate worries.
2. Emotional well-being is of paramount importance – the institution addressed the physical needs during the first week of the crisis, while the emotional needs were addressed with some delay.

    Potential solutions could be to offer a safe area with proper distancing/precautions right from the recognition of a health crisis, where HCWs can meet for short breaks and snacks, where they can share "stories" and offer peer support. Including "wellness carts" with relaxing single-use activities, such as coloring, aromatherapy, stress balls, etc., could have provided essential mental relief. Having mental health support staff directly call HCWs and assess wellness and need for individual interventions/support from the first weeks of the crisis, and in anticipation of the mounting COVID-19 illness, burden would have increased HCWs' access to emotional support resources. Broadcasting relaxing and soothing music through the hospital's PA system to help calm nerves and relieve tension, music interventions have demonstrated improvement of stress-related outcomes in a variety of settings [12].
3. Establish collaborative relationships with external programs and clinics to enhance the availability of mental health support for the workforce during crisis situations (some mental health programs volunteered their time and expertise to address the HCWs mental health needs, but the awareness of such resources was limited and consequently delayed).
4. Coordinate mental health efforts with spiritual/religious support offerings to address the level of comfort required for each individual impacted HCW.

References

1. Khetrapal S, Bhatia R. Impact of COVID-19 pandemic on health system & Sustainable Development Goal 3. Indian J Med Res. 2020;151(5):395–99. https://doi.org/10.4103/ijmr.IJMR_1920_20.
2. Moss M, Good VS, Gozal D, Kleinpell R, Sessler CN. A critical care societies collaborative statement: burnout syndrome in critical care health-care professionals. A call for action. Am J Respir Crit Care Med. 2016;194(1):106–13. https://doi.org/10.1164/rccm.201604-0708ST.
3. Guo WP, Min Q, Gu WW, Yu L, Xiao X, Yi WB, et al. Prevalence of mental health problems in frontline healthcare workers after the first outbreak of COVID-19 in China: a cross-sectional study. Health Qual Life Outcomes. 2021;19:103. https://doi.org/10.1186/s12955-021-01743-7.
4. The Mental Health of Healthcare Workers In COVID19 https://mhanational.org/mental-health-healthcare-workers-covid-19. Accessed 8 July 2021.
5. Feingold JH, Peccoralo L, Chan CC, Kaplan CA, Kaye-Kauderer H, Charney D, et al. Psychological impact of the COVID-19 pandemic on frontline health care workers during the pandemic surge in new York City. Chronic Stress (Thousand Oaks). 2021;5:2470547020977891. https://doi.org/10.1177/2470547020977891.
6. Epstein RM, Krasner MS. Physician resilience: what it means, why it matters, and how to promote it. Acad Med. 2013;88(3):301–3. https://doi.org/10.1097/ACM.0b013e318280cff0.
7. Bozdağ F, Ergün N. Psychological resilience of healthcare professionals during COVID-19 pandemic. Psychol Rep. 2020; https://doi.org/10.1177/0033294120965477.
8. Syed MP. Emotional Intelligence during a pandemic. NEJM Journal Watch. Emotional Intelligence During a Pandemic - Insights on Residency Training Insights on Residency Training (jwatch.org). Accessed 8 July 2021.
9. Emotional intelligence: 4 ways the pandemic is testing leaders – and how to respond. The Enterprisers Project. https://enterprisersproject.com/article/2020/9/emotional-intelligence-pandemic-challenges-leaders. Accessed 8 July 2021.
10. Fernandez CSP, Peterson HB, Holmström SW, Connolly AM. Developing emotional intelligence for healthcare leaders. In: Di Fabio A, editor. Emotional intelligence – new perspectives and applications. InTechOpen. 2012; p. 239–260. Accessed 30 Sept 2021.
11. U.S Department of Veterans Affairs. https://www.ptsd.va.gov/covid/COVID_healthcare_workers.asp. Accessed 8 July 2021.
12. de Witte M, Spruit A, van Hooren S, Moonen X, Stams GJ. Effects of music interventions on stress-related outcomes: a systematic review and two meta-analyses. Health Psychol Rev. 2020;14(2):294–324. https://doi.org/10.1080/17437199.2019.1627897.

Chapter 20
Recovery From Crisis

Ridwan Shabsigh and Joanne E. Nettleship

Introduction

COVID-19 has caused unprecedented global crisis, shocking public health systems, resulting in loss of millions of lives, and disrupting the entire economic and social fabric at a scale not witnessed for generations. The pandemic challenged administrations at local, regional, and global levels in their ability to respond to such a crisis. The effectiveness of this response depends on how healthcare systems are organised and governed and its preparedness for emergencies. An understanding of the impact the pandemic has had on healthcare systems worldwide may help identify core lessons to help strengthen their preparedness and respond more effectively to future challenges.

A resilient healthcare system has the capacity to prepare for, absorb the impact and recover from such disasters whilst maintaining core functions and serving the ongoing acute care needs of its communities. It effectively adapts to evolving situations and actively acts to reduce vulnerabilities when they arise. In this section, we will describe the worldwide impact of COVID-19 on the building blocks of health systems framework as described by the WHO [1] and draw lessons and recommendations for effective recovery post-pandemic. Finally, we will discuss the experience of SBH Health System's recovery process following the initial surge.

R. Shabsigh (✉)
Department of Surgery, SBH Health System, Bronx, NY, USA

Department of Urology, Weill Cornell Medical College of Cornell University, New York, NY, USA

CUNY School of Medicine, New York, NY, USA
e-mail: rshabsigh@sbhny.org

J. E. Nettleship
Astra Health, Sheffield, UK

© The Author(s), under exclusive license to Springer Nature Switzerland AG 2022
R. Shabsigh (ed.), *Health Crisis Management in Acute Care Hospitals*,
https://doi.org/10.1007/978-3-030-95806-0_20

Impact of COVID-19 on Health Systems

Impact on Health Service Delivery

In the face of COVID-19, there was a need to rapidly increase the healthcare infrastructure, and healthcare systems constructed new treatment facilities, converted public venues and reconfigured existing medical facilities. For instance, China were able to establish two specialty field hospitals in under 2 weeks [2], and NHS England configured seven public venues to into temporary 'Nightingale' hospitals to accommodate the increase in COVID-19 patients [3]. Other health systems with limited resources opted to modify their traditional healthcare facilities into COVID-19 specific centres. Most healthcare systems cancelled their elective surgeries to ensure capacity for care of COVID-19 patients. Additionally, changes were made worldwide in the way primary care was provided for routine and acute requirements within the communities, with rapid adoption of digital and telehealth services [4]. In some instances, services out of the reach of health systems were vulnerable, like in the case of aged individuals in long-term care homes [5]. Administrations were forced to prioritise such facilities for increased testing and surveillance and vaccine distribution.

Impact on the Health Workforce

As the health workforce were continuously at the forefront during the pandemic, they were disproportionately exposed to the virus and, in many cases, contracted SARS-CoV-2; in some cases, they died along with their patients [6]. The specific challenges faced by health systems regarding its workforce included low staffing levels, lack of training for a new emerging disease, erratic supply of personal protective equipment, and issues with psychological well-being [7]. To overcome staffing issues, many countries chose to reallocate their workforce from primary care providers to emergency care wards and ICUs [4]. In some cases, retired doctors and medical professionals were asked to rejoin clinical practice, under supervision, to compensate for staff shortages [8]. Furthermore, to protect the families of healthcare workforce, several health systems provided accommodation and childcare support near the workplace [9]. Many health systems made psychological support accessible to its workforce to maintain well-being and morale during the crisis. Much of this impact and adaptations are demonstrated at SBH throughout the previous chapters.

Impact on Finance

Health systems worldwide faced crippling financial losses during the pandemic that threatened their viability, particularly for those who were already vulnerable [10]. The substantial changes in the demand for health services has been one of the major causes for financial challenge. COVID-19 increased the demand for specialised acute care, which overwhelmed existing hospitals and brought with it unexpected costs. This, in conjunction with sharp decline in demand for routine services, has had a remarkable impact on revenues. Indeed, an American Hospital Association report suggests an expected loss of $323 billion in the year 2020 [11]. In Germany, hospital revenues dropped by an average of €2.5million during the first surge from March to May 2020 [12], and similar proportional losses can be seen around the globe. In most cases, governments provided assistance where possible to compensate for such financial losses so that the standard of healthcare was not compromised, albeit in in different ways based on the structure of the countries respective health systems.

Impact on Leadership and Governance

By the end of March 2020, most countries around the world had introduced public health measures to minimise the spread of COVID-19. Measures ranged from immediate lockdowns to business as usual, with dramatically varied health and economic outcomes [13]. In Europe and the USA, a combination of mitigation and suppression strategies were largely used, whilst in New Zealand, South Korea, China and Australia, efforts were made with contact tracing, isolation and quarantine, to rapidly exclude community transmission by a containment/elimination strategy [14]. This variation in response seems to stem from past experience in managing infectious outbreaks, societal values, healthcare infrastructures and, critically, the political will. At local levels, health systems were advised to set up incident management teams with clear chains of command. This would enable effective relaying of national directives and guidelines to clinical staff delivering care. Regional coordination between health systems, by pooling of resources, sharing clinical best practice and supporting the workforce, was also encouraged to effectively service closely linked populations or sparsely populated rural health systems.

Impact on Access to Treatment

Management of COVID-19 required ongoing development, production and sustained distribution of pharmaceutical products and technologies. The reliance on the production of medicines from only a few countries led to the disruption of supply chains and shortages globally. Some countries, such as Singapore, had drawn lessons from the past (SARS pandemic) and maintained a stockpile of medical products to the last 6 months [15]. Others, like in the case of Japan, boosted their manufacturing capacity to replenish the dwindling stockpiles [4]. In several countries, the increased demand of medications led to enactment of laws, to prevent hoarding and exploitative pricing, and policies, to promote imports and prohibit exports of pharmaceutical supplies. As we navigate our way out of the pandemic, vaccine procurement and equitable access still remains a concern.

Lessons Learned from the COVID-19 Pandemic

The magnitude of the COVID-19 pandemic challenged societies and infrastructure around the world. Unprecedented and drastic measures were taken at all levels to contain the spread of the virus. Although debates on the preparedness of various administrations and public health responses to COVID-19 will continue for some time, there are some vital lessons learned and knowledge gained that can help shape the future of healthcare in the day-to-day and in the face of future crises. Here, we outline some of the lessons learned which can help improve hospital services and healthcare delivery.

Establishing a Disaster Plan

All healthcare systems should develop a disaster plan that incorporates details regarding what areas of the hospital can be expanded and in what sequence, how to increase capacity to care for increased patient volumes (cancelling routine surgeries and appointments) and how to overcome staffing issues [16].

Supply Chains and Stocks

Generally, healthcare systems maintain minimal excess supplies to keep the running costs low. Furthermore, the supplies are sourced from limited vendors as consolidation of manufacturing further reduces costs. Whilst maintaining excess supplies may not be feasible, healthcare systems and hospitals could form a regional collaboration to maintain increased reserve supplies. Governments could also promote a basic level of manufacturing within the country by offering incentives and subsidies.

Improving Web-Based Primary Healthcare

The reduced access to primary healthcare below a certain threshold could itself be a significant health hazard and exacerbate the crisis. Whilst telemedicine with ad hoc remote consultations may be helpful in times of inadequate access, it cannot replace clinical advice informed by patient care history and knowledge of the patient. A digital healthcare revolution, which integrates personal histories and epidemiological evidence, can help reduce the stress on the health system without compromising on the standard of healthcare.

Infrastructural Alterations

During the pandemic when resources are stretched, it is essential to maximise staff utilisation. Strategies to improve the line of sight of primary care givers to the patients can help monitor them efficiently. These may include replacing walls with windows and upgrading communication devices to incorporate video monitoring. Increasing capacity of air-filtration units can also prove invaluable for managing air-borne infections [16].

Social Inequalities

The disproportionate impact of the pandemic on vulnerable groups and ethnic minorities laid bare the persistent disparities in healthcare. It gives an opportunity to refocus attention on how healthcare systems can ameliorate health inequities. A universal coverage of healthcare, especially in developed nations, could help bridge this gap. Increasing collaborations between the healthcare systems and the community-based agencies can help provide better access to these populations. These should also include effective means of communication with diverse communities. Furthermore, the healthcare systems should actively promote antiracism, equity and inclusion in-patient care [17].

Considerations for the 'Recovery' of Healthcare Systems

The recovery stage of a crisis such as the COVID-19 pandemic is highly capricious and requires balancing competing priorities, maintaining staff engagement and motivation and avoiding burnout within an environment which is, although less acute, still volatile and uncertain. In this section, we summarise some recommendations that could prove useful for the recovery of healthcare systems and hospitals.

Well-being of the Health Workforce Should Be of Paramount Importance

The recovery stage provides the first opportunity to acknowledge and celebrate the dedication and resilience showcased by staff. This is essential to keep morale high amongst the staff and reenergise and inspire individuals, teams and organisations. It also reinforces the fact that successful navigation through a crisis relies on contributions of every staff member.

The risk of psychological and physical exhaustion is a real issue during a crisis, especially amongst healthcare professionals who witness traumatic experiences regularly [7]. It is essential that during the recovery process, the staff have access to a support system that allows them to recover and heal. Furthermore, staff that do experience burnout should be allowed rest and receive adequate support or be transitioned to other roles whilst acknowledging their invaluable contributions. Teams and managers need to monitor the well-being of their staff with heightened acuity.

Clarity of Thought, Vision and Communication by Leadership

It is critical that leadership recognises the impact that the ever-evolving situation may have on their organisation and communities at both local and global level. This understanding is vital to developing effective strategies and navigating out of a crisis. This requires regular analysis of the information and keeping abreast with changes in policies and guidelines. Leadership should be prepared for setbacks and failures and be open to adapting to challenges in real time [18]. Clear, regular and unambiguous channels of communications with staff and other stakeholders are vital to engender trust and confidence in the leadership. They should actively aim to cultivate a culture of trust by being transparent and clarifying the process behind decision-making.

Reassessing Priorities, Optimising Performance and Management of Backlogs

It is likely that the pandemic has derailed any prior strategic plans, and it therefore provides an opportunity to reassess the priorities of the organisation and revaluate the services and needs of the communities that it serves. It also allows an opportunity to re-examine the management structure, staffing needs, costs and existing supply chains and collaborations. Furthermore, a strategic plan to carefully reintegrate paused or suspended services should be established based on the requirements of the population, organisational capacity and public health directives [19].

Preparation for Future Emergencies

To effectively prepare for any future emergencies, an introspective analysis and debriefing of individual, team, departmental and organisational performance is necessary. Understanding of what worked well, what the strengths and weaknesses were and what is required to be better prepared is essential to initiating the recovery process. An anonymous review could help identify areas that need optimisation, and this should be followed up by ensuring the required resources are in place to achieve those changes. Training requirements that equip staff with crisis specific skills should be identified and provided. Such introspection of performance and outcomes is likely to improve a health system's resilience, preparedness and viability during any future crisis. This reflection can be used alongside the documented triumphs and failures of other hospitals worldwide so that shared lessons can expand perspectives and allow broader considerations of healthcare improvements.

Recovery of SBH Health System from the Initial Surge

As detailed in the previous chapters, SBH Health System faced a dramatic first surge of COVID-19 patients during the pandemic in early 2020 and was considered the epicentre of the pandemic in the USA. After the peak of the surge and a subsequent decrease in-patient numbers, SBH Health System began the slow, arduous and long process of recovery.

Recovery Is Multifactorial

At SBH Health System, like with other hospital systems, the response to the pandemic involved a concerted effort from all departments, services and operations and the healthcare staff. The functioning of each departmental team or specialty, and their interactions with each other, had to adapt to the crisis. For effective functioning during the surge, certain departments at SBH Health System had to be merged like in the case of medical critical care, surgical critical care and anaesthesiology, which were all placed under joint leadership. Several discrete teams, including dental and podiatry residents and orthopaedists, were also integrated into one. Some healthcare workers were placed in a 'daily pool' and were assigned on a day-to-day basis as needs arose. As a result, there were significant alterations in the chains of command and reporting. It therefore becomes evident that returning to a non-crisis state will be a complex multifactorial process requiring careful coordination and institution-wide collaboration.

Recovery from Infectious Disease Is Unique

Whilst natural disasters, such as earthquakes or hurricanes, can result in high numbers of casualties and patients in need of hospital services, an infectious pandemic can affect the very healthcare workforce that delivers the critical services required to overcome the crisis. This presents a unique issue that needs careful consideration, especially when planning the gradual recovery from the initial surge of COVID-19. Although there was eagerness to return to non-crisis operations, reopen elective surgery and provide necessary healthcare services to the wider population, the recovery process needed to be gradual, keeping the concerns regarding the safety of the patients and the healthcare workers at the forefront.

Recovery of Clinical Services

At SBH Health System, the peak for patient admissions during the first surge was in the first half of April, and by early May, the hospital observed a slow decline in admissions and the number of accumulated patients with long length of stay (LOS). With this decrease in admissions of patients, a gradual process of recovery of non-critical care clinical services and departments was set in motion. This involved reducing the previously expanded intensive care units (ICUs), reopening elective surgery and reinstating the reduced outpatients' clinics. The recovery process also required restructuring the crisis teams and unmerging the departments to pre-crisis status. For instance, the medical critical care, surgical critical care, and anaesthesiology departments that were merged to form a hospital-wide critical care department during the surge were re-established as separate entities that attended to traditional roles and functions. Such unmerging could not be done abruptly and was governed by the rate of decrease in critically ill patients admitted. Recovery of each clinical service came with its own unique challenge; downsizing of the ICUs was significantly slower than expected due to slow recovery of some patients and bottlenecks in the patient workflow downstream. Additionally, a substantial number of patients required rehabilitation in chronic care facilities and therefore could not be discharged. Therefore, intermediate and regular care units needed to have beds available to accommodate them before the ICUs could be downsized. The availability of rehabilitation facilities was also a major challenge that further slowed the discharge process, and consequently downsizing, and recovery to normal functioning.

The reopening of elective surgery, which was initiated in June 2020, required meticulous planning and coordination to ensure that the maximum number of patients, whose surgeries had been delayed, benefited whilst preventing any intra-hospital transmission of the virus. A 'new normal' had to be established, which included processes for patient testing prior to surgery, prioritisation of surgery and procedures for managing asymptomatic COVID-19-positive patients. Similarly, reopening of outpatient clinics also required significant changes to pre-COVID-19 procedures by employing a hybrid practice of virtual and in-person visits to reduce crowding and allow for social distancing, in conjunction with measures to prevent transmission such as the use of masks and monitoring body temperatures.

Timeline for Recovery

The SBH Health System's timeline of the first surge in March 2020, and the recovery thereafter until the start of the second surge in November 2020, is illustrated in Fig. 20.1. The first surge, which lasted 4 months, was acute with large volumes of admission over a shorter time period. In comparison, the second surge was spread over a longer time period of 6 months with a less sharp increase in-patient volumes. Nevertheless, the number of admissions and patients requiring ventilation remained similar for both surges (Fig. 20.2). Additionally, the cumulative LOS for all patients was also similar in the two surges (Fig. 20.3), emphasising the need for continued vigilance, appropriate planning and relentless preparedness for any future surges. Fortunately, the need for mechanical ventilation and mortality rate were much lower for the second surge (Fig. 20.4), possibly due to a shift in the patient demographic

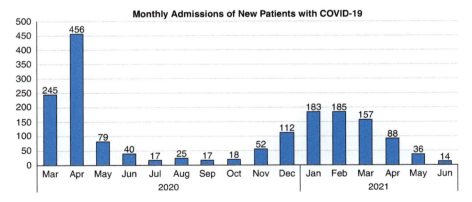

Fig. 20.1 Number of all admitted COVID-19 patients (monthly) from March 2020 through June 2021, showing the first surge of the COVID-19 pandemic in the period of March 2020 to June 2020 and the second surge in the period of November 2020 to May 2021

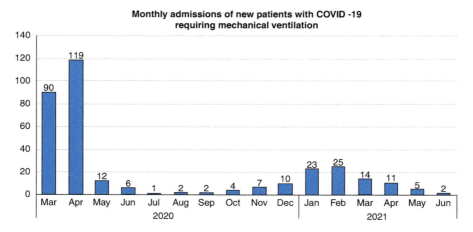

Fig. 20.2 Number of all ventilated COVID-19 patients (monthly) from March 2020 through June 2021, showing the first surge of the COVID-19 pandemic in the period of March 2020 to June 2020 and the second surge in the period of November 2020 to May 2021

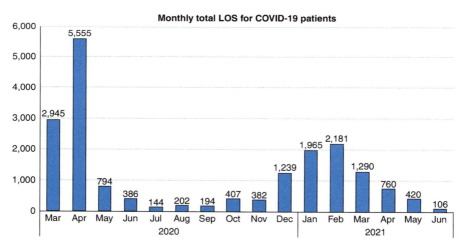

Fig. 20.3 Length of stay (LOS) of all admitted COVID-19 patients (monthly) from March 2020 through June 2021, showing the first surge of the COVID-19 pandemic in the period of March 2020 to June 2020 and the second surge in the period of November 2020 to May 2021

and a better understanding of the disease. From the perspective of health crisis planning, preparation and management, future surges would require a sustainable response over long periods of time without compromising on non-crisis-related services.

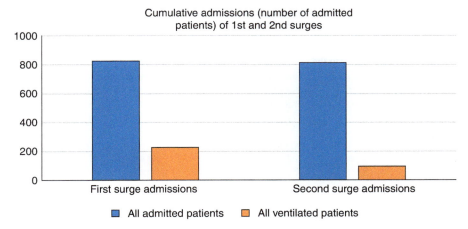

Fig. 20.4 Comparison of the total number of admissions and admissions requiring mechanical ventilation during the first surge of the COVID-19 pandemic from March 2020 to June 2021 and the second surge from November 2020 to May 2021

Recovering to a 'New Normal'

At SBH Health System, it quickly became apparent that many well-established operations, systems and processes will remain significantly altered from their pre-pandemic status. For instance, the scheduling of elective surgeries, pre-surgical screening and policies for cancellations has to be reviewed to accommodate COVID-19 testing in-patients for the foreseeable future. Furthermore, in cases with unknown COVID-19 status requiring emergency surgery that may release aerosols, the operating room always has to be placed under 'lockdown' post-surgery to lower the risk of viral transmission. The clinics and their waiting rooms will also continue to operate at reduced capacity to allow for social distancing. The use of telemedicine, with telephonic or virtual consultation, another vital adaptation during the surge to minimise transmission of the disease, will remain in some capacity to minimise patient footfall and risk of transmission. The health system responded dynamically by continuously evolving its processes and operations with changing scenarios, both within the hospital and at regulatory and policy levels. In hindsight, the sentiment of 'returning to normal' was undoubtedly nostalgic and developing a new post-surge normal was the need of the hour and encompassed expectations to be innovative, creative, adaptive and dynamic. Setting up the institution for the 'new normal' will indeed be the winning strategy (Table 20.1). Moreover, the lessons learned during the initial surge has provided invaluable confidence to the workforce in their ability to respond dynamically and adapt to the needs of any future surges or crisis.

Table 20.1 Comparison of 'return to normal' versus 'new normal'

	Return to normal	New normal
Expectations	Work will resume the way it was prior to the health crisis	Work will not be the same. There will be a need for innovation and creativity
Focus	Return to the comfort of the status prior to the health crisis	Adaptation to the new changes internally and externally. Learning lessons from the crisis
Priorities	Resumption of operations	Improvement over and beyond what was prior to the health crisis. Planning and preparation for future crises
Consequences	Frustration. Maladaptation. Slow recovery	Implementation of lessons learned, improvement of the hospital and better preparedness for future crisis

Establishing New Operations

In addition to the reopening of already existing services, the hospital had to establish new operations as it recovered from the initial surge. Here, we outline some of the new services initiated and the issues we encountered.

Testing for COVID-19

As COVID-19 was a novel virus, there were no established standardised tests, and those tests that did exist were under constant evolution. Each test differed in its sensitivity and specificity, and in the time it took to get the results, there were clinical and operational consequences. The erratic supply of testing kits and variable costs added a further level of complication, and they had to be rationed at times to ensure testing capabilities were not compromised.

Vaccination Program

The vaccination program involved a major educational campaign to raise awareness within the healthcare workforce, and being on the frontline, the vaccination of healthcare workers was set as a priority at SBH Health System. The supply of vaccines, storage requirements and personnel for administration needed to be managed acutely. Furthermore, the ambulatory care centre took on the responsibility of vaccinating members of the community in line with government recommendations.

Novel Treatments for COVID-19

Initially, the management of severely ill COVID-19 patients with ARDS was based on the general NIH guidance for patients with similar symptoms [20]. However, with better understanding of the disease, new treatment guidelines for ARDS specific to COVID-19 were developed and disseminated. Novel treatment options such as Sotrovimab received emergency authorisation from the FDA [21], and known antivirals such as Remdesivir were showing promising results in improving patient prognosis [22]. For the SBH Health System, it became necessary to acquire these new treatments, learn their indications, benefits, risks and participate in clinical trials. A special clinical guidelines committee was established to track the development of the new treatments and the emergence of new treatment guidelines and algorithms.

Managing Employee Health

Employee health management assumed special importance during the recovery from the COVID-19 surge. Protecting healthcare workers continued to be a top priority for the hospital. The post-surge time presented special demands, challenges and continuously evolving situations for employee health. From defining what was to be considered as exposure to COVID-19 to the home quarantining of healthcare workers who had tested positive, plus returning to work after illness – all of these were unprecedented issues and required new policies and procedures to be in place. The senior management worked tirelessly on the challenges of enforcing safety rules and assuring not only compliance but also conviction and adoption in the face of 'post crisis fatigue' – a known physical and psychological outcome of such crises [23].

Patient Visitation

At the time of the acute surge of COVID-19 patients in early 2020, visitation was disallowed for infection control reasons and to prevent the spread of the disease. The clinicians communicated with the patient families virtually, and audiovisual link was set up for the patients themselves. With the decline in COVID-19 cases, the visitation policy was modified and the rules gradually relaxed, allowing limited visitation with the necessary precautions and restrictions in place.

Learning from Clinical Outcomes

At SBH Health System, we give due importance to real-time learning and rapid-cycle improvement of our clinical outcomes to achieve excellence in-patient care. However, during the overwhelming acute surge of the COVID-19 crisis, there was no time or capacity to do so. Therefore, following the surge, SBH Health System launched the SBH COVID-19 clinical experience and outcomes study in collaboration with the CUNY School of Medicine. The main objective of the study was to create a de-identified database of all COVID-19 patients at SBH Health System during the first surge. The database would include the patient demographics,

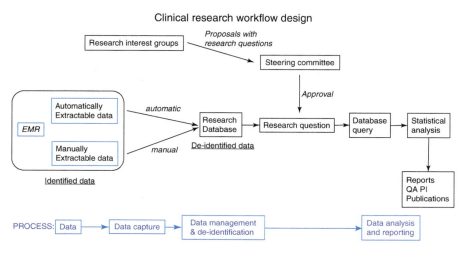

Fig. 20.5 The process of creation of a COVID-19 clinical experience and outcomes study with a de-identified database, approved by the SBH Health System Institutional Review Board (IRB), in collaboration with CUNY School of Medicine. EMR: Electronic Medical Record, QA PI: Quality Assurance and Performance Improvement

histories, test results, radiology reports, treatments and resultant outcomes, and this would facilitate clinical research into the disease. A process was put in place for the creation of the de-identified database and the mechanism of making it available to the research community at SBH Healthy System (Fig. 20.5).

Reflections, Learned Lessons and Formulation of an Improvement Plan

As we recovered from the initial COVID-19 surge, the SBH Health System senior management realised that there was an urgent need to draw lessons from and develop a constructive perspective of the crisis and they embarked on a major hospital-wide improvement effort. To initiate a plan for improving the hospital's ability to respond and manage such a health crisis, it was essential to identify the strengths and weaknesses of the SBH Health System and opportunities that inform of recommendations for the future. This comprehensive process involved all levels of management, clinical leaders as well as inputs frontline workers. Although there was recognition of the impressive selfless effort of all those at SBH, there was an institution-wide agreement in the fact that there were things the hospital could have done better and a strong resolve to improve before any future crisis. The summary of the key recommendations and reflections of this process are outlined in Box 20.1.

> **Box 20.1. Key Recommendations and Reflections**
> - SBH health system went through an unprecedented and challenging, highly transmissible and lethal infectious disease crisis.
> - All those who worked at SBH from the executive management to the front-line workers rallied heroically and collaboratively delivering an unimaginable volume and intensity of care.
> - The crisis showed points of significant strength and profound weakness.
> - This was a great opportunity for SBH to become the hospital that can 'quickly switch to a crisis mode and contribute to the vulnerable Bronx population'.
> - The physical facilities and equipment need significant upgrading and modernisation.
> - Continuation of handling non-crisis emergencies, trauma, MI, stroke, etc.
> - Investment in additional critical care personnel was vital.
> - Crisis preparedness efforts should be elevated.

Implementation of the Improvement Plan

Following reflection and crystallisation of the learned lessons and recommendations made for the future, the hospital embarked on the implementation of the improvement plan. The main areas identified for improvement and the corresponding objectives are outlined in Table 20.2. Subsequently, SBH Health System had to go through a meticulous process of prioritisation, taking into consideration the highest needs, projects with the highest impact and benefits to patients and affordability, as fulfilling each of them would not have been a feasible option. Lastly, implementation should cause minimal disruption to the ongoing functions and operations. Indeed, SBH Health System successfully conducted many improvement projects, including creating ICU-ready areas with central monitoring, enhancing mechanical ventilation and haemodialysis capacity, expanding capacity for ventilator alternatives, creating new negative pressure isolation rooms for infection control, improving staffing and equipment reserves and optimising supply chains. This was done in parallel to streamlining COVID-19 testing facilities, initiating vaccinations and managing employee well-being.

Conclusion

As we look ahead to a life after the COVID-19 pandemic, our progress will depend upon the lessons learned from our past and the changes we implement for our future. Whilst the COVID-19 pandemic exposed the current shortcomings of healthcare

Table 20.2 Goals for the improvement plan after the first surge of COVID-19

Item/area	Goals
Hospital units	Creation of large ICU-ready sections, isolation negative-pressure rooms, zoning sections for infected and non-infected, central monitoring, expanded haemodialysis readiness, tele-ICU, unified ventilator system with EMR integration, ventilator alternatives readiness
Emergency department	Infection control engineering, zoning, observation areas, triage for testing with rapid point-of-care diagnostics, barrier protections for airway procedures
Clinical care	Real-time outcomes data for rapid-cycle performance improvement, infrastructure for participation in clinical trials
Healthcare workers	Planning and training of integrated pooled tiered workforce to be activated efficiently at time of crises, preparation of a reserve workforce, planning phased deployment of the workforce, enhanced protection and communication protocols
Pharmacy	Anticipate alternative drug therapies, ensure orders are built in EMR and drug pump libraries, review concentrations of commonly used IV drips for critical care patients, ensure the concentrations and volumes are appropriate to accommodate most patient administration rate requirements for at least 12–24 hours, avoid spreading critical care patients on too many locations, increase staffing compliment to meet volume of physician orders
Disaster preparedness	Disaster preparedness for the entire institution with planning, education, training, continuous reinforcement and engagement of all departments and all ranks more seriously

systems worldwide, it can also serve as a catalyst for transformation, pushing reforms and changes that would have otherwise taken much longer to be realised. It has now become evident that it's not about returning to normal but to transition to a new improved normal gradually and cautiously, which is resilient to future crisis, provides better healthcare and is inclusive to all communities.

References

1. World Health Organization. Monitoring the building blocks of health systems: a handbook of indicators and their measurement strategies. 2010. p. 110. Accessed 26 Aug 2021.
2. Luo H, Liu J, Li C, Chen K, Zhang M. Ultra-rapid delivery of specialty field hospitals to combat COVID-19: lessons learned from the Leishenshan Hospital project in Wuhan. Autom Constr. 2020;119:103345. https://doi.org/10.1016/j.autcon.2020.103345. Epub 2020 Jul 4. PMID: 33311856; PMCID: PMC7334964.
3. Rimmer A. Sixty seconds on . . . nightingales. BMJ. 2020;368:m1290. https://doi.org/10.1136/bmj.m1290.
4. Haldane V, et al. Health systems resilience in managing the COVID-19 pandemic: lessons from 28 countries. Nat Med. 2021;27(6):964–80.
5. Dys S, Winfree J, Carder P, Zimmerman S, Thomas KS. Coronavirus disease 2019 regulatory response in united states-assisted living communities: lessons learned. Front Public Health. 2021;9:661042. https://doi.org/10.3389/fpubh.2021.661042. PMID: 34095066; PMCID: PMC8170034.

6. Bandyopadhyay S, et al. Infection and mortality of healthcare workers worldwide from COVID-19: a systematic review. BMJ Glob Health. 2020;5(12):e003097.
7. Greenberg N, et al. Managing mental health challenges faced by healthcare workers during COVID-19 pandemic. BMJ. 2020;368:m1211.
8. Dyer C. COVID-19: 15 000 deregistered doctors are told, "Your NHS needs you". BMJ. 2020;368.
9. Vimercati L, et al. The COVID-19 hotel for healthcare workers: an Italian best practice. J Hosp Infect. 2020;105(3):387–8.
10. Kaye AD, et al. Economic impact of COVID-19 pandemic on healthcare facilities and systems: international perspectives. Best Pract Res Clin Anaesthesiol. 2020;35:293.
11. AHA. Hospitals and health systems continue to face unprecedented financial challenges due to COVID-19. 2020;7. https://www.aha.org/system/files/media/file/2020/05/aha-covid19-financial-impact-0520-FINAL.pdf.
12. DKI, Krankenhaus Barometer Umfrage. 2020, Deutsches Krankenhaus Institut.
13. Han E, et al. Lessons learnt from easing COVID-19 restrictions: an analysis of countries and regions in Asia Pacific and Europe. Lancet. 2020;396(10261):1525–34.
14. Baker MG, Wilson and Blakely T. Elimination could be the optimal response strategy for COVID-19 and other emerging pandemic diseases. BMJ. 2020;371:m4907.
15. Chua AQ, et al. Health system resilience in managing the COVID-19 pandemic: lessons from Singapore. BMJ Glob Health. 2020;5(9):e003317.
16. Wei EK, Long T, Katz MH. Nine lessons learned from the COVID-19 pandemic for improving hospital care and health care delivery. JAMA Intern Med. 2021; https://doi.org/10.1001/jamainternmed.2021.4237.
17. Paremoer L, et al. COVID-19 pandemic and the social determinants of health. BMJ. 2021;372:129.
18. Narayan KMV, Curran JW, Foege WH. The COVID-19 pandemic as an opportunity to ensure a more successful future for science and public health. JAMA. 2021;325(6):525–6.
19. Appleby J. COVID-19: a V shaped recovery for the NHS? BMJ. 2020;370:3694.
20. NHLBI and NIH. 2020. Available from: http://www.ardsnet.org/.
21. Gupta A, et al. Early COVID-19 treatment with SARS-CoV-2 neutralizing antibody sotrovimab. medRxiv. 2021; https://doi.org/10.1101/2021.05.27.21257096.
22. Beigel JH, et al. Remdesivir for the treatment of COVID-19 — final report. N Engl J Med. 2020;383(19):1813–26.
23. Liu Q, et al. The experiences of health-care providers during the COVID-19 crisis in China: a qualitative study. Lancet Glob Health. 2020;8(6):e790–8.

Index

A
Acute respiratory distress syndrome (ARDS), 12
Admitted nutrition dashboard, 252
Agile project planning, 255
Air-filtration units, 319
Alternate care sites (ACS), 28
American Association of Respiratory Care (AARC), 166
American Thoracic Society criteria, 166
Angiotensin-converting enzyme 2 (ACE2), 147
Automated dispensing cabinets (ADC), 190

B
Bilevel positive airway pressure (BiPap), 230
Brief Resilience Scale (BRS), 303
Bronx, 278
    Black and Latino residents, 2
    isolation and social distancing, 3
    SBH health system, 5–7
    SBH patient community, 3–5
    SDOH, 1–3

C
Center for the Study of Traumatic Stress/Uniformed Services University, 310
Center for Disease Control and Prevention (CDC), 46, 132, 133, 232
City University of New York School of Medicine (CSOM), 259, 260
Clinical curriculum, 264, 265
Clinical nutrition services
    artificial preparations, 138
    aspect of, 137
    components, 137
    critical care expansion, 141
    critical illness, 138
    enteral nutrition, 138, 139
    nutritional care, 137, 138
    nutritional guidelines, 143–145
    parenteral nutrition, 138, 139
    PPE, 145
    recommendations, 138
    room revisions, 141
    SBH health system, 145
        enteral nutrition provision, 146
        micronutrients, 147
        parenteral nutrition provision, 146, 147
        strategy, 145
    staffing, 140, 141
    supply chain and procurement, 141–143
Communication, 26, 27
    and collaboration tools, 246
Continuous renal replacement therapy (CRRT), 54
COVID-19 crisis, 281
COVID-19 ESL (employee support line), 307

COVID-19 pandemic, 60, 61
　classification, 12
　definition, 9, 10
　origins of, 10
　screening questions, 244
　structure and genome, 10–12
　symptoms, 12
　timeline of pandemic
　　clinical effects, 13
　　emergency room visits, 15
　　hospital admissions, 15
　　hospitalizations, 14
　　mortality, 14
　　observations, 13, 16, 17
　　pathophysiology, 13
　　rapid surge in cases, 13
　　SBH health system, 17–19, 21, 22
　vaccine, 250, 251
Crisis standards of care (CSC), 87
Critical care
　advanced/complex hemodynamic monitoring, 54
　blood pressure monitoring, 54
　care, 54
　challenges, 83
　clinical interventions, 81
　components, 55
　contingency planning and management, 88, 89
　creative solutions
　　clinical practice adaptation, 76
　　crisis management, 76
　　staffing, 74, 75
　creativity and improvisation
　　anesthesiologists, 71
　　dental staff, 71, 72
　　medical school librarians, 72
　　medical students, 72
　　planning and preparedness, 68
　cross-training non-critical care physicians
　　challenges, 60, 61
　　COVID-19 pandemic, 60
　　didactic sessions, 61
　　follow-up program, 62
　　practical training, 61, 62
　　replacement and supplementary workforce, 62
　disabling conditions, 82
　emergent and urgent cases, continuation of, 82
　frontline workers
　　daily rounds, 79, 80
　　decision-making, 78
　　emotional and psychological support, 79
　　hospital system success, 77
　　material support, 79
　　overwork, long hours, intense situations, 78
　　team leadership, 77, 78
　health crisis
　　advantages, 59
　　disadvantages, 59
　　ICU-ready areas, 59
　　planning, 57–59
　health workers, 56
　ICU patients, 56
　information flow management, 81
　integrated tiered critical care team, 60
　intensive care, 56, 57
　intermediate care, 56, 57
　multidisciplinary committee
　　meetings, 64–70
　　mission, goals and composition, 62–65
　networking and information sharing, 90, 91
　neurosurgical education, 85
　neurotrauma, 84
　non-emergency neurosurgery, 84, 85
　nutrition support, 54
　overflow planning, 91
　patient scoring systems, 90, 91
　public health crisis, 85–88
　pulmonary dynamics, 54
　resources, 75, 80, 81
　respiratory monitoring, 54
　SBH Health System
　　expansion units, 93–94
　　re-purposing resources, 92, 93
　'splitting' ventilators, 73
　stroke care, 83, 84
　ventilator sharing, 72–74
Critical Care for Non-ICU clinicians, 61

D
Daily assessments, 255
Data reporting and analytics, 245
Data visualization tools, 29
Departmental communication, 27
Department of Pharmacy, 199
Digital transformation journey, 255, 256
Disaster plan, 318
Drive-through or make-shift COVID-19 testing center, 243
Dynamic decision-making, 281–283

Index

E
Ebola virus, 277
E-consults, 246
Effective collaboration, 291–292
Effective communication, 285
EHR downtime, contingency plan, 254, 255
Electronic health records (EHR), 244
Emergency medicine
    departmental reconfiguration
        diversion status, 107, 108
        patient transfers, 106, 107
        physical space, staff and supporting supplies, 104, 105
        reluctance of, 103
        tent process, 105, 106
        time and energy, 103
        visitation by family, 108
        zones, 103, 104
    global crisis, 99, 100
    governance and communication, 100–102
    initial crisis, 120
    nursing staff, 111, 112
    physician staff, 112
    resident staffing, 114, 115
    resources and infrastructure
        pharmacy, 110, 111
        PPE, 108, 109
        ventilators, 109
    risk awareness, staff in, 113, 114
    staff sickness, 116
    staff wellness, 112, 113
Emotional and social intelligence, 303–305
Emotional support, 302
Employee health management, 327
End-tidal CO_2 ($ETCO_2$), 54
Enhanced information security, 248–253
Enteral nutrition, 138, 139
Environmental crises, 23
Extracorporeal membrane oxygenation (ECMO), 54

F
Facial recognition, 244
Fair-process model, 287–289
Federal Emergency Management Agency (FEMA), 242
Financial challenge, 317
Food services, *see* Clinical nutrition services

G
Greater New York Hospital Association (GNYHA), 228

H
Healthcare workers (HCWs), 301
    in China, 302
    collaborative relationships, 312
    communication, 312
    emotional and psychological problems, 303
    emotional wellbeing, 312
    fear of contamination, 305
    leadership, 312
    level of stress/burnout, 305
    physical and psychological wellness, 302
    psychological impact, 302
    resilience of, 303
    schedule for psychiatrist rounds, 310
    spiritual/religious support, 312
    support groups, 307–309
    under non-pandemic conditions, 302
    virtual meeting, 305
    wellbeing, 310, 312
Health crisis management
    HICS (*see* Hospital incident command system)
    preparation and planning, 23, 24
Health service delivery, impact on, 316
Health workforce, impact on, 316
Hemodialysis (HD), 54
High efficiency particulate air (HEPA) filters, 230
HIPAA-compliant collaborative tool, 242
Hospital incident command system (HICS)
    activation, 24
    clinical leadership, 32
    clinical volunteers, 33–35
    communication, 24–27
    daily safety call, 27, 28
    dashboard, 29
        crisis management, 31
        daily meetings (teleconference), 30
        data visualization tools, 29
        employee morale, 31
        timely actions, 30
        transparency, 30
    definition, 24
    emergency operations plan, 28, 29
    float pool, 28
    frontline teams, 32
    leadership, 31, 32
    role of, 25, 26
    transfer process, 28

I
Incident command system (ICS), 242
Infection control (IC), 46–48

Infectious crises, 24
Information technology, 241
Integrated tiered critical care team, 60
Intensive care unit (ICU), 54
Internal medicine, 37
    beds, 38–40
    discharging patients with COVID-19, 45, 46
    hospitalist service, 37, 38
    infection control, 46–48
    morbidity/severity and mortality, 19, 20
    OHS, 48, 49
    physician shortages, 43, 44
    physician staff, 40, 41
    residents role, 41–43
    SBH health services, 50, 51
    treatment protocols, 44, 45
Intracranial pressure (ICP) monitoring, 55
Intravenous (IV) access, 55
Invasive mechanical ventilation (IMV), 166
ISCO WebEx virtual conferencing platform, 242
IT Customer and technical support, 254–255

J
Jacob Javitz Center (JJC), 45, 46

L
Laboratory
    ambulatory laboratory services, 203
    committee conference calls, 205
    communication and reporting plan, 205
    comprehensive risk assessment, 202
    crisis and continuity management plan, 202
    dedicated laboratory team and capacity building, 203
    disruption mitigation, 202
    emergency succession plan
        access and phlebotomy area, 207
        anatomic pathology, 207
        blood bank, 208
        core laboratory, 208
        development, 206
        instructions, 206
        microbiology, 208
        during partial shutdown of services, 206, 207
        point-of-care testing, 208, 209
        recovery processes, 209
        shutdown of laboratory services, 209
        during temporary disruption of services, 206
    incident command or coordination set up, 203
    linkages development, 205
    mass fatality management, 209, 210
        case management/tracking, 213
        family management, 213, 214
        fuel management, 212
        handling, and transport of human remains, 211
        infection control procedures, 211, 212
        managing of body collection points, 211
        morgue census survey, 213
        personal effects, 213
        release cases to funeral homes, 214
        request and preparation of body collection points, 210, 211
        retrieval of body collection point, 214
        security, 213
        staffing, 211
        storage of bodies, 212
        temperature monitoring, 212
    mobilization of staff, 204
    patient nearside testing services, 203
    point of care testing (POCT), 203
    prioritized test menu, 203
    rapid diagnostics, 203
    resource management, 204
    role, response, and continuity plan, 201
    SBH Health System Laboratory, 202, 205
    SWOT analysis, 202
Leadership and governance, 317
Lean daily management (LDM), 292, 294
    beginning, 296
    changes, 296, 297
    collaborative servant leadership, 297
    contributions, 297
    definition, 294
    goal, 294
    healthcare workers, 295
    planning and preparation, 298
    recovery stages, 298
    steps, 295
    trained organization, 298
Liaison Committee on Medical Education, 271
Lives of courage, 268

M
Macro-management *vs.* micro-management, 283–285
Medicaid, 156
Medical education
    clinical curriculum, 264, 265
    community service, 270

Index 337

COVID-19 pandemic long-term impact and reflections, 271, 272
COVID-19 patient chart reviews, 269, 270
curricular changes and innovations, 260, 261
educational setting, 259–260
graduation and residency, 266, 267
research and community service activities, 268, 269
service learning/value-added education, 263, 264
teaching environment, 261–263
wellness needs, 267, 268
Medical Reserve Corporation (MRC), 43–44
Medicare, 156
Mental Health America (MHA), 302
Mental health and support resources, 307, 308
Middle East respiratory syndrome (MERS), 277
Mobile Army Surgical Hospital (MASH), 57
MRN-specific mortality status, 248
Multidisciplinary critical care teams, 56

N

National Board of Medical Examiners (NBME), 266
National Center for PTSD/US Department of Veterans Affairs, 310
National Institute of Occupational Safety & Health (NIOSH), 232
New York State Department of Health (NYSDOH), 45
Nightingale hospitals, 316
Nursing
  education, 132, 133
  hospital nursing leadership, 124
  morale-boosting huddles, 124, 125
  morale, engagement, and support, 133, 134
  nurse director, 130, 131
  nursing union leadership, 124
  OEM, 135
  patient capacity
    collaboration, 127, 128
    nursing units, 127
  quality differentiation, 126
  SBH health system
    challenges, 129, 130
    nursing staff ratios, 128, 129
    reflective practice, 134, 135

O

Occupational Health Service (OHS), 46, 48, 49

Office of Emergency Management (OEM), 135
Organizational deployment, 257

P

Pandemics
  classification, 12
  definition, 9, 10
Parenteral nutrition, 138, 139
Patient care monitoring solutions, 253–254
Patient safety Friday, 296
Peritoneal dialysis (PT), 54
Personal protective equipment (PPE), 47, 48, 108, 109, 145
Persons under investigation (PUI), 46
Pharmacy
  automated dispensing cabinets, 190
  clinical services, 192
    health information systems, 192, 193
    health workforce, 193, 194
    knowledge-based medication barcoding system, 193
    multidisciplinary pharmacy committee, 193
  crisis management plan, 184, 185, 187
  critical care unit expansion, 190, 191
  distressed supply chains, 189, 190
  distribution/security of medications, 184
  leadership/governance, 183, 184
  mitigation phase, 186
  monitoring, 184
  operational services and clinical services, 184, 185
  ordering and prescribing, 184
  practice elements, 185, 186
  preparation/administration, 184, 187, 188
  recovery phase, 188, 189
  response phase, 188
  SBH pharmacy response
    critical care patient care units, 195–197
    gaining access to essential medications, 196
    remarkable success, 198
    senior leadership, 195
    staffing levels, 197, 198
  secure medication, 190
  services and operations, 189
  staffing concerns, 191, 192
  STAT IV orders, 191
  supply chain/procurement, 184
  WHO health system framework, 183, 184
Pharmacy Critical Care Services, 193
Pharmacy Emergency Services, 194
Pharmacy Transition of Care Services, 194

Phases of pandemic, 317
Plan, do, study, and act (PDSA), 27
Positive and negative affect schedule (PANAS), 303
Post anesthesia care unit (PACU), 71
Powered air purifying respirator (PAPR), 108
PPE, *see* Personal protective equipment (PPE)
Problem-based learning (PBL), 261, 262
Proning, 174–176
    complication, 173
    final padding, 177
    mortality reduction, 170
    Nursing Department and Hospital Leadership, 170
    oxygenation, 170
    post-proning procedure and maintenance, 174–179
    pre-proning procedure, 172
    proning team assembly, 173
    SBH Health System, 170
    staffing and education, 170
    standard principles, 170
    supine position, 170
    "time out" safety checklist, 173
Psychological burden, 301, 302
Pulse oximeter orders dashboard, 252
Pulse oximetry, 54

R
Radiology
    anxiety, assurance and recognition, 221
    communication, 222
    dynamic reorganization of resources and processes, 221, 222
    early testing and isolation/quarantine, 221
    effectiveness of communication, 224
    electronic medical record (EMR), 224
    history of medical imaging, 218
    magnetic resonance imaging (MRI), 218
    nuclear medicine studies, 219
    organization of modern-day radiology department, 219
    personal protective equipment (PPE), 220
    protecting staff and patients, 220
    psychiatric support, 223
    radiologist's reflection, 217–218
    super spreader event, 220
Rapid cycle PDSA methodology, 247
Rapid-sequence intubation (RSI), 110
Real time outcome dashboards, 247
Recommended daily intake (RDI), 138
Recovery of healthcare systems
    leadership, 320
    preparation for future emergencies, 321
    strategic plan, 321
    wellbeing of health workforce, 320
Registered nurses (RNs), 55, 111
Rehabilitation
    in acute care
        acute care setting, 158
        clinical management, 157
        comorbidities and challenges, 158, 159
        immobility and bed rest, 157
        patient prone position, 156
    frontline staff protection, 156
    hospital administration, 161
    initial response, 151
    inpatient rehabilitation, 152, 153
    integrated discharge planning process, 161
    manual therapy, 160
    outpatient rehabilitation, 152–154
    in-patient bed management, 151–152
    physical rehabilitation, 154
    post-acute care, 159, 160
    protective personal equipment (PPE), 151
    resilience of rehabilitation staff, 161
    SBH health system, 160
    social distancing, 160
    step-by-step movements, 155
    telehealth, 155
Remote patient monitoring (RPM), 246
Resilience, 302, 303
Respiratory therapists (RTs), 56
Respiratory therapy
    challenges faced at SBH, 179
    in COVID-19 crisis, 166, 167
    emotional and psychological support, 169
    equipment, 167, 168
    personal protective equipment (PPE) challenges, 169, 170
    proning, 174–176
        complication, 173
        final padding, 177
        mortality reduction, 170
        Nursing Department and the Hospital Leadership, 170
        oxygenation, 170
        post-proning procedure and maintenance, 174–179
        pre-proning procedure, 172
        proning team assembly, 173
        SBH Health System, 170
        staffing and education, 170
        standard principles, 170
        supine position, 170
        "time out" safety checklist, 173

Index

respiratory therapists role, 165, 166
staffing concerns, 168, 169, 180
training and education of staff, 179, 180

S
SARS, 277
Satisfaction with life scale (SWLS), 303
SBH health system, 167, 223
  additional storage space, 237, 238
  allocations and backorders, 234
  CDC and NIOSH certified products, 237
  challenges, 235, 236
  chief financial officer (CFO), 236
  clinical outcomes, 327, 328
  comprehensive process, 328
  COVID-19 testing, 326
  culture, 293, 294
  daily meetings, 229, 230
  disaster plan, 281
  during pandemic, 229
  employee health management, 327
  'fair-process' model, 287–289
  gray markets, 237
  group purchasing organization, 231, 232
  improvement plan implementation, 329, 330
  international sourcing, 237
  leadership, 292
  lean daily management (LDM), 292, 294
    beginning, 296
    changes, 296, 297
    collaborative servant leadership, 297
    contributions, 297
    definition, 294
    goal, 294
    healthcare workers, 295
    planning and preparation, 298
    recovery stages, 298
    steps, 295
    trained organization, 298
  managing shortage of supplies, 233
  material management, 238–239
  new operations, 326
  non-exclusive possibilities, 292
  patient care, list of items, 232, 233
  patient-centered excellence, 294
  patient interest first, 292
  patient visitation, 327
  patient workflow, 285
  readiness, 278, 280, 281
  recommendations and reflections, 329
  recovery, 322

  of clinical services, 322, 323
  from infectious disease, 322
  to new normal, 325, 326
  timeline, 323–325
  resource allocation and expansion planning, 285
  senior management, 328
  staff and patients, 293
  supply chain, 227, 228, 232, 238–239
  surveys and meetings, 230, 231
  treatments for COVID-19, 326, 327
  for underserved population, 278
  vaccination program, 326
Sequential organ failure assessment (SOFA), 90, 91
Service learning/value-added education, 263, 264
SmartNotes, 241
Social determinants of health (SDOH), 1–3
Social inequalities, 319
Society of Critical Care Medicine (SCCM), 193
Strategic decisions, 278, 279
Stress and trauma
  during week 1, 305
  during week 2, 305, 307
  during week 3, 307, 308
  during week 4, 309
  during week 6, 310, 311
  onsite intervention, 310
Supply chain management, 80
  and stocks, 318
Survey of perceived organizational support (SPOS) brief form, 303
Swan-Ganz catheters, 54

T
Technology and communication infrastructure, 242–243
Tele-ICU, 246

U
United States Medical Licensing Exam (USMLE), 266

V
Virtual care platform, 246–247
Virtual care scorecard dashboard, 249
Virtual command center (VCC), 242

Virtual laboratories, 262
Virtual platforms, 263, 271
Visit-specific mortality status, 247
Voice over internet protocol (VoIP), 242

W
Web-based primary healthcare, 319
Wi-Fi access implementation, 243
World Health Organization (WHO), 183